# CAUSES OF CONDUCT DISORDER
# AND JUVENILE DELINQUENCY

# Causes of Conduct Disorder and Juvenile Delinquency

*Edited by*

Benjamin B. Lahey
Terrie E. Moffitt
Avshalom Caspi

Foreword by David P. Farrington and Rolf Loeber

THE GUILFORD PRESS
New York    London

©2003 The Guilford Press
A Division of Guilford Publications, Inc.
72 Spring Street, New York, NY 10012
www.guilford.com

Printed in the United States of America

This book is printed on acid-free paper.

Last digit is print number:  9  8  7  6  5  4  3  2  1

**Library of Congress Cataloging-in-Publication Data**

Causes of conduct disorder and juvenile delinquency / edited by Benjamin
B. Lahey, Terrie E. Moffitt, Avshalom Caspi ; foreword by David P.
Farrington and Rolf Loeber.
    p.   cm.
Includes bibliographical references and index.
  ISBN 1-57230-881-8
  1. Conduct disorders in children. I. Lahey, Benjamin B. II. Moffitt,
Terrie E. III. Caspi, Avshalom.
  RJ506.C65C38 2003
  618.92′89—dc21
                                                    2003000812

# About the Editors

Benjamin B. Lahey, PhD, is Professor of Psychiatry and Chief of Psychology at the University of Chicago. His research addresses three related aspects of developmental epidemiology: (1) the childhood origins of serious conduct problems, (2) the validity of diagnostic criteria for ADHD and other mental disorders of childhood, and (3) the integration of structural models of child and adolescent psychopathology with structural models of temperament. Dr. Lahey served as President of the International Society for Research in Child and Adolescent Psychopathology and is President-Elect of the Society for Child and Adolescent Clinical Psychology (Division 53 of the American Psychological Association). He served on the Child Disorders Work Group of the Task Force for DSM-IV and conducted the DSM-IV field trials for the disruptive behavior disorders. In 1991, he received the Research Prize of the National Academy of Neuropsychology, and in 2002, he received the Distinguished Research Contributions Award from the Society for Child and Adolescent Clinical Psychology.

Terrie E. Moffitt, PhD, is Professor of Social Behavior and Development at the Institute of Psychiatry at King's College, London, and Professor of Psychology at the University of Wisconsin. In her research, she studies the interplay between nature and nurture in the genesis of psychopathology, particularly antisocial behavior. Currently, Dr. Moffitt directs the Medical Research Council-funded Environmental-Risk Study (E-risk), which follows 1,100 pairs of twins from birth to age 7 to test effects of family adversity and heritable risk on children's behavior problems. She has served for 10 years as Associate Director of the NIMH-funded Dunedin Multidisciplinary Health and Development Study at the University of Otago in New Zealand, which is conducting a 32-year longitudinal study of a birth cohort of 1,000 individuals. This study is described in her recent book, *Sex Differences in Antisocial Behaviour: Conduct Disorder, Delinquency and Violence in the Dunedin Study.* For her research, she received the Distin-

guished Scientific Award for Early Career Contribution to Psychology in
the area of psychopathology from the American Psychological Association
in 1993. Dr. Moffitt is also a fellow of the United Kingdom Academy of
Medical Sciences and holds a Royal Society–Wolfson Merit Award. She is a
licensed clinical psychologist and received her hospital training at the University of California, Los Angeles, Neuropsychiatric Institute.

**Avshalom Caspi, PhD,** is Professor of Personality and Social Psychology at
the Institute of Psychiatry at King's College, London, and Professor of Psychology at the University of Wisconsin. His research focuses on the measurement, development, and implications of personality differences in children and adolescents. For his research, he received the Distinguished
Scientific Award for Early Career Contribution to Psychology in the area of
developmental psychology from the American Psychological Association in
1995, and the John P. Hill Memorial Award for contributions to the understanding of adolescent development from the Society for Research on Adolescence in 2002.

# Contributors

**Patricia A. Brennan, PhD,** Department of Psychology, Emory University, Atlanta, Georgia

**Kenneth A. Dodge, PhD,** Center for Child and Family Policy, Duke University, Durham, North Carolina

**Emily R. Grekin, MA,** Department of Psychology, Emory University, Atlanta, Georgia

**Cynthia L. Huang-Pollock, PhD,** Department of Psychiatry, University of California–San Francisco, San Francisco, California

**Sharon S. Ishikawa, PhD,** Department of Psychology, University of Southern California, Los Angeles, California

**Kate Keenan, PhD,** Department of Psychiatry, University of Chicago, Chicago, Illinois

**Benjamin B. Lahey, PhD,** Department of Psychiatry, University of Chicago, Chicago, Illinois

**Sarnoff A. Mednick, PhD,** Department of Psychology and Social Science Research Institute, University of Southern California, Los Angeles, California

**Terrie E. Moffitt, PhD,** Social, Genetic, and Developmental Psychiatry Research Centre, Institute of Psychiatry, King's College, London, United Kingdom; University of Wisconsin–Madison, Madison, Wisconsin

**Joel T. Nigg, PhD,** Department of Psychology, Michigan State University, East Lansing, Michigan

**Gerald Patterson, PhD,** Oregon Social Learning Center, Eugene, Oregon

**Adrian Raine, PhD,** Department of Psychology, University of Southern California, Los Angeles, California

**John Reid, PhD,** Oregon Social Learning Center, Eugene, Oregon

**Soo Hyun Rhee, PhD,** Department of Psychology and Institute for Behavioral Genetics, University of Colorado, Boulder, Colorado

**Michael Rutter, MD,** Social, Genetic, and Developmental Psychiatry Research Centre, Institute of Psychiatry, King's College, London, United Kingdom

**Robert J. Sampson, PhD,** Department of Sociology, Harvard University, Cambridge, Massachusetts; Center for Advanced Study in the Behavioral Sciences, Stanford, California

**Daniel S. Shaw, PhD,** Department of Psychology, University of Pittsburgh, Pittsburgh, Pennsylvania

**James Snyder, PhD,** Department of Psychology, Wichita State University, Wichita, Kansas

**Stephen J. Suomi, PhD,** Laboratory of Comparative Ethology, National Institute of Child Health and Human Development, National Institutes of Health, Bethesda, Maryland

**Richard E. Tremblay, PhD, FRSC,** Groupe de recherche sur l'inadaptation psychosociale chez l'enfant (GRIP), University of Montreal, Montreal, Quebec, Canada

**Irwin D. Waldman, PhD,** Department of Psychology, Emory University, Atlanta, Georgia

**Per-Olof H. Wikström, PhD,** Department of Ecological and Developmental Criminology, Institute of Criminology, University of Cambridge, Cambridge, United Kingdom; Center for Advanced Study in the Behavioral Sciences, Stanford, California

# Foreword

The aim of this book is extremely noble: to make significant progress toward an understanding of the causes of conduct disorder and serious juvenile delinquency. The authors have been asked to advance testable hypotheses about causes and to describe critical studies that could confirm or disconfirm these hypotheses. The challenge to the field is to carry out these critical tests.

After reading the book's excellent contributions, it struck us that the editors of this volume achieved a third, unstated goal. All of the chapters, by addressing key hypotheses in different ways, focus on several critical choices in the scientific investigation of conduct disorder and serious juvenile delinquency. Foremost is the taxonomy of conduct disorder and serious delinquency, which covers a wide variety of different antisocial acts. Variations in the taxonomy of antisocial behavior among studies are likely to produce differences in insights on what is causally related to antisocial behavior. An overarching set of questions are: What is the best way to measure and conceptualize antisocial behavior? Which constructs based on the taxonomy can best be used across development, and how can this knowledge best be used to address causality? To what extent are there different types of offenders and different pathways to antisocial behavior?

Strongly related to taxonomy is the issue of what is the underlying concept that can explain different behavioral manifestations of antisocial acts. The chapters argue for different underlying concepts such as antisocial propensity (Lahey and Waldman, Chapter 4) and self-regulatory processes (Moffitt, Chapter 3; Keenan and Shaw, Chapter 6; Nigg and Huang-Pollock, Chapter 8). Hypotheses about causality are closely tied to conceptualizations and choices of underlying concepts. The volume alerts the reader that the scientific discussion about these underlying concepts is ongoing and that progress about causation can be achieved by comparisons between concepts and, possibly, the formulation of a hierarchy of underlying concepts (e.g., Lahey and Waldman, Chapter 4; Nigg and Huang-Pollock, Chapter 8).

All of the chapters address crucial questions about the causes of antisocial behavior. However, the chapters vary in their assumption about whether causes apply equally to all forms of antisocial problems. This is illustrated by several chapters that specifically (but sometimes not exclusively) focus on aggression (e.g., Keenan and Shaw, Chapter 6; Tremblay, Chapter 7; Nigg and Huang-Pollock, Chapter 8; Dodge, Chapter 9; Ishikawa and Raine, Chapter 10; Suomi, Chapter 13). Given this concentration of knowledge, hypotheses about the causes of covert antisocial acts and property crime are much needed (see Snyder, Reid, and Patterson, Chapter 2).

The volume also illustrates how each author postulates causes on different levels, including individual temperament, social information processing, social interactions, neighborhood factors, psychophysiology, and genetics. In some of the chapters, interactions between causes at more than one level are considered (e.g., Lahey and Waldman, Chapter 4). Many important theoretical issues are raised in these chapters. For example, should theories focus on the learning of aggression (Snyder, Reid, and Patterson, Chapter 2) or on learning to inhibit aggression (Tremblay, Chapter 7)? The chapters especially advance knowledge about the explanation of gender differences in offending. Many theories are put forward, including faster nervous system maturation of girls, better language development of girls, and the greater importance of peer influence for girls, but there is surprising concordance among most of the theorists. After reading this book, we had a real sense of excitement about the value and potential contributions of these theories.

Many of the authors also link causes to interventions and give important examples of how it may be possible to learn about causality through manipulation and experimentation. Conversely, it is important that interventions to reduce offending and antisocial behavior are based on well-validated theories. In making significant progress toward better theories, this volume not only advances knowledge but also holds out the promise of significantly reducing crime and associated social problems. We are delighted to recommend it to all readers who are interested in the explanation and prevention of conduct disorder and serious juvenile delinquency.

DAVID P. FARRINGTON, PHD
*Cambridge University*

ROLF LOEBER, PHD
*University of Pittsburgh and
Free University, Amsterdam*

# Preface

A great deal is known about the correlates of serious conduct problems, but we have made much less progress toward understanding their causes. Because understanding causation will undoubtedly lead to improvements in prevention and treatment, it is essential that future research focus more on causal factors and causal mechanisms (Hinshaw, 2002). In this volume, many of the world's top researchers in developmental psychopathology and developmental criminology have advanced specific and testable *hypotheses* about the *causes* of conduct disorder and serious juvenile delinquency. The explicit mission of this volume is to entice other researchers to test these hypotheses to advance knowledge about causation.

We are very pleased that the chapter authors responded to our encouragement to be bold but specific in stating their causal hypotheses. Following philosopher of science Karl Popper (1963), we believe that the job of the scientist is to boldly conjecture, to conjecture in disconfirmable terms, and to expose our conjectures to severe risk of refutation in empirical studies. Hence, we asked the chapter authors (1) to advance explicit, disconfirmable causal hypotheses; and (2) to provide specific descriptions of the crucial studies needed to disconfirm their hypotheses. When appropriate to their topics, we also asked the chapter authors to provide hypotheses regarding the causes of differences in conduct problems as a function of age, gender, race–ethnicity, and socioeconomic status. Because some of these differences are large, it is essential that we eventually understand their causes.

The authors for this volume were selected across disciplines because of their significant accomplishments in research and their well-known respect for data. Some of the chapter authors had previously advanced causal hypotheses, but most had not. This book provides a forum for all of the chapter authors to advance causal hypotheses in the full understanding that they may or may not be supported by future studies. That is, we all agreed to go out on a limb together in inviting other researchers to take our hypotheses to task. As Popper (1963) said, in science, we learn the most from our mistakes (refuted hypotheses).

The volume opens with a chapter by Michael Rutter, providing an overview of the research paths that must be taken to understand the causes of serious conduct problems and the obstacles that lie along the way. The next part provides four general and integrative causal models of conduct disorder and serious delinquency: a social learning model, a developmental pathways model, an integrative antisocial propensity model, and an integrative ecological–developmental model. The remainder of the volume is devoted to chapters that provide causal models that focus on specific aspects of the origins of conduct problems. These chapters cover early childhood influences, cognitive factors, and genetic and other biological influences. The volume closes with a chapter on the important role of animal models in understanding environmental and biological causes of aggression.

We are deeply indebted to the chapter authors for finding time in their busy schedules to write their chapters. Each chapter is an eloquent scientific jewel that is important in its own right. Together, these chapters constitute a remarkable summary of leading thinking across disciplines regarding the many causal factors, and the many levels of analysis, that must be considered in eventually understanding the causes of conduct disorder and serious juvenile delinquency.

## REFERENCES

Hinshaw, S. P. (2002). Process, mechanism, and explanation related to externalizing behavior in developmental psychopathology. *Journal of Abnormal Child Psychology, 30,* 431–538.
Popper, K. (1963). *Conjectures and refutations.* London: Routledge & Kegan Paul.

# Contents

# PART I

# RESEARCH AND THEORETICAL STRATEGIES

# Crucial Paths from Risk Indicator to Causal Mechanism

MICHAEL RUTTER

## WHY AREN'T THE CAUSES OF ANTISOCIAL BEHAVIOR ALREADY WELL UNDERSTOOD?

Given the vast number of systematic empirical studies of antisocial behavior, using a range of effective research strategies (Hill & Maughan, 2001; Loeber & Farrington, 1998; Rutter, Giller, & Hagell, 1998; Stoff, Breiling, & Maser, 1997), it might be supposed that these should have provided a reasonably firm understanding of the causes of antisocial behavior. Undoubtedly, they have provided a set of well-replicated risk indicators for antisocial behavior. There is every reason to suppose that many, perhaps most, of these are implicated in some way or another in the causal processes leading to antisocial behavior. Nevertheless, that is a far cry from an understanding of the precise nature of the causal mechanisms and of the ways in which they operate.

Part of the difficulty is that many of the risk factors have to be considered as *indicators* rather than as *mechanisms*. Thus, for example, low socioeconomic status (SES), membership of certain ethnic groups, and male sex are all associated with an increased risk for antisocial behavior, but, on their own, are completely uninformative about the nature of the risk process. For example, being male might be associated with an increased risk because of a hormonal effect during either the prenatal period or adolescence, because a gene on a sex chromosome is associated with a risk variable, or because of the ways in which society responds to boys—to name three very different alternatives among a larger array of possibilities. Equally, the association between maleness and antisocial behavior might be mediated through some associated characteristic such as reading difficulties or hyperactivity, rather than through any direct effect on an antisocial tendency. Similar considerations apply to most other risk features. There are, however, other reasons why the existing evidence is not enough for us to draw any firm conclusions on causal processes. Six issues may serve to illustrate some of the key issues that need to be dealt with in providing a rigorous test of any causal hypothesis.

## Failure to Incorporate the Range of Different Causal Questions

Almost all research has focused on the question of mechanisms that might underlie individual differences in the liability to engage in antisocial behavior. This is an important question but it is far from the only one that needs to be addressed. Three other rather different causal issues may be noted as examples of the diversity of causal questions.

First, there are group differences in the level of antisocial behavior. For example, it is well documented that males are much more likely than females to engage in most (but not all) forms of antisocial behavior (Moffitt, Caspi, Rutter, & Silva, 2001). Similarly, during the second half of the last century, there was a massive increase in crime in most industrialized countries (Rutter & Smith, 1995). Area differences in rates of crime are quite large (Mayhew, Aye, Maung, & Mirless-Black, 1993; Reiss, 1995). There are also large differences among nations in certain sorts of crime. For example, the homicide rate in the United States is exceptionally high (Snyder, Sickmund, & Poe-Yamagata, 1996). In this case, the high homicide rate is largely attributable to killings with firearms, which are much more readily available in the United States than in Europe. It is noteworthy, however, that the differential ease of access to firearms does not account for variations in homicide rates *within* the United States. Within countries too there are large variations in crime among different ethnic groups (Sampson & Lauritsen, 1997; Smith, 1997a, 1997b). It is important to note that, although the causes of individual differences in liability and the causes of group differences in level may reflect similar risk factors, that need not be the case. For example, it is obvious that the reasons why one person may be out of work whereas another one is in a stable job are quite different from the political and economic factors responsible for the huge rises and falls in the unemployment rate that take place from time to time (see Rutter, 1994a).

Second, there is a need to determine the causal mechanisms that underlie age trends in antisocial behavior. Why does crime tend to reach a peak in adolescence, with the rate of antisocial activity falling again during early to midadult life? Is this because the liability to antisocial behavior follows this developmental pattern or is it rather because the antisocial propensity is less likely to lead to overt criminal acts for reasons that are unassociated with variations in individual liability? Age trends in psychopathological progression must also be considered. In middle childhood this involves the transition (in some individuals) from oppositional-defiant behavior to overt conduct disorder or to delinquency and in adolescence a transition from conduct problems to drug taking in some people (Rutter, 2002b).

Third, there is the question of why and how, in some circumstances, a preexisting propensity to engage in antisocial behavior is translated into the commission of actual delinquent acts. The available evidence suggests that this translation is influenced by a range of situational factors (Clarke, 1980, 1995; Rutter et al., 1997). The factors involved include young people's perceptions of criminal opportunities and their ability to create or take advantage of them, together with their appraisal of the risks of being caught and the consequences that would follow if they were apprehended. Through its effects in causing disinhibition (Ito, Miller, & Pollock, 1996) alcohol use is associated with an increased likelihood of disorderly behavior and of driving offenses.

## Inadequate Attention to Likely Heterogeneity

Although it has been obvious for very many years that antisocial behavior takes many forms, it is only relatively recently that there has been evidence of meaningful heterogeneity in varieties of antisocial behavior (Rutter et al., 1998). Two differentiations have a substantial amount of supporting evidence, although key questions remain to be answered. First, antisocial behavior that is associated with hyperactivity tends to be characterized by early onset, accompanying difficulties in peer relationships, somewhat below-average cognitive skills, poor scholastic achievement, and a marked tendency to persist into adult life (Rutter et al., 1998). The pattern is also more strongly influenced by genetic factors than is the case with antisocial behavior unaccompanied by hyperactivity and other associated problems (Nadder, Rutter, Silberg, Maes, & Eaves, 2002; Silberg, Meyer, et al., 1996a; Silberg, Rutter, et al., 1996b).

The second validated differentiation is that between life-course-persistent and adolescence-limited antisocial behavior (Moffitt, 1993a; see also Moffitt, Chapter 3, this volume). Research findings in several longitudinal studies (Fergusson, Lynskey, & Horwood, 1996; Moffitt, Caspi, Dickson, Silva, & Stanton, 1996; Patterson, 1996; Patterson & Yoerger, 1997) have shown that the life-course-persistent group is associated not only with unusually early onset, but with a very high level of both individual risk factors (such as lower cognitive skills, hyperactivity, and adverse temperamental features during the preschool years) and family risk factors (such as parental antisocial behavior and poor discipline). The adolescence-limited group tends to show a much lower rate of these risk factors but, possibly, a more important association with negative peer group influences. As is evident from this description, there is considerable uncertainty as to whether this differentiation is synonymous with that involving an association with early-onset hyperactivity.

There is also some evidence that violent crime, antisocial behavior accompanied by psychopathy, and antisocial behavior that arises out of serious mental disorder may also define meaningful subgroups. Possibly too pedophilia may constitute a pattern that is rather different in cause and course from other varieties of antisocial behavior, although systematic evidence on this point is almost entirely lacking.

Research that has made use of these differentiations has been usefully informative, but serious questions remain on the defining characteristics of these patterns, on whether the differentiations are dimensional or categorical in form, and especially on the implications for causal mechanisms. The evidence so far is almost entirely descriptive. Moreover, genetic studies have yet to use these differentiations in a satisfactory fashion.

### One Causal Path or Many?

Although it is generally agreed that antisocial behavior has a multifactorial origin that involves both genetic and environmental factors (and probably multiple types of each), much less attention has been paid to what this might mean in terms of causal pathways. Thus, for example, do genetic and environmental risk factors operate on the same personal risk factors associated with individual differences in liability to engage in antisocial behavior? It is generally assumed that genetic factors are likely to operate indirectly through temperamental features (e.g., hyperactivity, sensation seeking, or impulsivity), or through cognitive features (e.g., low IQ or impaired executive planning [Moffitt, 1993b]) rather than on an antisocial propensity as such. Does the same apply to psychosocial risk factors in the family? Is their association with antisocial behavior mediated through these early-onset personal risk factors or do they operate in rather different ways? For example, are they less concerned with individual differences in temperament and cognitive features than in creating the circumstances in which those personal features may lead to antisocial behavior? Can genetic factors predispose individuals to antisocial behavior in the absence of psychosocial risks? Similarly, can environmentally mediated risks operate in the absence of an individual's genetic susceptibility?

Many theorists seek to reduce risk mechanisms to one basic underlying causal process (although they differ in what that one process might comprise). Although that could prove to be the case, it seems rather unlikely. Even with well-circumscribed diseases in internal medicine, it is quite common to find that several rather different pathways may lead to the same end point pathophysiological process (see Rutter, 1997). Given the diversity of antisocial behavior, and its likely heterogeneity, it must be expected that several rather different causal pathways may be involved. However, if these are to be delineated and understood, it will be essential to move from the identification of risk indicators to the creation of specific hypotheses on the mechanisms involved in risk mediation.

## Inadequate Attention to Possible Confounding Factors

Four issues stand out as of particular importance. First, as Bell (1968) pointed out over 30 years ago, with respect to the study of socialization experiences, it is crucial to use research designs that can differentiate between *person effects on the environment* and *environmental effects on the person* (Bell & Chapman, 1986). Through their behavior, children will elicit or evoke different responses from other people. Accordingly, it is essential to ask questions such as whether parental negativity toward a child is causing the child to behave in antisocial ways or, instead, is the child's oppositional-defiant behavior eliciting negative responses from the parents? Of course, in any social situation, influences are likely to be bidirectional, but the crucial point is that it is necessary to test for the direction of causal influence if a causal hypothesis is to be tested in adequate fashion.

A variant on the same issue is provided by the need to differentiate between *social selection* and *social causation* (Dohrenwend et al., 1992). Environments are not randomly distributed, and through their behavior people shape and select their own environments and those of their children. The consequence is that an association between a putative environmental risk factor and antisocial behavior may reflect the effects of either the child's antisocial behavior or of family features (see Borge, Rutter, Côté, & Tremblay, in press) on social selection or the effects of the social experience on the liability to engage in antisocial behavior. Thus, for example, in studies of possible school influences on children's behavior, it has been necessary to determine whether the variations among schools in rates of disruptive behavior could be a function of variations in their intake of pupils with high-risk characteristics or from high-risk family backgrounds (Rutter, Maughan, Mortimore, Ouston, & Smith, 1979). The same issues apply to possible area influences on delinquency (Brooks-Gunn, Duncan, & Aber, 1997; Sampson, Raudenbush, & Earls, 1997). In resolving this issue, the need is not only to examine possible social selection factors, but also to test for possible social causation mediating variables and to examine the timing of associations, using longitudinal data. *Social selection* would lead to an expectation that associations would be most marked at the time individuals entered the risk situation, whereas (if the effects are enduring) *social causation* would expect associations to be stronger after a period of time in the putative risk situation. This would not necessarily apply if the effects of risk experience are both immediate and short-lived, but this is not applicable in the case of persistent antisocial behavior.

A third variety of confound is provided by the need to differentiate between *proximal* and *distal* risk factors. Thus, at one time, parental loss and parent–child separations were viewed as a major risk factor for psychopathology (including, but not confined to, antisocial behavior). However, empirical research showed that the risks were largely mediated through the effects of loss or separation in leading to poor parenting or other family adversities (Harris, Brown, & Bifulco, 1986; Fergusson, Horwood, & Lynskey, 1992; Rutter, 1971). The family adversities and poor parenting led to psychopathology even if parental loss or parent–child separation were not involved; conversely, there was little risk from loss or separation if family adversities were not brought about. The implication is that loss may be important because, at an early point in the causal chain, it increases the likelihood of proximal risk factors, but it does not in itself bring about risk. Rather similar issues have been evident in studies of poverty. Economic pressure has a distal effect on antisocial behavior but the risks are mediated by parental depression, marital conflict, and parental hostility, with little direct effect that is independent of these mediators (Conger et al., 1992; Conger, Conger, Elder, & Lorenz, 1993; Conger, Ge, Elder, Lorenz, & Simons, 1994). In comparable fashion, Rutter and Quinton (1977) showed that increased risks for childhood psychopathology associated with a depriving inner-city environment were largely mediated through the effects on the family and through school influences, with little direct impact of the city environment on the children themselves.

A fourth important confound is provided by the effect of *genetic influences* on individual differences in *environmental risk exposure* (Plomin & Bergeman, 1991; Plomin, 1994). This gene–environment correlation arises passively through the fact that parents pass on genes as well as create the rearing environment for their children, and actively because children's behavior serves to shape and select the environments they experience (Plomin, DeFries, & Loehlin, 1977; Rutter et al., 1997). Accordingly, it is important to use designs (such as twin and adoptee strategies) that can differentiate between genetic and environmental risk mediation; such designs have been employed by very few psychosocial researchers.

### Inadequate Attention to the Need to Test for Mode of Risk/Protective Mediation

Despite Baron and Kenny's (1986) conceptual distinction between *moderating* and *mediating* risk factors, together with an outline of how these may be examined statistically (see also Kraemer, Stice, Kazdin, Offord, & Kupfer, 2001), there have been relatively few systematic attempts to determine whether postulated risk or protective factors could account for the differences between individuals who do and those who do not exhibit antisocial behavior. For example, it has often been argued that intervention studies provide a powerful test of environmental risk mediation. There are two major problems with this line of argument. First, the fact that a treatment alleviates some form of problem behavior does not in itself indicate that a lack of the environmental feature that the treatment purports to right constituted the cause of the problem in the first place. Second, because almost all treatments, whether pharmacological or psychological, involve multiple elements, the finding that a treatment is effective is completely uninformative about the mechanism unless it has been demonstrated that a change in the postulated mediating mechanism is associated systematically in a dose–response fashion with a change in the target behavior. There have been a few studies that have attempted to do this (see, e.g., Forgatch & DeGarmo, 1999), but such attempts have been few and far between. Moreover, even when this has been done, the findings have been somewhat inconclusive. Thus, in the Forgatch and De Garmo (1999) study, the intervention led to a significant improvement in parenting practices (the postulated mediating variable for the effects on child behavior), but no significant change in child behavior, whether measured by teacher, mother, or child report. Accordingly, following the usual conventions (Baron & Kenny, 1986; Kraemer et al., 2001), there was no effect to be mediated. The implication of possible mediation derived only from path analyses showing that changes in parenting were associated with changes in the child's school adjustment. A further important need, however, is to test competing hypotheses on mode of risk mediation. When this has been done, the findings have sometimes run counter to the original claims (see Scarr, 1997). Thus, De Baryshe, Patterson, and Capaldi (1993) used their findings from comparing competing models of mediation to argue that the effects of parental IQ/education on their children's academic achievement were due to the mediating role of antisocial behavior and ineffective discipline. Scarr (1997), through further analyses undertaken by De Baryshe, showed that the previously untested model of a direct effect of parental IQ/education on child achievement plus an indirect effect via academic engagement was superior to the published model implicating antisocial behavior and parental discipline.

Although it has become widely recognized that causal processes often involve a series of stepping-stones (Farrington, 1986), or indirect causal chains involving several rather different links (Rutter, 1989: Rutter & Rutter, 1993), there have been rather few attempts to undertake systematic analyses to test hypotheses on different phases in the causal developmental process. In particular, there have been few studies that have set out to examine whether different risk factors operate at different points in the causal chain (but see Robins, Davis, & Wish, 1977, and Robins, 1993, for an example in relation to narcotic addiction).

It has been known for a long time that there is huge individual variation in different people's responses to what appear to be the same risk factors (Rutter, 2000a). This has led to an interest in the concept of *resilience*, the phenomenon of relatively good functioning despite the experience of major risks. Although research has provided a number of valuable leads, rather little is known about the mechanisms involved in these individual differences in response to adversity. However, it is clear that one factor involves genetic effects on susceptibility to environmental stressors (Rutter & Silberg, 2002; Rutter, 2003). Although the available empirical evidence is sparse, it suggests that the main environmental effects on antisocial behavior are evident only in those who are genetically vulnerable. Clearly, that finding should have major implications for a theory of causation but up to now there has been very little attention paid to the possibility of gene–environment interaction in relation to antisocial behavior (or indeed other forms of psychopathology).

In principle, it seems obvious that attention must be paid to the possibility of factors that protect against antisocial behavior as well as to those that predispose to it. Sometimes this has been conceptualized in terms of a need to examine the effects of the positive role of some feature. However, if the risk and protective factors operate dimensionally, nothing much is to be gained by, say, focusing on the beneficial effects of family harmony rather than the harmful effects of family discord and conflict. In essence, the two are providing the same message. On the other hand, there is real value in examining the possibility of factors that provide protection in the presence of risk, even though they have little effect in the absence of such risk (see Rutter, 1990). Thus, adoption of children from a high-risk background may bring substantial benefits, even though it does not improve the outcome for children from a low-risk background (see Duyme, Dumaret, & Tomkiewicz, 1999), although the possibility that it has this protective effect in relation to the risk of antisocial behavior has yet to be put properly to the test. If the field of possible protective factors is to be moved forward, however, we need a much better conceptualization of putative protective processes.

Until relatively recently, there has tended to be an implicit assumption that events or experiences that are brought about by people's own behavior need to be excluded as possible causal influences. For example, life events research has predominantly focused on events that are supposedly independent of a person's own behavior. However, the assumption that the origin of a risk experience necessarily indicates the mode of risk mediation is clearly false (Rutter, Silberg, & Simonoff, 1993). Moreover, as already noted, all social experiences are likely to be influenced to some degree by a person's own behavior and, as also already noted, that behavior will involve some genetic influence. The use of longitudinal data, of multiple measures of behavior and of risk factors, and of appropriate statistical techniques has made it possible to show convincingly that experiences brought about by people themselves can nevertheless have major effects on their subsequent behavior. This has been shown, for example, with respect to incarceration (Rutter et al., 1998; Sampson & Laub, 1993), a harmonious supportive marriage in adult life (Laub, Nagin, & Sampson, 1998; Zoccolillo, Pickles, Quinton, & Rutter, 1992), and military service (Sampson & Laub, 1996; Elder, 1986).

## Weak Concepts and Measures of Putative Mediating Mechanisms

Over the years, theories of causation and antisocial behavior have taken several rather different forms (Farrington, 1994; Rutter & Giller, 1983). Some have emphasized some supposed general social process such as *status frustration*, or the *strain* that derives from the disparity between people's goals and what they can actually achieve, or bonding to society. Others have focused on a general psychological mechanism, such as social learning or social information processing. But many too have used as their starting point some specific risk factor such as low IQ, temperamental difficulty, or broken homes. Because none of these has been seen to provide an adequate explanation of antisocial behavior, there has been an increasing tendency to develop integrated theories that encompass a range of mechanisms. A key problem, however, stems from the huge number of risk factors that have been identified. Farrington (1994) argued that future theories need to be wide ranging, including individual, family, peer, school, and neighborhood factors, as well as energizing, directing, inhibiting, and decision-making processes. He went on to point out, however, that there is a danger that theories become so complex that *they can explain everything but predict nothing*. He also noted that most theories focused on the adolescent years when crime rates tend to be at their peak, rather than on the preschool years when disruptive behavior first becomes manifest, or on adulthood when crime rates drop. The history of science clearly indicates that as the understanding of causal processes develops, what initially appears extremely complex ultimately proves to reduce to a relatively small number of mediating mechanisms. Clearly, this reduction is needed in the field of antisocial behavior, but it is essential that the hypotheses about mediating mechanisms are put in a form that makes them susceptible to potential falsification, and it is equally necessary that the testing involve contrasting competing hypotheses about causal processes.

In that connection, as well as the problems that derive from rather general hypotheses, there are constraints that derive from the weakness of so many of the measures that are available. It is not just that it has proved difficult to create quantified operationalized measures of constructs such as social bonding but also that the measures of risk factors (particularly when they need to be used on large samples) are most unsatisfactory. For example, there is a paucity of discriminating measures of people's peer groups, of possible community influences, of school features, and of child-specific socialization experiences.

## POSSIBLE WAYS FORWARD

### Clear Specification of the Supposed Causal Process

As follows from the above, any adequate causal concept will have to be explicit on what it purports to cover. Does it, for example, deal with what is involved in the origins of antisocial behavior during the preschool years or, rather, the translation of these precursors into actual criminal acts? Does it account for the occasional delinquent acts undertaken by most people at some time in their lives, or just life-course-persistent varieties of antisocial behavior, or the increase in criminal activities during the adolescent years in individuals who show little engagement in antisocial behavior in either childhood or adult life? Does the causal hypothesis depend on an interaction between some individual susceptibility and some social experience, and, if so, how is that specified? If not, there needs to be specification of why there are individual differences in response.

With respect to individual variations in response, two somewhat different distinctions need to be made. First, there is the distinction between individual differences in response to exposure to a *risk factor* and individual differences in response to a *risk process*. Throughout the whole of medicine, and the whole of biology, it is usual to find that most people exposed to a risk factor do not develop a disorder. That would be so, for example, with exposure to infectious agents, carcinogens, and smoking. There is an interest in why some people respond and others do not (genetic factors may well be relevant in that connection: see Rutter & Silberg, 2002; Rutter, 2003), but the finding that only some people succumb in no way threatens the causal hypothesis. On the other hand, if direct measurement of the causal process (e.g., the early stage of carcinogenesis) shows that in many cases this does not lead to the predicted outcome, that finding does challenge the causal hypothesis, unless there is some testable hypothesis about why that might be the case. So far as hypotheses about the causation of antisocial behavior are concerned, this distinction requires, in the case of environmental risk mediation, specification of what exposure to the risk factor does to the organism, and therefore the circumstances in which this exposure leads to antisocial behavior. This process might involve mechanisms as various as cognitive processing, neuroendocrine changes, changes in brain structure/function, or altered patterns of interpersonal interaction. Any hypothesis that does not go on to specify how the effects of risk are carried forward (either through changes in the organism or changes in the interaction between the organism and its environment) falls short.

The second type of distinction is that between variations in response to risk and variations in whether or not the dependent outcome (in this case, antisocial behavior) is associated with the specified risk mechanism. If antisocial behavior (of the kind covered by the hypothesis) arises in the absence of the postulated causal process, that challenges the hypothesis. Note that the expectation is *not* that there will be a single risk factor; that would be completely inconsistent with the concept that antisocial behavior is a multifactorial trait. However, even when multiple risk factors are involved, the expectation from biology is that a limited number of causal pathways are likely to be involved.

In that connection, it is often helpful to predict when an effect should *not* be found (Rutter, 1974). For example, if the hypothesis is that the personal experience of interpersonal conflict in the family constitutes a key risk mechanism, it would be predicted that parental loss, or poverty, or social disadvantage should not predispose to antisocial behavior if such conflict is not involved. Equally, the prediction would be that, in the context of overall family conflict, there should not be a risk if that does not impinge on, or involve, the particular child being considered.

## Testing Hypotheses about the Causes of Individual Differences in Liability

Most information on risk factors necessarily derives from some kind of case–control comparison—either as part of a broader epidemiological study or from a deliberate choice of groups that have and that do not have the specified behavior. That constitutes quite an efficient way of obtaining a list of potentially important risk factors but, on its own, it is not likely to provide an adequate test of a hypothesis on a causal process. The first problem is that it is usual to find substantial intercorrelations among many of the possible risk factors. Appropriate multivariate statistical methods are helpful in sorting out which of the possible risk factors might actually be operative. However, showing that there is a significant effect after taking other variables into account is not synonymous with showing that there is an effect in the absence of other variables (see Rutter, 1983). Also, inevitably, the statistical manipulations involve extrapolation to situations other than those reflected in the particular data set being analyzed (see Rutter, Pickles, Murray, & Eaves, 2001). That is, mathematical adjustments are made to infer what would happen if, for example, family conflict was *not* accompanied by poverty, or limited education, or parental psychopathology. But that is not the case in the sample studied. Causal inferences are thereby shaky. The research need is for some form of "natural experiment" in which the combination of appropriate samples, critical research designs, and appropriate methods of statistical analysis "pull apart" variables that ordinarily go together. Thus, the various forms of twin and adoptee design do just that with respect to the differentiation of genetic and environmental influences (Rutter et al., 1990; Rutter et al., 1999). However, in testing hypotheses about causal processes, the mere separation of genetic and environmental influences does not get one very far. So far as environmental risk factors and environmentally mediated risk processes are concerned, the need is to use genetically sensitive designs that are environmentally informative with respect to specific postulated risk factors. There are several twin and adoptee designs that can be used for this purpose—for example, differences within monozygotic (MZ) pairs, or the study of the offspring of twins, or effects within adoptive families (Rutter et al., 2001). In addition, however, there is a substantial range of other types of natural experiments that also serve to "pull apart" variables that ordinarily go together—such as migration, or major environmental change, or different patterns of rearing following parenting breakdown (see Rutter et al., 2001).

It is often claimed that studies of treatment provide a particularly effective way of testing causal hypotheses. Undoubtedly, they are valuable in that connection, but there are three important limitations (see above). First, and most crucially, the finding that a treatment has benefits is completely uninformative about risk mediation unless it can be shown that variations in response to the treatment are systematically associated with the degree to which the postulated mediating process has been altered. Second, treatments may be effective for reasons that are unconnected with the causal process. Third, although the demonstration that treatment-induced change in a postulated mediating mechanism reduces antisocial behavior constitutes a good test of its role in the risk process, nevertheless a failure to bring about change may mean that the processes involved in the initial causation of antisocial behavior are not quite the same as those involved in its persistence over time. As a result, treatment studies constitute one good element in the overall program of testing causal hypotheses, but they are far from sufficient on their own.

However, separation of genetic and environmental mediation, together with the separation of the effects of different risk variables, constitute only two of the needs. Thus, attention has already been drawn to the need to separate possible social selection from social causation. Two other considerations are important. First, most studies rely on between-group differences to infer causal processes within the individual. Various statistical methods are available to test the validity of this extrapolation, but the test is inevitably an indirect one. Wherever possible, studies of within-individual change in relation to the onset of exposure to a risk variable constitute a stronger research strategy (Farrington, 1988; Rutter, 1994b; Rutter et al., 2001). Of course, such testing is only possible in relation to risk exposure that has an onset after a period of previously normal development. Second, it is necessary to differentiate between person effects on the environment and environmental effects on the person. That too requires longitudinal data and the study of within-individual change.

It will be appreciated that the natural experiments referred to above all involve designs that in some way have as their starting point the postulated risk factor, rather than the outcome of antisocial behavior. This constitutes an essential step in testing hypotheses about risk mechanisms.

On their own, however, although these designs go a long way in the rigorous testing of hypotheses about risk features, they do not deal with the essential stage of testing hypotheses about the risk process itself. There have been only a few attempts to deal with that issue. One of the few examples is provided by the longitudinal studies undertaken by Dodge and his colleagues (Dodge, Bates, & Pettit, 1990; Dodge, Pettit, Bates, & Valente, 1995). They tested the hypothesis that the process by which the experience of child abuse led to antisocial behavior was through the mechanism of altered cognitive processing. Their findings provided only limited support for the hypothesis and, unfortunately, they did not pit competing hypotheses against one another (e.g., biased cognitive processing vs. altered attachment relationships or changed neuroendocrine functioning). Nevertheless, the research strategy is one that warrants much wider application.

Although what is needed with respect to testing genetic hypotheses differs in detail, similar principles apply to those involved in testing environmental mediation. Thus, hypotheses on genetic mediation need to specify the genetically influenced traits that mediate the risk for antisocial behavior. Thus, the hypothesis might specify effects on some temperamental or cognitive feature. Whether or not this is so can be tested through both quantitative genetic and molecular genetic strategies. The former can be informative on the intervening mediating variable, but only the latter can identify the particular genes concerned. But even this is not enough. Genes do not affect behavior directly. Rather, genes have effects on proteins and these protein products have downstream effects on behavior. There is also the further need to specify how, and under what circumstances, the behaviors that mediate risk lead to the phenotype in question (namely, antisocial behavior). A range of different types of science will be required to provide understanding of the variety of interlinked steps in this causal chain (Rutter, 2000a, 2002b).

As already noted, it is likely that many genetic effects rely on gene–environment correlations and interactions. These need to be specified and tested as part of the causal hypothesis. By the same token, many environmental effects will only be found, or will be mainly evident, in genetically susceptible individuals. Once more, this needs to be part of what is specified and tested.

Finally, attention needs to be paid, in both hypothesis making and hypothesis testing, to whether or not the causal processes are specific to antisocial behavior or whether they involve a broader range of outcomes of which antisocial behavior is just one. If the latter is postulated, it is necessary that the causal hypothesis specifies reasons why antisocial behavior might be the outcome in some individuals whereas some other forms of psychopathology develop in others exposed to the same risk factors. One of the few studies to tackle this issue is that undertaken by Quiggle, Garber, Panak, and Dodge (1992), in which they compared social information processing in aggressive and depressed children.

## Testing Hypotheses about the Causal Processes Involved in Group Differences

The principles involved in testing causal hypotheses about the processes responsible for group differences in antisocial behavior are much the same as those already discussed in relation to individual differences in liability. That is to say, there are the same needs to find means of putting hypotheses to the test, of pitting competing hypotheses against one another, and of considering the range of possible confounds that need to be taken into account. Similarly, there is a need to move on to testing for risk mediation, using the model put forward by Baron and Kenny (1986) and expanded by Kraemer et al. (2001), but with the crucial difference that the dependent variable has to be the group difference, rather than individual variation within the group. For obvious reasons, the specifics of how this may best be done will vary with the kind of group comparison required.

For example, ethnic differences may often be examined most effectively by making use of migration research strategies (see Rutter et al., 2001). For example, the finding that schizophrenia was much commoner in Afro-Caribbeans living within the United Kingdom than in Caucasians also living in the United Kingdom was initially investigated by comparing rates of schizophrenia in Afro-Caribbeans in the United Kingdom with those of Afro-Caribbeans living in the West Indies. The finding that the rate was raised only among those living in the United Kingdom pointed clearly to the likely operation of some risk factor that was concerned with life in the United Kingdom. Cross-ethnic comparisons on familial loading for schizophrenia also indicated that a genetic explanation was unlikely to be correct. The research has been effective in ruling out several plausible environmental risk factors, but, to date, it has not identified the key causal mechanism. The same strategy has proved effective in the study of various medical conditions, and, in principle, it could also be applied to the investigation of the causes of ethnic differences in antisocial behavior. However, this approach has yet to be followed. In examining the possible reasons for ethnic differences in the rate of antisocial behavior, it will be important to differentiate between the causal processes concerned with variations in levels and those that apply to individual differences, but to consider the possibility that the developmental processes are the same in the two cases and to test for this possibility (see Rowe, Vazsonyi, & Flannery, 1994).

Elucidation of the causes of the major rise in the rate of antisocial behavior during the last 50 years or so has not proceeded very far, although it has been possible to rule out several possibilities (Rutter & Smith, 1995). Several research needs will have to be met. First, it is necessary either to find countries that have not shown the rise in crime, or to focus on time periods in which crime rates have gone down before or after a period in which they have risen, or both. Alternatively, internation comparisons may be useful if the rise in crime in different countries has taken place at different times. The need, of course, is to specify what causal processes might have been responsible for these differences in timing. Second, the causal hypothesis must concern some feature that has changed over time in populations as a whole. Third, there must be measures available to quantify changes over time in these risk features in order that these may be related to the changes in rates of crime. In that connection, it is crucial that the measures are able to determine whether the population-wide changes have actually impinged on the age group under consideration. Thus, for example, it is of limited value to chart changes over time in, say, unemployment or poverty unless it is possible to determine whether these applied to the age group in which antisocial behavior occurs.

The study of the possible causal processes underlying sex differences in antisocial behavior provides a somewhat different challenge. In essence, however, the requirement is to test the main alternatives that (1) there are risk or protective factors that differ between the sexes; (2) that the risk factors are similar but one sex has more of them (or has them more severely); and (3) that one sex is more susceptible to the same risk factors (Moffitt et al., 2001). In order to undertake such a study, it is necessary to examine the operation of risk factors in both sexes separately; to test for sex differences in rates of risk factors; to check that the sex difference in antisocial behavior is not an artifact of measurement; and to determine whether the features that appear to account for the sex difference actually do mediate it. That is, if they are introduced into an overall regression model, do they remove the sex difference that constituted the starting point? Much the same strategy has been used to good effect to examine competing hypotheses on causes for the twin–singleton difference in language development (Rutter, Thorpe, Greenwood, Northstone, & Golding, 2003; Thorpe, Rutter, & Greenwood, 2003). The findings from the study of sex differences in antisocial behavior (Moffitt et al., 2001) indicated that the likely mediator was the higher rate of neurodevelopmental difficulties in males as compared with females, and that this primarily affected lifespan-persistent antisocial behavior. That leaves open, of course, the question of why such neurodevelopmental impairment is more common in males. Genetic hypotheses will certainly be among those that need to be considered in that connection.

Up to now the study of sex differences has been based on comparisons between singleton males and singleton females. Inevitably, that leaves uncertainties as to whether or not the risk factors truly operated similarly, and impinged similarly, on males and females. It would be preferable to make comparisons either between brothers and sisters in the same family or within opposite-sex twin pairs (which would have the advantage that they are of the same age). For obvious reasons, it would be necessary to build in a direct comparison of the findings with same-sex male and same-sex female pairs (Kendler, Thornton, & Prescott, 2001).

Possible sex differences in genetic liability can be examined by determining whether there are sex differences in familial loading as they apply to the risks for antisocial behavior (see, e.g., Merikangas, Weissman, & Pauls, 1985; Reich, Winokur, & Mullaney, 1975). The possibility that genetic effects on sex differences may derive from protective genes on the X chromosome or risk genes on the Y chromosome may be examined by studying sex chromosome anomalies. Although the sample size is small, the evidence suggests that an extra Y chromosome may be associated with a higher rate of hyperactivity that predisposes to antisocial behavior (see Rutter et al., 1998).

Molecular genetic strategies will also be very important insofar as they may lead to the identification of risk or protective influences associated with genes on one or the other of the sex chromosomes. So far, there have been few findings of this kind. Nevertheless, one study did suggest that a gene may serve to make women more susceptible to the carcinogenic effects of smoking (Shriver et al., 2000). Also, Skuse (2000) used findings from XO females to postulate that a gene on the X chromosome affecting social responsiveness may provide females with a relative protection against autism.

A rather different sort of group effect is implied by the evidence showing the importance of situational influences on antisocial behavior (Clarke, 1995; Pease, 1997). Similar principles to the testing of causal hypotheses apply. That is, it is necessary to specify the putative feature that creates the situational effect, to pit this hypothesis against competing alternatives, and to determine whether changes in the key situational mediation (in either direction) have the predicted effects on the level of antisocial behavior in that situation.

Yet another different type of group effect concerns psychopathological progressions over particular age periods. Thus, for example, a key issue in relation to depression has concerned the rise in the rate of depressive disorder during adolescence and the emergence of a female preponderance during the same age period. The evidence suggests that both gene–environment correlations and gene–environment interactions play a crucial mediating role (Silberg et al., 1999; Silberg, Rutter, Neale, & Eaves, 2001a; Silberg, Rutter, & Eaves, 2001b). Similar attention to the possibility of gene–environment interplay may be needed in relation to age changes in antisocial behavior (e.g., the reduction in criminal activities that ordinarily takes place in early adult life). The developmental progression from, say, oppositional-defiant behavior to conduct problems to overt crime requires strategies that span those used for testing individual liability and those used for testing group differences. Thus, it is necessary to consider both why this is a general pattern of progression that is seen in the population as a whole, and also the fact that only some individuals proceed down this pathway. What is different, for example, in the individuals showing early oppositional-defiant behavior who do not go on to develop conduct problems? Are their personal characteristics relevant, or is it their experiences, or is it some combination of the two?

## CONCLUSIONS

In considering how causal hypotheses may be tested most effectively, a wide range of conceptual, strategic, sampling, and analytic challenges have to be met. At first sight, these seem daunting and it might be thought that the level of demands has been set too high. However, the research task is a doable one, and, as the remainder of the chapters in this volume show, there are many good leads to be followed. Behavioral scientists are all too well aware of the hazards involved in inferring causation from statistical correlations but epidemiological longitudinal methods can go far in testing causal hypotheses (Rutter, 1981; Rutter et al., 2001). Both criminologists and clinical scientists often draw back from tightly conceptualized causal hypotheses on the grounds that because a variety of causal questions are involved, because risk factors are so many and various and span so many domains, and because multistep causal chains are involved, an integrative causal theory has got to have bits of everything in it. This is a counsel of despair. The main argument of this chapter has been that the histories of biology and of medicine indicate that it is usually possible to reduce complex multifactorial causation to a much more limited set of causal mechanisms. That is the challenge that we must meet.

## REFERENCES

Baron, R. M., & Kenny, D. A. (1986). The moderator–mediator variable distinction in social psychological research: Conceptual, strategic, and statistical considerations. *Journal of Personality and Social Psychology, 51,* 1173–1182.

Bell, R. Q. (1968). A reinterpretation of the direction of effects in studies of socialization. *Psychological Review, 75,* 81–95.

Bell, R. Q., & Chapman, M. (1986). Child effects in studies using experimental or brief longitudinal approaches to socialization. *Developmental Psychology, 22,* 595–603.

Borge, A. I. H., Rutter, M., Côté, S., & Tremblay, R. E. (in press). Early childcare and physical aggression: Differentiating social selection and social causation. *Journal of Child Psychology and Psychiatry.*

Brooks-Gunn, J., Duncan, G. J., & Aber, J. L. (1997). *Neighborhood poverty: Vol. 1. Context and consequences for children.* New York: Russell Sage Foundation.

Clarke, R. V. (1980). Situational crime prevention: Theory and practice. *British Journal of Criminology, 20,* 136–147.

Clarke, R. V. (1995). Situational crime prevention. In M. Tonry & D. P. Farrington (Eds.), *Crime and justice* (Vol. 19, pp. 91–149). Chicago: University of Chicago Press.

Conger, R. D., Conger, K. J., Elder, G. H., & Lorenz, F. O. (1993). Family economic stress and adjustment of early adolescent girls. *Developmental Psychology, 29,* 206–219.

Conger, R. D., Conger, K. J., Elder, G. H. Jr., Lorenz, F. O., Simons, R. L., & Whitbeck, L. B. (1992). A family process model of economic hardship and adjustment of early adolescent boys. *Child Development, 63,* 526–541.

Conger, R. D., Ge, X., Elder, G. H. Jr., Lorenz, F. O., & Simons, R. L. (1994). Economic stress, coercive family process, and developmental problems of adolescents. *Child Development, 65,* 541–561.

DeBaryshe, B. D., Patterson, G. R., & Capaldi, D. M. (1993) A performance model for academic achievement in early adolescent boys. *Developmental Psychology, 29,* 795–804.

Dodge, K. A., Bates, J. E., & Pettit, G. S. (1990). Mechanisms in the cycle of violence. *Science, 250,* 1678–1683.

Dodge, K. A., Pettit, G. S., Bates, J. E., & Valente, E. (1995). Social information-processing patterns partially mediate the effect of early physical abuse on later conduct problems. *Journal of Abnormal Psychology, 104,* 632–643.

Dohrenwend, B. P., Levav, I., Shrout, P. E., Schwartz, S., Naveh, G., Link, B. G., Skodol, A. E., & Stueve, A. (1992). Socioeconomic status and psychiatric disorders: The causation–selection issue. *Science, 255,* 946–952.

Duyme, M., Dumaret, A.-C., & Tomkiewicz, S. (1999). How can we boost IQs of "dull children"?: A late adoption study. *Proceedings of the National Academy of Sciences USA, 96,* 8790–8794.

Elder, G. H. Jr. (1986). Military times and turning points in men's lives. *Developmental Psychology, 22,* 233–245.

Farrington, D. P. (1986). Stepping stones to adult criminal careers. In D. Olweus, J. Blockand, & M. R. Yarrow (Eds.), *Development of antisocial and prosocial behavior* (pp. 359–384). New York: Academic Press.

Farrington, D. P. (1988). Studying changes within individuals: The causes of offending. In M. Rutter (Ed.), *Studies of psychosocial risk: The power of longitudinal data* (pp. 158–183). Cambridge, UK: Cambridge University Press.

Farrington, D. P. (1994). *Psychological explanations of crime.* Aldershot, UK: Dartmouth.

Fergusson, D. M., Horwood, L. J., & Lynskey, M. T. (1992). Family change, parental discord and early offending. *Journal of Child Psychology and Psychiatry, 33,* 1059–1075.

Fergusson, D. M., Lynskey, M. T., & Horwood, J. (1996). Factors associated with continuity and changes in disruptive behavior patterns between childhood and adolescence. *Journal of Abnormal Child Psychology, 24,* 533–554.

Forgatch, M. S., & DeGarmo, D. S. (1999). Parenting through change: An effective prevention program for single mothers. *Journal of Consulting and Clinical Psychology, 67,* 711–724.

Harris, T., Brown, G. W., & Bifulco, A. (1986). Loss of parent in childhood and adult psychiatric disorder: The role of lack of adequate parental care. *Psychological Medicine, 16,* 641–659.

Hill, J., & Maughan, B. (Eds.). (2001). *Conduct disorders in childhood and adolescence.* Cambridge, UK: Cambridge University Press

Ito, T., Miller, N., & Pollock, V. E. (1996). Alcohol and aggression: A meta-analysis on the moderating effects of inhibitory cues, triggering events, and self-focused attention. *Psychological Bulletin, 120,* 60–82.

Kendler, K. S., Thornton, L. M., & Prescott, C. A. (2001). Gender differences in the rates of exposure to stressful life events and sensitivity to their depressogenic effects. *American Journal of Psychiatry, 158,* 587–593.

Kraemer, H. C., Stice, E., Kazdin, A., Offord, D., & Kupfer, D. (2001). How do risk factors work together?: Mediators, moderators and independent, overlapping and proxy risk factors. *American journal of Psychiatry, 158,* 848–856.

Laub, J. H., Nagin, D. S., & Sampson, R. J. (1998). Trajectories of change in criminal offending: Good marriages and the desistance process. *American Sociological Review, 63,* 225–238.

Loeber, R. L., & Farrington, D. P. (Eds.). (1998). *Serious and violent juvenile offenders: Risk factors and successful interventions.* Thousand Oaks, CA: Sage.

Mayhew, P., Aye Maung, N., & Mirrlees-Black, C. (1993). *The 1992 British Crime Survey*. London: Her Majesty's Stationery Office.

Merikangas, K. R., Weissman, M. M., & Pauls, D. L. (1985). Genetic factors in the sex ratio of major depression *Psychological Medicine*, 15, 63–69.

Moffitt, T. E. (1993a). Adolescence-limited and life-course-persistent antisocial behavior: A developmental taxonomy. *Psychological Review*, 100, 674–701.

Moffitt, T. E. (1993b). The neuropsychology of conduct disorder. *Development and Psychopathology*, 5, 135–152.

Moffitt, T. E., Caspi, A., Dickson, N., Silva, P., & Stanton, W. (1996). Childhood-onset versus adolescent-onset antisocial conduct problems in males: Natural history from ages 3 to 18 years. *Development and Psychopathology*, 9, 399–424.

Moffit, T. E., Caspi, A., Rutter, M., & Silva, P. A. (2001). *Sex differences in antisocial behaviour: Conduct disorder, delinquency and violence in the Dunedin Longitudinal Study*. Cambridge, UK: Cambridge University Press.

Nadder, T. S., Rutter, M., Silberg, J. L., Maes, H. H., & Eaves, L. J. (2002). Genetic effects on the variation and covariation of attention deficit-hyperactivity disorder (ADHD) and oppositional-defiant disorder/conduct disorder (ODD/CD) symptomatologies across informant and occasion of measurement. *Psychological Medicine*, 32, 39–53.

Patterson, G. R. (1996). Some characteristics of a developmental theory for early onset delinquency. In M. Lenzenweger & J. J. Haugaard (Eds.), *Frontier of developmental psychopathology* (pp. 81–124). New York: Oxford University Press.

Patterson, G. R., & Yoerger, K. (1997). A developmental model for late-onset delinquency. In R. Dienstbier (Series Ed.) & D. W. Osgood (Vol. Ed.), *The Nebraska Symposium on Motivation: Vol. 44. Motivation and delinquency* (pp. 119–177). Lincoln: University of Nebraska Press.

Pease, K. (1997). Crime prevention. In M. Maguire, R. Morgan, & R. Reiner (Eds.), *The Oxford handbook of criminology* (2nd ed., pp. 963–995). Oxford, UK: Clarendon Press.

Plomin, R. (1994). *Genetics and experience: The interplay between nature and nurture*. Thousand Oaks, CA: Sage.

Plomin, R., & Bergeman, C. S. (1991). The nature of nurture: Genetic influences on "environmental" measures. *Behavioral and Brain Sciences*, 10, 1–15.

Plomin, R., DeFries, J. C., & Loehlin, J. C. (1977). Genotype–environment interaction and correlation in the analysis of human behavior. *Psychological Bulletin*, 84, 309–322.

Quiggle, N. L., Garber, J., Panak, W. F., & Dodge, K. A. (1992). Social information processing in aggressive and depressed children. *Child Development*, 63, 1305–1320.

Reich, T., Winokur, G., & Mullaney, J. (1975). The transmission of alcoholism. In R. R. Fieve, D. Rosenthal, & H. Brill (Eds.), *Genetic research in psychiatry* (pp. 261–271). Baltimore: Johns Hopkins University Press.

Reiss, A. J. (1995). Community influences on adolescent behavior. In M. Rutter (Ed.), *Psychosocial disturbances in young people: Challenges for prevention* (pp. 305–332). Cambridge, UK: Cambridge University Press.

Robins, L. N. (1993). Vietnam veterans' rapid recovery from heroin addiction: A fluke or normal expectation? *Addiction*, 88, 1041–1054.

Robins, L. N., Davis, D. H., & Wish, E. (1977). Detecting predictors of rare events: Demographic family and personal deviance as predictors of stages in the progression towards narcotic addiction. In J. S. Strauss, H. M. Babigian, & M. Roff (Eds.), *The origins and course of psychopathology* (pp. 379–406). New York: Plenum Press.

Rowe, D. C., Vazsonyi, A. T., & Flannery, D. J. (1994). No more than skin deep: Ethnic and racial similarity in developmental process. *Psychological Review*, 101, 396–413.

Rutter, M. (1971). Parent–child separation: Psychological effects on the children. *Journal of Child Psychology and Psychiatry*, 12, 233–260.

Rutter, M. (1974). Epidemiological strategies and psychiatric concepts in research on the vulnerable child. In E. Anthony & C. Koupernik (Eds.), *The child in his family: Children at psychiatric risk* (Vol. 3, pp. 167–179). New York: Wiley.

Rutter, M. (1981). Epidemiological/longitudinal strategies and causal research in child psychiatry. *Journal of the American Academy of Child Psychiatry, 20,* 513–544.

Rutter, M. (1983). Statistical and personal interactions: Facets and perspectives. In D. Magnusson & V. Allen (Eds.), *Human Development: An interactional perspective* (pp. 295–319). New York: Academic Press.

Rutter, M. (1989). Pathways from childhood to adult life. *Journal of Child Psychology and Psychiatry, 30,* 23–51.

Rutter, M. (1990). Psychosocial resilience and protective mechanisms. In J. Rolf, A. S. Masten, D. Cicchetti, K. N. Neuchterlein, & S. Weintraub (Eds.), *Risk and protective factors in the development of psychopathology* (pp. 181–214). Cambridge, UK, and New York: Cambridge University Press.

Rutter, M. (1994a). Concepts of causation, tests of causal mechanisms, and implications for intervention. In A. C. Petersen & J. T. Mortimer (Eds.), *Youth unemployment and society* (pp. 147–171). New York: Cambridge University Press.

Rutter, M. (1994b). Beyond longitudinal data: Causes, consequences, changes and continuity. *Journal of Consulting and Clinical Psychology, 62,* 928–940.

Rutter, M. (1997). Comorbidity: Concepts, claims and choices. *Criminal Behaviour and Mental Health, 7,* 265–286.

Rutter, M. (2000a). Resilience reconsidered: Conceptual considerations, empirical findings, and policy implications. In J. P. Shonkoff & S. J. Meisels (Eds.), *Handbook of early childhood intervention* (2nd ed., pp. 651–682). Cambridge, UK: Cambridge University Press.

Rutter, M. (2000b). Genetic studies of autism: From the 1970s into the millennium. *Journal of Abnormal Child Psychology, 28,* 3–14.

Rutter, M. (2002a). Nature, nurture and development: From evangelism through science towards policy and practice. *Child Development, 73,* 1–21.

Rutter, M. (2002b). Substance use and abuse: Causal pathways considerations. In M. Rutter & E. Taylor (Eds.), *Child and adolescent psychiatry* (4th ed., pp. 455–462). Oxford, UK: Blackwell Scientific.

Rutter, M. (2003). Genetic influences on risk and protection: Implications for understanding resilience. In S. Luthar (Ed.), *Resilience and vulnerability* (pp. 489–509). New York and Cambridge, UK: Cambridge University Press.

Rutter, M., Bolton, P., Harrington, R., Le Couteur, A., Macdonald, H., & Simonoff, A. (1990). Genetic factors in child psychiatric disorders: I. A review of research strategies. *Journal of Child Psychology and Psychiatry, 31,* 3–37.

Rutter, M., & Giller, H. (1983). *Juvenile delinquency: Trends and perspectives.* Harmondsworth, UK: Penguin Books.

Rutter, M., Giller, H., & Hagell, A. (1998). *Antisocial behavior by young people.* New York and London: Cambridge University Press.

Rutter, M., Maughan, B., Meyer, J., Pickles, A., Silberg, J., Simonoff, E., & Taylor, E. (1997). Heterogeneity of antisocial behavior: Causes, continuities, and consequences. In D. W. Osgood (Ed.), *Nebraska Symposium on Motivation: Vol. 44. Motivation and delinquency* (pp. 45–118). Lincoln: University of Nebraska Press.

Rutter, M., Maughan, B., Mortimore, P., Ouston, J., & Smith, A. (1979). Fifteen thousand hours: Secondary schools and their effects on children. Cambridge, MA: Harvard University Press.

Rutter, M., Pickles, A., Murray, R., & Eaves, L. (2001). Testing hypotheses of specific environmental risk mechanisms for psychopathology. *Psychological Bulletin, 127,* 291–324.

Rutter, M., & Quinton, D. (1977). Psychiatric disorder: Ecological factors and concepts of causation. In H. McGurk (Ed.), *Ecological factors in human development* (pp. 173–187). Amsterdam: North-Holland.

Rutter, M., &, Rutter, M. (1993). *Developing minds: Challenge and continuity across the lifespan.* New York: Basic Books.

Rutter, M., & Silberg, J. (2002). Gene–environment interplay in relation to emotional and behavioral disturbance. *Annual Review of Psychology, 53,* 463–490.

Rutter, M., Silberg, J., O'Connor, T., & Simonoff, E. (1999). Genetics and child psychiatry: I. Advances in quantitative and molecular genetics. *Journal of Child Psychology and Psychiatry, 40*, 3–18.

Rutter, M., Silberg, J., & Simonoff, E. (1993). Whither behavior genetics?: A developmental psychopathology perspective. In R. Plomin & G. E. McClearn (Eds.), *Nature, nurture, and psychology* (pp. 433–456). Washington, DC: American Psychological Association Books.

Rutter, M., & Smith, D. J. (Eds.). (1995). *Psychosocial disorders in young people: Time trends and their causes.* Chichester, UK: Wiley.

Rutter, M., Thorpe, K., Greenwood, R., Northstone, K., & Golding, J. (2003). Twins as a natural experiment to study the causes of mild language delay: I. Design, twin singleton differences in language, and obstetric risks. *Journal of Child Psychology and Psychiatry, 44*, 326–341.

Sampson, R. J., & Laub, J. H. (1993). *Crime in the making: Pathways and turning points through life.* Cambridge, MA: Harvard University Press.

Sampson, R. J., & Laub, J. H. (1996). Socioeconomic achievement in the life course of disadvantaged men: Military service as a turning point, circa 1940–1965. *American Sociological Review, 61*, 347–367.

Sampson, R. J., & Lauritsen, J. L. (1997). Racial and ethnic disparities in crime and criminal justice in the United States. In M. Tonry (Ed.), *Crime and justice* (Vol. 21, pp. 311–374). Chicago: University of Chicago Press.

Sampson, R. J., Raudenbush, S. W., & Earls, F. (1997). Neighborhoods and violent crime: A multilevel study of collective efficacy. *Science, 277*, 918–924.

Scarr, S. (1997). Behavior–genetic and socialization theories of intelligence: Truth and reconciliation. In R. J. Sternberg & E. L. Grigorenko (Eds.), *Intelligence, heredity, and environment* (pp. 3–41). Cambridge, UK: Cambridge University Press.

Shriver, S. P., Bourdeau, H. A., Gubish, C. T., Tirpak, D. L., Davis, A. L. G., Luketich, J. D., & Siegfried, J. M. (2000). Sex-specific expression of gastrin-releasing peptide receptor: Relationship to smoking history and risk of lung cancer. *Journal of the National Cancer Institute, 92*, 24–33.

Silberg, J., Meyer, J., Pickles, A., Simonoff, E., Eaves, L., Hewitt, J., Maes, H., & Rutter, M. (1996). Heterogeneity among juvenile antisocial behaviours: Findings from the Virginia Twin Study of Adolescent Behavioural Development. In G. R. Bock & J. A. Goode (Eds.), *Genetics of criminal and antisocial behaviour: Ciba Foundation Symposium 194* (pp. 76–86). Chichester, UK: Wiley.

Silberg, J. L., Pickles, A., Rutter, M., Hewitt, J., Simonoff, E., Maes, H., Carbonneau, R., Murrelle, L., Foley, D., & Eaves, L. (1999). The influence of genetic factors and life stress on depression among adolescent girls. *Archives of General Psychiatry, 56*, 225–232.

Silberg, J., Rutter, M., & Eaves, L. (2001). Genetic and environmental influences on the temporal association between earlier anxiety and later depression in girls. *Biological Psychiatry, 49*, 1040–1049.

Silberg, J. L., Rutter, M., Meyer, J., Maes, H., Hewitt, J. K., Simonoff, E., Pickles, A., Loeber, R., & Eaves, L. J. (1996). Genetic and environmental influences on the covariation between hyperactivity and conduct disturbance in juvenile twins. *Journal of Child Psychology and Psychiatry, 37*, 803–816.

Silberg, J., Rutter, M., Neale, M., & Eaves, L. (2001). Genetic moderation of environmental risk for depression and anxiety in girls. *British Journal of Psychiatry, 179*, 116–121.

Skuse, D. H. (2000). Imprinting, the X-chromosome and the male brain: Explaining sex differences in the liability to autism. *Pediatric Research, 47*, 1–8.

Smith, D. J. (1997a). Race, crime and criminal justice. In M. Maguire, R. Morgan, & R. Reiner (Eds.), *The Oxford handbook of criminology* (2nd ed., pp. 703–759). Oxford, UK: Clarendon Press.

Smith, D. J. (1997b). Ethnic origins, crime and criminal justice in England and Wales. In M. Tonry (Ed.), *Ethnicity, crime and immigration: Comparative and cross-national perspectives* (pp. 101–182). Chicago: University of Chicago Press.

Snyder, H. N., Sickmund, M., & Poe-Yamagata, E. (1996). *Juvenile offenders and victims: 1996 update on violence.* Washington, DC: Office of Juvenile Justice and Delinquency Prevention.

Stoff, D., Breiling, J., & Maser J. D. (Eds.). (1997). *Handbook of antisocial behavior.* New York: Wiley.

Thorpe, K., Rutter, M., & Greenwood, R. (2003). Twins as a natural experiment to study the causes of mild language delay: II. Family interaction risk factors. *Journal of Child Psychology and Psychiatry, 44,* 342–355.

Zoccolillo, M., Pickles, A., Quinton, D., & Rutter, M. (1992). The outcome of childhood conduct disorder: Implications for defining adult personality disorder and conduct disorder. *Psychological Medicine, 22,* 971–986.

# PART II

# GENERAL AND INTEGRATIVE CAUSAL MODELS

# 2

# A Social Learning Model of Child and Adolescent Antisocial Behavior

JAMES SNYDER
JOHN REID
GERALD PATTERSON

Developmental trajectories for antisocial behavior are the end result of multiple causes that change with age and are interrelated in complex ways. These causes operate at ecological (e.g., socioeconomic status [SES], neighborhood), social-relational (e.g., family members, teachers, peers), and individual (e.g., temperament, sex) levels, and unfold on the backdrop of maturation and age-related social-developmental conventions. According to social learning theory, processes occurring in daily social interaction provide the proximal nexus at which these causal factors converge to exert their influence. Social relationships provide recurring learning experiences that cumulatively engender antisocial behavior as it unfolds with age. The effect of broader ecological variables on child antisocial behavior is mediated by their impact on social interactions. As such, contextual variables have a more distal and indirect causal role in the genesis of antisocial behavior.

This chapter provides a brief account of the core social causes of antisocial development from early childhood through adolescence. We first consider empirically derived growth trajectories that describe interindividual variation in the frequency and form of antisocial behavior. While these trajectories can be construed as largely descriptive, current accounts are intrinsically theory-laden and not entirely congruent with a social learning model. We then describe the social processes that serve as core engines in the evolution and shaping of antisocial trajectories. These core processes include coercive exchange, social contingencies, the evocative effects of behavior, monitoring, and environmental selection. We also examine how cognitive-attentional and emotion regulatory processes modulate social experiences. Finally, we describe the relationships of ethnicity, social status, and gender to antisocial development in terms of their impact on proximal core social processes. Longitudinal and random assignment interventions are described that link key causal variables to antisocial trajectories at various developmental periods.

## DEVELOPMENTAL TRAJECTORIES FOR ANTISOCIAL BEHAVIOR

Antisocial behavior can be described by a set of developmental trajectories that unfold over time. To define such trajectories, global reports (e.g., checklists, rating scales) are typically collected from multiple informants (e.g., parent, teacher, child) at annual intervals and combined to form constructs, and then analyzed using autocorrelational methods. The resulting correlations show high stabilities over periods of 2–4 years. While such trait-like information is useful, a more developmental perspective also emphasizes age-related changes in mean level. Our working perspective is that changes in the form and frequency of antisocial behavior come about as a function of qualitative and quantitative shifts in social interaction and in the settings in which it occurs. In terms of theory, antisocial behavior is placed "in social interaction" rather than "in the person."

The primary focus of the coercion model is on mechanisms that bring about changes in the form of and growth in antisocial behavior. It is a theory about *why* things change. Trait theory is relatively silent about this key issue. Stronger causal theories will evolve as models are developed that describe the conditions and processes that account for temporal and setting variations in antisocial behavior. We need to understand how persistent and serious antisocial behavior evolves from simple noncompliance and early oppositional behavior. The causes of antisocial behavior vary according to behavioral form, setting, and time. Growth in antisocial behavior occurs in a given setting, or a particular form emerges insofar as such behavior is found to be functional—that is, "it works."

We offer two empirical exemplars of this functional approach to describing development. Consider the propositions that growth trajectories for antisocial behavior in different settings may be unrelated *or* that initial levels in one setting may be related in unexpected ways to growth in that setting or in other settings. This hypothesis was tested by measuring antisocial behavior in each of three settings at four 6-month intervals beginning at kindergarten entry, using data from 250 at-risk boys and girls from the School Transition Project (Snyder, Stoolmiller, & Patterson, 2001). Antisocial behavior at home was measured by parent ratings, in the classroom by teacher ratings, and on the playground by behavioral observations. There was no source overlap in measures of antisocial behavior across settings. As a first step, cross-setting constructs for antisocial behavior were derived at each age, and stability correlations were calculated. The constructs fit the data well. The loading of indicators on their respective constructs was greater than .45; the average loading was .68. There was substantial continuity in antisocial behavior at the construct level. The shared variance among antisocial constructs measured 6 months apart averaged 46%; among constructs measured 1 year apart, 41%; and between kindergarten-entry and first-grade-exit constructs, 34%, even with changes in teachers and observers from kindergarten to first grade. This consistency across settings and over time is congruent with a "trait" model, even at this young age. However, even given stability, changes in mean level of antisocial behavior may occur during the same time intervals.

Applying a functional approach to these data, separate best-fitting growth models were derived for antisocial behavior at home, in the classroom, and on the playground. Each univariate trajectory fit a linear growth model (mean level increases, or a positive slope) with the exception of parent reports (nonlinear increases with age). All three models showed significant interindividual variation in antisocial behavior at kindergarten entry and in age-related change during kindergarten and first grade. A multivariate model was then used to ascertain correlations between the intercepts and growth parameters for antisocial behavior in each setting. The intercepts (antisocial behavior at kindergarten entry) for the three settings were reliably intercorrelated (home–classroom = .46, home–playground = .25, classroom–playground = .75). Correlations among the growth parameters across the three settings were statistically nonsignificant. Growth was specific to setting. At home and on the playground, individuals who initially displayed higher levels of antisocial behavior evidenced more growth over the subsequent 2 years (home $r$ = .28; playground $r$ = .47), but this was not the case in the classroom ($r$ = −.31, NS). The correlation between playground intercept and classroom slope was significant (−.68); children initially most antisocial on the playground showed the largest declines in classroom antisocial behavior.

The functional approach indicates substantial individual differences in the direction of growth in antisocial behavior across settings even though the initial rank order of individuals was moderately consistent across those settings. The degree to which distinct causal factors influence growth in antisocial behavior at different developmental periods and in different settings, and the conditions by which growth in one setting influences growth in another setting, are important open empirical questions. From a functional perspective, growth in antisocial behavior in each setting reflects the social contingencies encountered in that setting. Similarly modest cross-setting consistency (correlations from .20 to .25) has been reported in previous research (e.g., Dishion, Duncan, Eddy, Fagot, & Fetrow, 1994; Ramsey, Patterson, & Walker, 1990) using common observational methods to measure antisocial behavior in each setting.

The next set of analyses focus on the question of why these differences in growth occur. The coercion model would suggest that, at this age, growth in covert and overt forms of antisocial behavior is a function of contingencies supplied by peers. Presumably, trait theory would be silent on this crucial issue. The importance of situational variables and immediate contingencies is readily apparent in the data from a recent intervention to reduce peer aggression on the school playground (Stoolmiller, Eddy, & Reid, 2000). Significant reductions in the absolute rate of aggressive behavior were observed in children targeted by a group-level behavioral contingency intervention relative to a nonintervention group. Effects within the intervention group varied significantly according to preintervention rates of aggressive behavior. Children who were most aggressive at preintervention showed the largest reductions at postintervention. No changes in rates of aggression were found in the control condition. The stability correlation for children in the control condition was .89; the natural state appears to facilitate very high stability. In contrast, the stability coefficient for the contingency management group was .08. The environmental determinants manipulated by the intervention nearly eliminated all of the stability in naturally occurring peer aggression on the playground. This implies that a large portion of variance in aggression is accounted for by time-specific determinants—the ambient social conditions experienced by a child on the playground. What appears to be "trait-like" stability may in fact be situational, relationship-specific, and "functional." The advantage of the functional approach is that it specifies environmental variables that can be manipulated to foster change.

This functional explanation could be extended to current findings concerning developmental changes (negative slope) in overt antisocial behavior from early childhood to adolescence (Nagin & Tremblay, 1999; Shaw et al., 1994). It is congruent with the emergence of covert forms of antisocial behavior in the peer setting during the early elementary school years (Snyder, Suarez, & Brooker, 2001), and with its rapid growth (positive slope) and differentiation during adolescence (Patterson & Yoerger, 2002). Though overt and covert forms are correlated with each other, they are "growing" in opposite directions (Patterson, Forgatch, Yoerger, & Stoolmiller, 1998)! The "functional" hypothesis is that proximal causes of normative and individual differences in the development of specific forms of antisocial behavior will be found in the behavior–environment contingencies encountered by individuals in the various settings and relationships that comprise their social ecology.

## CORE CAUSAL PROCESSES IN THE DEVELOPMENT OF ANTISOCIAL BEHAVIOR

Social learning theory hypothesizes that antisocial development is driven by two core causal processes. The first process involves the social and material contingencies that are engendered by aggressive, oppositional, and stealthy behavior. The second process entails the selection of environmental niches that strongly influence the experiences and contingencies to which children are exposed and the manner in which adults manage such exposure via monitoring.

### Core Function 1: Coercion, Social Reinforcement, and Response Choice

Developmental trajectories for antisocial behavior are initiated, maintained, and diversified as a result of cumulative daily social experiences with parents, siblings, and peers that are highly aversive, inconsistent, and unsupportive. Coercive behavior is shaped by short-term social contingencies, or its functional value in turning off aversive events and control by others (negative reinforcement) and in attaining attention and access to desired activities and materials (positive reinforcement) (Patterson, 1982). Such overt coercive behavior is readily apparent to others. Covert forms of antisocial behavior have similar social-functional properties. They provide access to material or activity reinforcers that are denied by others or are otherwise unavailable, or serve as a means of undetected retribution. The emergence of covert forms of antisocial behavior arises, in part, from discrimination learning about setting conditions associated with detection and punishment. Persistent and serious antisocial behavior is typically accompanied by children's failure to acquire an increasingly sophisticated array of skills that bridge the gap between short- and long-term contingencies (Conger & Simons, 1999). Social contingencies and experiences that foster antisocial behavior often simultaneously mitigate the acquisition of capacities to self-regulate emotions, deploy attention, problem solve, engage in autonomous rule following, and relate effectively to others. Antisocial and skilled behaviors are "opposite sides of the same coin."

Parents and siblings provide one set of critical experiences and contingencies involved in shaping antisocial and skilled behaviors during early development (Snyder & Patterson, 1995). As additional social agents (e.g., teachers, peers) and settings (e.g., classroom, playground, neighborhood) are encountered, increasingly complex networks of reinforcers and punishers for coercive-antisocial behavior or for constructive-skilled behavior are encountered, further shaping and elaborating these alternate trajectories according to their functional value (Reid & Eddy, 2002). Antisocial behavior is not inert; it powerfully impacts other people. Coercive and antisocial behaviors often meet with countercoercion, rejection, and exclusion by others. These reactions provide social experiences and contingencies that further elaborate the coercive antisocial child behavior from which they arose (Dodge, 1983; Patterson, Reid, & Dishion, 1992). As constructive skillful behavioral alternatives remain underdeveloped, the antisocial child is less able to access activities and relationships requisite to the development of self-regulation, social skills, and educational advancement. Thus two types of reciprocal behavior–environment transactions serve as causal processes: (1) coercive behavior and countercoercive reactions and (2) skills deficits and diminished access to skill-enhancing experiences.

Current evidence suggests that coercive processes operate as early as the preschool years (Garcia, Shaw, Winslow, & Yaggi, 2000) and continue through adolescence (Dishion, Patterson, & Griesler, 1994). The prospective association of coercive exchange and associated reinforcement contingencies for aggressive and antagonistic behavior in family, classroom, and peer settings has been replicated in a number of longitudinal studies (Bank, Burraston, & Snyder, in press; Dodge, 1983; Kellam, Ling, Merisca, Brown, & Ialongo, 1998). The impact of iterative and continuing exposure to these causal coercive processes in multiple social settings on the development of antisocial behavior may be dynamic, conditional, and interactive rather than additive in nature.

One particular advantage of social learning theory is its emphasis on malleable social processes that can be put to strong experimental test in random assignment prevention and clinical trials. The causal role of daily social experiences in the development of antisocial behavior is supported by randomized assignment interventions that systematically alter social contingencies for antisocial and skillful behavior in family (Webster-Stratton & Hammond, 1997), classroom (Kellam et al., 1998), and playground (Reid & Eddy, 2002; Stoolmiller et al., 2000) environments. Typically, these changes are clinically significant and persist over time. That the observed change in antisocial behavior is mediated, at least in part, by changes in social contingencies is clearly evident in the previously described impact of playground contingency management on peer aggression (Stoolmiller et al., 2000). Intervention-induced reductions in parental coercion and harsh punishment account for declines in child antisocial behavior from pre- to posttreatment (Dishion, Patterson, & Kavanaugh, 1992; Schrepferman & Snyder, 2002). These studies test for the causal status of specific mechanisms as they maintain or exacerbate antisocial behavior during the targeted developmental period. Such studies do not speak directly to the causal status of these mechanisms in origins or early etiology of antisocial behavior.

Given that the critical period for the development of overt forms of antisocial behavior may occur as early as 24 months of age, a randomized design to test the etiological role of these mechanisms would require a large-scale prevention study with a sample of at-risk 12- to 18-month-old toddlers. In keeping with correlational research (Kingston & Prior, 1995; Martin, 1981; Shaw & Winslow, 1997), such a prevention effort should target parents' contingent responsiveness to both socially competent and oppositional child behavior. Presumably, by the age of 2 or 3, children in the parenting intervention condition would evidence significant reductions in overt forms of antisocial behavior, and their caretakers would be observed to be more responsive and less coercive during parent–child interaction. Intervention versus control group differences in parent–child interaction and in child outcomes would speak directly to the status of social contingencies as critical etiological mechanisms in the development of antisocial behavior.

In summary, substantial data from both longitudinal and intervention-experimental designs support the hypothesis that coercive social processes and associated contingencies play a causal role in antisocial development. Additional longitudinal and field-experimental research is needed to expose this hypothesis to even more stringent causal tests. In intervention research, an increased emphasis should be placed on specifying and measuring the mechanisms that map onto the social experiences and contingencies posited as causal by social learning theory in addition to measuring the impact of intervention on short- or long-term child outcomes. This will require increased reliance on real-time behavioral observation of social processes in the home, on the playground, and in classroom settings, and less exclusive reliance on global reports or ratings of those processes. The causal status of core variables will be advanced insofar as we learn how and why interventions work as well as whether they have an effect (Kazdin & Weisz, 1998).

Clearer support for the causal status of core variables will also be advanced by applying interventions in more focused and discrete ways to specific settings and developmental periods. Multicomponent and multisetting preventive interventions delivered repeatedly across developmental periods are ideally suited to maximize the efficacy of intervention, but mitigate clear inferences concerning which component (causal mechanism) altered at what developmental period in which setting contributes to favorable outcomes. Focused discrete interventions that explicitly measure and manipulate the specific processes hypothesized to be causal by a given theory provide an important complementary research strategy.

Forgatch and DeGarmo (1999) provide an example of a carefully focused intervention that assessed and manipulated very specific processes thought to increase risk for child antisocial behavior. Newly divorced mothers with 6- to 8-year-old sons (specific developmental period) were randomly assigned to a family intervention (specific settings) or a no-intervention control. The intervention focused on improving the parental tracking, limit setting, and contingent responding needed to discourage problem child behavior. It also focused on problem solving, communication, and reinforcement of skillful child behaviors (specific causal mechanisms). Using family observational methods, these mechanisms were explicitly measured before intervention and again at 6- and 12-month intervals after the intervention was initiated. Teacher, parent, and child reports were used to assess the impact of the intervention on child adjustment. Parental contingencies and family processes hypothesized to be causal were reliably altered in the intervention. Baseline- to 12-month improvements in boys' adjustment (as reported by all three informants) were either partly or fully mediated by changes in the processes (causal variables) manipulated in the intervention. More recent reports (Martinez & Forgatch, 2001) indicate that this intervention had increasingly powerful effects on boys' adjustment at 18 and 24 months postbaseline, and that these long-term benefits were also specifically tied to changes in parental contingencies.

The social contingencies and experiences hypothesized to maintain or exacerbate antisocial behavior during childhood and adolescence vary across its behavioral forms, across settings, and over time. An adequate causal explanation for the emergence and growth of covert antisocial behavior requires a second set of interrelated core processes, adult monitoring, niche selection by the child, and peer reinforcement of deviant activities.

### Core Function 2: Monitoring, Environmental Selection, and Peer Deviancy Training

The shaping and elaboration of coercive and antisocial versus constructive behavior are played out against the backdrop of ongoing maturation and age-related transitions to new social environments and activities that comprise the social-developmental conventions of a particular social class or culture. Based on the assumption of increased cognitive, physical, self-regulatory, and social capacities, children spend decreasing time in mandatory caretaking relationships with adults, and increasing time in elective peer relationships and activities. As socialization by adults diminishes and children's relationships and activities become increasingly elective, parents, teachers, and other adults monitor and intervene to influence children's activity and affiliative choices, titrating elective experiences to the growing capacity of the child to problem solve and self-regulate. Monitoring entails a complex set of parent–child relational processes that evolve during the elementary school years, including (1) information exchange in which parents evoke and children disclose information about activities and associates at school and in the neighborhood (or parents seek information by other means such as talking to teachers and neighbors); (2) parent–child problem solving and agreement about rules concerning child activities, associates, and whereabouts; and (3) applying consequences for adherence to the rules (Chamberlain, 1994). These processes evolve from earlier discipline, communication, and problem-solving processes at home, now extended to activities not immediately under parents' (and other adults') purview (Kerr & Stattin, 2000).

Children's choice of environments is not random. Children gravitate toward settings, activities, and people that are compatible with their own background, characteristics, and behavior. Niches are selected to maximize positive (reinforcement) and minimize aversive (punishment) experiences beginning in preschool (Snyder, West, Stockemer, Gibbons, & Almquist-Parks, 1996) and continuing into adolescence (Poulin, Dishion, & Haas, 1999). Choice is not unilateral. Given the differential impact of coercive behavior on persons who are candidates for elective relationships and on the graded skills requirements for various activities and affiliations, access to specific individuals and learning opportunities may become selectively unavailable (Cairns & Cairns, 1994). Unskilled antisocial children seek out niches that involve association with antisocial peers and environments with minimal adult supervision. Niche selection also occurs on the basis of positive characteristics and can enhance constructive skilled behavior (Kindermann, 1993). Selective peer affiliation plays an important role in the development of antisocial behavior as early as the elementary school years (Snyder et al., 1996).

The complementarity of children's ecological choices and behavior results in rich opportunities for the shaping of overt and covert antisocial behavior, especially in the absence of effective adult monitoring. Both direct and vicarious reinforcement of antisocial behavior by peers increases risk. Peers' talk about and endorsement of antisocial activities provide prescriptions for such activities—such exchanges are more likely to occur among children who are already antisocial. The rate of deviant talk and its endorsement by peers at age 10 are prospectively associated with growth in antisocial behavior, drug use, and precocious sexual activity during adolescence (Patterson, Dishion, & Yoerger, 2000). This process appears to begin earlier in development. Our current hypothesis is that the emergence of covert antisocial behavior (i.e., changes in form from overt to covert) and initial growth in that behavior originates in peer interaction during the early elementary school years, especially in contexts with minimal adult supervision.

Many school playgrounds offer a venue ripe for experiences that promote and elaborate overt and covert antisocial behavior. Data from the School Transitions Project indicate that the rate at which adult playground supervisors direct positive attention to child nonaversive (.25) and aversive behavior (.26) are indistinguishable. Comparable rates of negative attention for aversive (.09) and nonaversive (.04) behavior are similarly noncontingent. Only 1.7% of children's aversive behavior and only 3% of their physical aggression toward peers result in time-out or similar backup consequences. There is really little adult tracking and few adult contingencies operating in the playground environment. We have observed high rates of deviant talk (mean rate per minute = .30) among kindergarten children in this sample; the rates at which children engage in deviant talk are correlated with covert (.58) and overt (.43) antisocial behavior 1 year later. Finally, there was reliable growth in observed overt and covert antisocial behavior on the playground from entry to kindergarten to the end of first grade. Children actively coparticipate in antisocial acts and reinforce deviant talk, implicating both modeling and direct reinforcement as important social processes. Playground aggression frequently receives peer encouragement. Adolescent delinquent acts are committed in groups. Similar collusion processes operate in sibling relationships (Bullock & Dishion, 2002).

The causal role of monitoring is supported by random assignment intervention trials. At-risk fifth graders involved in a family- and school-based intervention (including monitoring) relative to a nonintervention control group evidenced reliable reductions (by an odds ratio of 1.5:2.5) in early arrest, use of alcohol and marijuana, and association with deviant peers during the 3 years after intervention (Reid & Eddy, 2002). Family-focused intervention for at-risk sixth graders that enhances parental monitoring leads to reduced growth in child self-reported alcohol and tobacco use over the subsequent 3 years, relative to a nonintervention control group (Dishion, Kavanagh, Kaufman, Schneiger, & Dorham, in press). However, because these interventions involve multiple components, limited inferences can be made about the specificity with which monitoring played a causal role in beneficial outcomes. The causal role of peer deviancy training is supported by the iatrogenic effects of interventions that are delivered in groups that aggregate antisocial children (Dishion, McCord, & Poulin, 1999).

Clearer support for the causal role of monitoring requires that it be measured in more detailed social relational terms in daily parent–child exchanges (Kerr & Stattin, 2000). The degree to which intervention-induced changes in monitoring is an active, effective ingredient in altering antisocial behavior needs to be explicitly documented. Eddy and Chamberlain (2000) provide an exemplary initial effort. Boys with a substantial history of antisocial behavior were assigned to intensive therapeutic foster care or to a community intervention. Monitoring, discipline, and contact with deviant peers were assessed using detailed daily parent and school reports. Monitoring and discipline were improved and deviant peer association was reduced in family foster care but not in the community intervention. Good monitoring and discipline, and reduced deviant peer association, mediated the effects of the foster care condition, and were reliably associated with reduced arrests and self-reported delinquency during the year after exit from placement, even after controlling for preplacement arrests.

Monitoring does not arise *de novo* in adolescence. More effort is needed to identify how monitoring is affected by and evolves from other familial social processes, and how it operates during earlier developmental periods. We have several testable hypotheses to offer. Frequent coercive exchange may disrupt family social processes by which monitoring is implemented, including child self-disclosure, problem solving, rule setting, and contingency contracting. Monitoring, as reflected in parental contingencies for child truth telling, tracking neighborhood playmates, and putting limits on TV viewing, may influence antisocial development as early as kindergarten (Kilgore, Snyder, & Lentz, 2000).

Early monitoring, selective peer affiliation, and peer deviancy training are closely linked with the emergence of covert antisocial behavior. The frequency of overt oppositional and aggressive behavior normatively decreases from its peak during early childhood. A small subset of children (early starter or life-course-persistent trajectories) continue to display such behavior at high rates and in multiple settings, and are at considerable risk for progression into more serious forms of antisocial behavior and other problems. While overt antisocial behavior is undergoing a normative decline, covert antisocial behavior emerges and then shows dramatic growth during adolescence. This growth in covert antisocial behavior is displayed not only by early starters but also by a very large number of adolescents, often called "late starter" and "adolescence-limited" (Moffitt, 1993; Patterson et al., 1996). The emergence and initial growth of covert antisocial behavior during the elementary school years is poorly documented and poorly understood. We hypothesize that antisocial behavior undergoes a *normative* transformation from overt into increasingly covert forms during the elementary school years. This is a result of contingencies that adults successfully apply for easily discernable, overt forms. As a result, antisocial behavior "goes underground" and is increasingly expressed in its more surreptitious forms, especially in playground and neighborhood settings where peer interaction is subject to minimal adult monitoring and contingencies. These venues are the site of early peer deviancy training. Early starters, in particular, develop increasing confidence in their ability to evade adult supervision in order to carry out antisocial and aggressive acts during the early elementary school years.

Prevention experiments are needed to test the role of peer contingencies and deviant talk in the emergence and origins of covert antisocial behavior during the early elementary school years. Such interventions might usefully be instigated on school playgrounds during kindergarten and first grade. The intervention might expand group-contingency interventions already demonstrated as effective in reducing physical aggression to focus on deviant talk and covert antisocial behavior as well. The causal, perhaps etiological, status of peer contingencies in relation to the emergence of covert antisocial behavior would be supported insofar as children targeted in such an intervention showed later emergence or less growth in covert antisocial behavior relative to a control group.

Current developmental theory and intervention practice are primarily organized around the early- versus late-starter distinction. During earlier childhood, the primary focus is on altering coercive processes in family (e.g., discipline, warmth, responsiveness) and peer settings (e.g., playground aggression, classroom oppositional behavior, peer rejection) to mitigate overt antisocial behavior. In adolescence, the focus is on parental monitoring to minimize deviant peer affiliation, collusion, and deviancy training. This conceptualization has considerable empirical support and provides a useful formula for intervention. But it is too simple and limits the efficacy and effectiveness of current interventions. A more detailed causal picture is hidden in this conceptualization. Covert and overt forms of antisocial behavior grow at different rates and in different directions in different settings. Different processes are associated with the decline in overt antisocial behavior and the emergence and initial growth in covert antisocial behavior. These processes themselves transform and evolve. Monitoring grows out of and extends earlier efforts at discipline. Peer deviancy training moves from reinforcement of overt aggression and opposition to early forms of peer deviant talk, to extensive affiliation with deviant peers, and finally to coparticipation in delinquent acts. This more differentiated developmental picture of antisocial behavior and associated social processes suggests that the early elementary school years may provide a sensitive period for interventions targeting covert antisocial behavior and early initiation to drug use.

The social learning tradition has focused on malleable, observable social–environmental processes as core causes of antisocial behavior. These microlevel processes can be manipulated to address pressing social problems, but also to provide experimental tests of their causal status. However, social experiences change the characteristics of the developing child and are reciprocally influenced by those characteristics. This linkage of microsocial experiences and individual characteristics are now considered in relation to antisocial development.

## INDIVIDUAL CHARACTERISTICS AND ANTISOCIAL BEHAVIOR: COGNITIONS, EMOTIONS, AND SELF-REGULATION

Social learning theory has relied heavily on observable family and peer social processes as proximal causes of antisocial behavior. As such, the theory might be accused of taking an empty organism or "black box" perspective. While we assert that such processes are the core causes, "person" variables work in concert with social–environmental experiences to determine antisocial development. A wide array of person variables have been offered as risk factors for antisocial behavior (Coie & Dodge, 1998; Rothbart & Bates, 1998). Of this array, three interrelated, organismic self-regulation variables are relevant to antisocial development and compatible with social learning theory: executive attentional control, motivational inhibition, and negative emotional reactivity (Barkley, 1997; Nigg, 2000; Mezzacappa, Kindlon, Saul, & Earls, 1998). These forms of self-regulation hold considerable promise for several reasons. First, neuropsychological research suggests that they are tied to activity in specific neural networks. Second, objective, psychometrically sound, behavioral marker tasks independent of self-report and parent or teacher ratings are available to ascertain individual differences in each of these self-regulatory capacities (Kindlon, Mezzacappa, & Earls, 1995). Third, though such capacities come "on line" at an early age and show considerable temporal continuity, they are malleable and affected by social experience into adolescence (Davidson, Jackson, & Kalin, 2000).

These child self-regulatory capacities and their hypothesized contribution to antisocial behavior are briefly described. Executive attentional control is associated with activity in the midline prefrontal neural network, and ties emotions, cognitions, and attention together to facilitate planful action and goal-directed behavior. This network functions as a "top-down" cognitive system involving effortful inhibition of irrelevant responses, and is requisite to sustained task orientation in the face of stimulus or resource competition (Posner & Rothbart, 2000; Nigg, 2000). Performance deficits in marker tasks for executive attentional control are related to externalizing disorders and reduced social competence, even after controlling for IQ, age, sex, and reading level (Kindlon et al., 1995). Motivational inhibition is mediated by the limbic system, and entails the suppression of responses under contingencies for punishment and extinction. It is a "bottom-up" form of behavioral inhibition critical to passive avoidance learning (Nigg, 2000). Antisocial behavior has been associated with reduced sensitivity to aversive feedback, especially in the presence of reward (Mezzacappa et al., 1998). Negative emotional reactivity reflects the frequency and intensity with which negative emotions are experienced and expressed. Normally adaptive emotions contribute to disordered behavior when their experience and expression do not fit the context, are out of proportion to events, or unduly persist (Davidson et al., 2000). Negative emotional reactivity or emotion dysregulation increase vulnerability for externalizing behavior problems (Bates, 2000). The limbic system is implicated in emotional experience and expression, in part via modulation of peripheral nervous (resting heart rate and vagal tone), motor (facial expression), and endocrine (cortisol secretion) functions. Prefrontal networks associated with executive attentional control are also involved in emotional anticipation and in preparatory behavioral approach and withdrawal. Negative emotionality, deployment of attention, and sensitivity to punishment involve functionally overlapping neural systems and behavioral functions.

Although there is some empirical support for the role of these self-regulatory capacities in the development of antisocial behavior, additional research using prospective longitudinal and field-experimental designs are needed to more stringently test their causal status. First, the degree to which self-regulatory capacities are associated with antisocial behavior must be examined in prospective longitudinal designs, using measurement methods that minimize overlap in source variance. This association should be examined during the elementary school years because it is during this period that children are progressively exposed to new environments, activities, and people while adult tracking and contingencies simultaneously diminish. Given these conditions, antisocial development, especially in its covert form, is likely to reflect children's capacity to manage emotional distress in response to challenge, inhibit behavioral choices driven by immediate environmental contingencies, and attend to relevant information in order to formulate and execute plans consistent with goal-directed behavior under delayed reinforcement contingencies. Second, it is important to test how and how much children's self-regulatory capacities are shaped by social processes in the family during early child development, and thereafter are elaborated in less supportive and more challenging experiences in school and peer settings. The degree to which such capacities are malleable in response to environmental manipulation is critical to examining their causal status and to their incorporation as targets of intervention. Third, the mediator and moderator relationships among child self-regulatory capacities and social–environmental influences should be examined. Parents, peers, and teachers are impacted by a child's capacity to self-regulate behavior and emotions. Self-regulatory capacities may influence how the ambient social environment is experienced by the child. A more complete understanding of the reciprocal and conjoint roles of child self-regulatory and social–environmental processes in the development of antisocial behavior may facilitate more precise targeting and adaptation of standard medical and psychosocial interventions. Child self-regulatory and family environmental profiles may provide information about what works well for whom (in contrast to a "one size fits all" method), and guide prioritizing and efficient resource allocation in primary and secondary prevention efforts. We anticipate that efforts to alter self-regulatory mechanisms using interventions that target the child in the absence of changes in natural environmental contingencies will have modest effects on antisocial behavior, but may be useful adjuncts to such contingency-based programs.

## INDIVIDUAL CHARACTERISTICS AND ANTISOCIAL BEHAVIOR: CHILD GENDER

Gender differences in the rate of opposition are observed as early as 18 months of age (Shaw & Winslow, 1997). Gender differences in aggressiveness are well in place by age 5 (McFadyen-Ketchum, Bates, Dodge, & Pettit, 1996) and persist throughout childhood and adolescence. Moffitt, Caspi, Rutter, and Silva (2001) report that fewer girls (1%) than boys (5–

10%) evidence persistent and serious antisocial behavior associated with early-onset or life-course-persistent trajectories. Males account for more adolescent and adult crimes (especially those involving violence), and males have a higher lifetime prevalence for antisocial disorders. An exception to this general developmental pattern occurs in early adolescence, during which time females' offending approaches that of males. Females' increasing display of antisocial behavior during this period is congruent with later onset, life-course-limited trajectories (Moffitt, 1994). The adolescent burst in antisocial activity is tied to early timing of pubescence in females but not in males. Thus, causal explanations for two types of gender differences in antisocial behavior may be sought. One refers to mean-level group differences. The other concerns gender differences in variability and distribution of antisocial behavior—particularly at the high end of the distribution. The two types of differences may or may not share common causes.

The early origins of gender differences in opposition and aggression may reflect average gender-related variation in rates of nervous system maturation (Maccoby, 1998). Male infants lag behind females in behavioral inhibition, emotion regulation, attention deployment, and verbal development. These regulatory differences extend into the second and third years of life. As a result, boys and girls may evoke different responses from parents, and may respond differently to the same parenting conditions (Martin, 1981). Boys and girls are exposed to different social contingencies. Mothers are more coercive toward boys than girls, and this difference is even more pronounced for highly aggressive boys and girls (McFayden-Ketchum et al., 1996). Variation in the frequency of coercive exchanges may reflect gender differences in child self-regulation, parents' gender-biased attitudes about how to socialize children, acquired differences in boys' and girls' responsiveness to aversive social stimuli, or some combination thereof. We hypothesize that girls display less antisocial behavior because they are less frequently involved in coercive parent–child interaction, and also less frequently reinforced for oppositional and countercoercive responding. We hypothesize that, on the average, parents value and more frequently reinforce the positive social behavior of girls than boys.

Peer socialization processes contribute even more powerfully to gender differences in opposition and aggression as children move into preschool and kindergarten. Boys and girls show a robust preference for interaction with same-gender children beginning at age 3. The dyadic and group play of boys and girls have markedly different behavioral characteristics. There is more verbal challenge, noncompliance, and rough-and-tumble play, plus a more clearly articulated dominance ranking, in male groups. There is more cooperation, verbal exchange, compliance, and mutual accommodation in girls' groups (Maccoby, 1998). Peer reactions to male and female aggression differ. Based on extensive observation in preschool groups, Fagot, Hagan, Leinbach, and Kronsberg (1985) found that boys' physical aggression led to negative peer responses 40% of the time, and were ignored 15% of the time. In contrast, girls' physical aggression led to negative peer responses 15% of the time and were ignored 48% of the time. Boys also ignore girls who attempt to enter their play groups. Boys receive substantially more peer playground training for aggression than girls. A girl who is socialized to engage in frequent opposition and aggression by her family is not likely to find such behavior very functional in the peer group. She would have difficulty finding other highly coercive females with whom to interact, and also would be relatively unable to access boys' groups (Offord, Boyle, & Racine, 1991). In summary, average gender differences in social contingencies and in self-regulation operate conjointly to increase boys' risk relative to girls' risk for persistent antisocial behavior during the elementary school years (i.e., for early-starter or life-course-persistent trajectories).

Less is known about gender differences in the origins, emergence, and growth of covert antisocial behavior. High rates of overt antisocial behavior during childhood increase risk for early onset and growth in covert antisocial behavior for males. We hypothesize that the same risk-transformation process applies to females, implying more delayed emergence and slower growth in covert antisocial behavior as a result of their lower average rates of overt antisocial behavior during childhood. There are also fewer highly antisocial, same-sex peers with whom younger girls can associate and exchange deviant talk. Gender differences in emergence and growth in covert behavior are the result of the different environmental experiences and contingencies encountered by boys and girls.

There are two developmental periods or settings in which the typical gender differences in antisocial behavior are dramatically diminished. One occurs in early adolescence. Contingencies change as preference for same-gender peer associates diminishes, a broad array of potential peer affiliates becomes available, association with opposite-gender individuals increases (especially for early maturing females), and monitoring decreases. We hypothesize that these transitions result in systematic changes in social contingencies and experiences that diminish previous gender-differentiated environmental support for antisocial behavior, and that these changes are responsible for the growth burst in antisocial behavior by females in adolescence. Similar gender-leveling social processes may explain the reciprocal involvement of both men and women in partner-directed violence (Capaldi, Dishion, Stoolmiller, & Yoerger, 2001).

The same core, causal variables that account for individual differences in aggression and antisocial behavior more generally also account for gender differences in that behavior, including its more extreme and persistent forms. Aggressive antisocial behavior is displayed insofar as it is socially functional in a specific setting and in a specific development period. It varies across settings and over time in predictable ways, changing with ambient social environmental contingencies. The moderating effect of child self-regulatory capacities on social experience is similarly involved in individual and gender differences in antisocial behavior. The causes of antisocial behavior in females have been less well specified than antisocial behavior in males. An important research agenda is to ascertain whether the same causal variables operate across gender, or operate in the same way or to the same degree. Field-experimental and prospective longitudinal research are both relevant to this agenda. Gender, even as an ascribed social classification, is not very malleable. The differential effectiveness of interventions for boys and girls and the need for gender-sensitive interventions should be ascertained.

## SOCIAL CONDITIONS: ECONOMIC STATUS AND ETHNICITY

Macrolevel contexts and social classifications, such as SES and ethnicity, do not directly incur liability for antisocial behavior, but rather are catalytic and set into motion an indirect causal chain. Macrolevel variables impact proximal day-to-day social relational (microlevel) experiences of individuals by biasing the frequency and nature of adverse and supportive events to which individuals are exposed. Living in a dangerous and impoverished neighborhood and being African American leads to a different set of daily experiences and contingencies than living in a safe and affluent area and being European American. Such experiential biases are often not a matter of choice, but rather are socially constructed realities imposed on individuals. This is often termed a "social causation model." The relationship between macrolevel contexts and development is reciprocal. As described earlier, an individual's own developmental trajectory sets constraints on access to relationships, activities, and settings (macrolevel contexts) that affect subsequent developmental opportunities. In this social selection model, environments are actively selected in terms of compatibility with an individual's current repertoire or "credentials." The causal status of macrolevel variables will remain ambiguous in that they are not easily manipulated or are derived from enduring social ascriptions and biases associated with immutable individual characteristics.

SES is usefully construed as a marker variable for the "social address" or social-organizational characteristics of the environment in which individual development unfolds. The impact of these characteristics is strongly mediated by proximal, social-relational processes. Hart and Risely's (1995) exquisite longitudinal study on the covariation between family SES and the linguistic environment experienced by children is an excellent example. Intensive and repeated home observation indicated that, by age 4, children in "welfare" families were cumulatively exposed to adult speech at one-half (estimated 17 million words) the rate of children in middle-class families (estimated 32 million words), and at one-third the rate of children in professional families (estimated 48 million words). Dramatic differences in the quality of linguistic environments were also apparent. Parents who were professionals affirmed, extended, repeated, and elaborated child utterances at eight times the rate as parents on welfare and at four times the rate of working-class parents. Parents on welfare directed discouragement and prohibitions (don't, stop, bad, wrong) toward children at over twice the rate as parents with professional occupations. The impact of family SES on children's language development and intelligence at age 10 was powerfully mediated by the early linguistic environment provided by parents. These findings have profound implications for school readiness and educational performance, communication, problem solving, and child self-regulation, all in turn linked to risk for antisocial behavior. Childrearing is only one task among many competing demands encountered by parents. Economically disadvantaged parents faced with multiple daily challenges and few resources are less able to provide environments that optimize children's development (Bugental & Goodnow, 1998).

Race and ethnicity are often inextricably confounded with SES. Because of systemic discrimination, ethnic and racial minorities are overrepresented at the lower end of the educational, employment, and economic continuum. Race and ethnicity are proxies for SES, exposure to a greater number of adverse environmental experiences, and exclusion from access to resources, activities, and settings that optimize child development. Race and ethnicity may operate in additional complicated ways. Racial and ethnic groups may develop unique solutions for social tasks, and unique views of self and the world that are communicated across generations, based on the functional value of those solutions in the group's recent historical experience. The uniqueness of these solutions and representations are further complicated by variations in language that may accompany race and ethnicity. Individuals of minority status are often confronted with a difficult dual developmental task that encompasses the acquisition of competence within their own racial or ethnic group and also accommodates the majority culture.

One important question is whether unique adaptive solutions and representations occur according to race and ethnicity independent of SES. The evidence is unclear. For example, McLoyd (1998) found that poverty was associated with coercive harsh discipline and interfered with effective monitoring in poor, single-parent, African American families, similar to the impact of comparable contextual conditions in European American families. Some research suggests that punitive parental discipline is differentially associated with the development of antisocial behavior in African American relative to European American children (Deater-Deckert, Dodge, Bates, & Pettit, 1997), whereas other research suggests that harsh discipline is linked to child antisocial behavior in African American families as well (Kilgore et al., 2000).

One research agenda is to delineate how proximal, microlevel social causal processes operate when race and ethnicity are "unstacked" from socioeconomic context and acculturation. It is likely that adverse experiences and exclusion from opportunity are compounded when minority status is added to socioeconomic disadvantage, but current research does not provide very definitive answers. Some progress has been made in discerning how social-relational causes of antisocial behavior may be moderated by ethnicity and SES, but additional research is needed. This should include field-experimental efforts. Even though social class and ethnicity as ascribed social classifications are not very malleable, the differential effectiveness of interventions under varying macrocontextual conditions bear further study.

## ACKNOWLEDGMENTS

This chapter was written with support to Drs. Snyder and Patterson from National Institute of Health Grant No. R01 MH57342, "Child Conduct Problems: Competing Theories of Socialization," and to Dr. Reid from National Institute of Health Grant No. P30 MH4469, "Oregon Prevention Research Center."

## REFERENCES

Bank, L., Burraston, B., & Snyder, J. (in press). Sibling conflict and unskilled parenting as predictors of adolescent antisocial behavior and peer relations: Additive and interactional effects. *Journal of Adolescence.*

Barkley, R. A. (1997). Behavioral inhibition, sustained attention, and executive functions: Constructing a unifying theory for ADHD. *Psychological Bulletin, 121,* 65–94.

Bates, J. E. (2000). Temperament as an emotion construct: Theoretical and practical issues. In M. Lewis & J. M. Haviland-Jones (Eds.), *Handbook of emotions* (2nd ed., pp. 382–396). New York: Guilford Press.

Bugental, D. B., & Goodnow, J. J. (1998). Socialization processes. In N. Eisenberg (Ed.), *Handbook of child psychology: Vol. 5: Social emotional and personality development* (5th ed., pp. 389–461). New York: Wiley.

Bullock, B. M., & Dishion, T. J. (2002). Sibling collusion and problem behavior in early adolescence: Toward a process model for family mutuality. *Journal of Abnormal Child Psychology, 30,* 143–153.

Cairns, R. B., & Cairns, B. D. (1994). *Lifelines and risks: Pathways of youth in our time.* New York: Cambridge University Press.

Capaldi, D. M., Dishion, T. J., Stoolmiller, M., & Yoerger, K. (2001). Aggression toward female partners by at-risk young men: The contribution of male adolescent friendships. *Developmental Psychology, 37,* 61–73.

Chamberlain, P. C. (1994). *Family connections: A treatment foster care model for adolescents with delinquency.* Eugene, OR: Castalia.

Coie, J., & Dodge, K. A. (1998). Aggression and antisocial behavior. In W. Damon (Series Ed.) & N. Eisenberg (Vol. Ed.), *Handbook of child psychology (5th ed.): Vol. 3. Social, emotional, and personality development* (pp. 779–862). New York: Wiley.

Conger, R. D., & Simons, R. L. (1999). Life course contingencies in the development of adolescent antisocial behavior: A matching law approach. In T. P. Thornberry (Ed.), *Developmental theories of crime and delinquency: Life span perspectives* (pp. 183–209). New Brunswick, NJ: Transaction Books.

Davidson, R. J., Jackson, D. C., & Kalin, N. H. (2000). Emotion, plasticity, context, and regulation: Perspectives from affective neuroscience. *Psychological Bulletin, 126,* 890–909.

Deater-Deckard, K., Dodge, K. A., Bates, J. E., & Pettit, G. S. (1996). Discipline among African-American and European-American mothers: Links to children's externalizing behaviors. *Developmental Psychology, 32,* 1065–1072.

Dishion, T. J., Duncan, T., Eddy, J. M., Fagot, B. I., & Fetrow, R. (1994). The worlds of parents and peers: Coercive exchanges and children's social adaptation. *Social Development, 3,* 255–268.

Dishion, T. J., Kavanagh, K., Kaufman, N. K., Schneiger, A., & Dorham, C. (in press). Longitudinal effects on substance use for a tiered-family intervention within the middle school ecology. *Prevention Science.*

Dishion, T. J., McCord, J., & Poulin, F. (1999). When interventions harm: Peer groups and problem behavior. *American Psychologist, 54,* 755–764.

Dishion, T. J., Patterson, G. R., & Griesler, P. C. (1994). Peer adaptations in the development of antisocial behavior: A confluence model. In L. R. Heusmann (Ed.), *Aggressive behavior: Current perspectives* (pp. 61–95). New York: Plenum Press.

Dishion, T. J., Patterson, G. R., & Kavanaugh, K. (1992). An experimental test of the coercion model: Linking theory, measurement and intervention. In J. McCord & R. Tremblay (Eds.), *Preventing antisocial behavior* (pp. 253–282). New York: Guilford Press.

Dodge, K. A. (1983). Behavioral antecedents of peer social status. *Child Development, 54,* 1386–1399.

Eddy, J. M., & Chamberlain, P. C. (2000). Family management and deviant peer association as mediators of treatment condition on youth antisocial behavior. *Journal of Consulting and Clinical Psychology, 68,* 857–863.

Fagot, B. I., Hagan, R., Leinbach, M. D., & Kronsberg, S. (1985). Differential reactions to assertive and communicative acts of toddler boys and girls. *Child Development, 56,* 1499–1505.

Forgatch, M. S., & DeGarmo, D. S. (1999). Parenting through change: An effective prevention program for single mothers. *Journal of Consulting and Clinical Psychology, 67,* 711–724.

Garcia, M., Shaw, D. S., Winslow, E. B., & Yaggi, K. E. (2000). Destructive sibling conflict and the development of conduct problems in young boys. *Developmental Psychology, 36,* 44–53.

Hart, B., & Risley, T. R. (1995). *Meaningful differences in the everyday experiences of young American children.* Baltimore: Brookes.

Kazdin, A. E., & Weisz, J. R. (1998). Identifying and developing empirically supported child and adolescent treatments. *Journal of Consulting and Clinical Psychology, 66,* 19–36.

Kellam, S. G., Ling, X., Merisca, R., Brown, C. H., & Ialongo, N. (1998). The effect of the level of aggression in the first grade classroom on the course and malleability of aggressive behavior into middle school. *Development and Psychopathology, 10,* 165–185.

Kerr, M., & Stattin, H. (2000). What parents know, how they know it, and several forms of adolescent adjustment: Further support for a reinterpretation of monitoring. *Developmental Psychology, 36,* 366–380.

Kilgore, K., Snyder, J., & Lentz, C. (2000). The contribution of parental discipline, parental monitoring, and school risk to early-onset conduct problems in African-American boys and girls. *Developmental Psychology, 36,* 1–11.

Kindermann, T. A. (1993). Natural peer groups as contexts for individual development: The case for children's motivation in school. *Developmental Psychology, 29,* 970–977.

Kindlon, D., Mezzacappa, E., & Earls, F. (1995). Psychometric properties of impulsivity measures: Temporal stability, validity and factor structure. *Journal of Child Psychology and Psychiatry, 36,* 645–661.

Kingston, L., & Prior, M. (1995). The development of patterns of stable, transient, and school-age onset aggressive behavior in young children. *Journal of the American Academy of Child and Adolescent Psychiatry, 34,* 348–357.

Maccoby, E. E. (1998). *The two sexes: Growing up apart, coming together.* Cambridge, MA: Harvard University Press.

Martin, J. A. (1981). A longitudinal study of the consequences of early mother–infant interaction: A microanalytic approach. *Monographs of the Society for Research in Child Development, 46* (3, Serial No. 190).

Martinez, C. R., & Forgatch, M. S. (2001). Preventing problems with boys' noncompliance: Effects of a parent training intervention for divorcing mothers. *Journal of Consulting and Clinical Psychology, 69,* 416–428.

McFayden-Ketchum, S. A., Bates, J. E., Dodge, K. A., & Pettit, G. S. (1996). Patterns of change in early childhood aggressive-disruptive behavior: Gender differences in predictions from early coercive and affectionate mother–child interactions. *Child Development, 67,* 2417–2433.

McLoyd, V. C. (1998). Socioeconomic disadvantage and child development. *American Psychologist, 53,* 185–204.

Mezzacappa, E., Kindlon, D., Saul, J. P., & Earls, F. (1998). Executive and motivational control of performance task behavior, and autonomic heart-rate regulation in children: Physiologic validation of two-factor solution inhibitory control. *Journal of Child Psychology and Psychiatry, 39,* 525–531.

Moffitt, T. E. (1993). Adolescence-limited and life-course-persistent antisocial behavior: A developmental taxonomy. *Psychological Review, 100,* 674–701.

Moffitt, T. E. (1994). Natural histories of delinquency. In E. Weitekamp & H. J. Kerner (Eds.), *Cross-national longitudinal research on human development and criminal behaviour* (pp. 3–61). Dordrecht, The Netherlands: Kluwer Academic Press.

Moffitt, T. E., Caspi, A., Rutter, M., & Silva, P. A. (2001). *Sex differences in antisocial behavior, conduct disorder, delinquency and violence in the Dunedin Longitudinal Study.* New York: Cambridge University Press.

Nagin, D. S., & Tremblay, R. E. (1999). Trajectories of boys' physical aggression, opposition and hyperactivity on the path to physically violent and non-violent juvenile delinquency. *Child Development, 70,* 1181–1196.

Nigg, J. T. (2000). On inhibition/disinhibition in developmental psychopathology: Views from cognitive and personality psychology and a working taxonomy. *Psychological Bulletin, 126,* 220–246.

Offord, D. R., Boyle, M. C., & Racine, Y. (1991). The epidemiology of antisocial behavior. In D. Pepler & K. Rubin (Eds.), *The development and treatment of childhood aggression* (pp. 31–54). Hillsdale, NJ: Erlbaum.

Patterson, G. R. (1982). *Coercive family process.* Eugene, OR: Castalia.

Patterson, G. R., Dishion, T. J., & Yoerger, K. (2000). Adolescent growth in new forms of problem behavior: Macro- and micro-peer dynamics. *Prevention Science, 1,* 3–13.

Patterson, G. R., Forgatch, M. S., Yoerger, K., & Stoolmiller, M. (1998). Variables that initiate and maintain early onset trajectory for juvenile offending. *Development and Psychopathology, 10,* 541–547.

Patterson, G. R., Reid, J. B., & Dishion, T. J. (1992). *Antisocial boys.* Eugene, OR: Castalia.

Patterson, G. R., & Yoerger, K. (2002). A developmental model for early and late onset delinquency. In J. B. Reid, G. R. Patterson, & J. Snyder (Eds.), *Antisocial behavior in children and adolescents: A developmental analysis and model for intervention* (pp. 147–172). Washington, DC: American Psychological Association Press.

Posner, M. I., & Rothbart, M. K. (2000). Developing mechanisms of self-regulation. *Development and Psychopathology, 12,* 427–442.

Poulin, F., Dishion, T. J., & Haas, E. (1999). The peer influence paradox: Friendship quality and deviancy training within male adoelscent friendships. *Merrill-Palmer Quarterly, 48,* 42–61.

Ramsey, E., Patterson, G. R., & Walker, H. M. (1990). Generalization of antisocial trait from home to school settings. *Journal of Applied Developmental Psychology, 11,* 209–223.

Reid, J. B., & Eddy, J. M. (2002). Preventive efforts during the elementary school years: The Linking the Interests of Families and Teachers Project. In J. B. Reid, G. R. Patterson, & J. Snyder (Eds.), *Antisocial behavior in children and adolescents: A developmental analysis and model for intervention* (pp. 219–234). Washington, DC: American Psychological Association Press.

Rothbart, M. K., & Bates, J. E. (1998). Temperament. In N. Eisenberg (Ed.), *Handbook of child psychology: Vol. 3. Social, emotional and personality development* (5th ed., pp. 105–175). New York: Wiley.

Schrepferman, L., & Snyder, J. (2002). Reinforcement mechanisms in behavioral parent training associated with long-term alteration of child antisocial behavior. *Behavior Therapy, 33,* 339–359.

Shaw, D. S., & Winslow, E. B. (1997). Precursors and correlates of antisocial behavior from infancy to preschool. In D. M. Stoff, J. Breiling, & D. Maser (Eds.), *Handbook of antisocial behavior* (pp. 148–158). New York: Wiley.

Shaw, D. S., Winslow, E. B., Owens, E. B., Vondra, J. I., Cohn, J. F., & Bell, R. Q. (1994). The development of early externalizing problems among children from low income families: A transformational perspective. *Developmental Psychology, 30,* 355–364.

Snyder, J., & Patterson, G. R. (1995). Individual differences in social aggression: A test of a reinforcement model of socialization in the natural environment. *Behavior Therapy, 26,* 371–391.

Snyder, J., Stoolmiller, M., & Patterson, G. R. (2001). *The School Transitions Project: Situational variation in early developmental trajectories for antisocial behavior.* Unpublished manuscript, Wichita State University, Wichita, Kansas.

Snyder, J., Suarez, M., & Brooker, M. (2001, April). *Growth, continuity and correlations among direct and relational aggression in 5 to 7 year old boys and girls.* Paper presented at the annual conference of the Society for Research in Child Development, Minneapolis, Minnesota.

Snyder, J., West, L., Stockemer, V., Gibbons, S., & Almquist-Parks, L. (1996). A social learning model of peer choice in the natural environment. *Journal of Applied Developmental Psychology, 17,* 215–238.

Stoolmiller, M., Eddy, J. M., & Reid, J. B. (2000). Detecting and describing preventive intervention effects in a universal school-based randomized trial targeting delinquent and violent behavior. *Journal of Consulting and Clinical Psychology, 68,* 296–306.

Webster-Stratton, C., & Hammond, M. (1997). Treating children with early-onset conduct problems: A comparison of child and parent training interventions. *Journal of Consulting and Clinical Psychology, 65,* 93–109.

# 3

# Life-Course-Persistent and Adolescence-Limited Antisocial Behavior

## A 10-Year Research Review and a Research Agenda

TERRIE E. MOFFITT

This chapter reviews 10 years of research on a developmental taxonomy of antisocial behavior that proposed two primary hypothetical prototypes: life-course-persistent versus adolescence-limited offenders. According to the theory, life-course-persistent offenders' antisocial behavior has its origins in neurodevelopmental processes, begins in childhood, and continues worsening thereafter. In contrast, adolescence-limited offenders' antisocial behavior has its origins in social processes, begins in adolescence, and desists in young adulthood. According to the theory, life-course-persistent antisocials are few, persistent, and pathological. Adolescence-limited antisocials are common, relatively transient, and near normative (Caspi & Moffitt, 1995; Moffitt, 1990, 1993, 1994, 1997).

Discussions in the literature have pointed out that if the taxonomic theory is proven accurate, it could usefully improve classification of subject groups for research (Nagin, Farrington, & Moffitt, 1995; Silverthorn & Frick, 1999; Zucker, Ellis, Fitzgerald, Bingham, & Sanford, 1996), focus research into antisocial personality and violence toward the most promising causal variables (Brezina, 2000; Lahey, Waldman, & McBurnett, 1999; Laucht, 2001; Osgood, 1998), and guide the timing and strategies of interventions for delinquent types (Howell & Hawkins, 1998; Scott & Grisso, 1997). The taxonomy of childhood-onset versus adolescent-onset antisocial behavior has been codified in the DSM-IV (American Psychiatric Association, 1994), invoked in the National Institute of Mental Health (2000) *Child and Adolescent Violence Research* and the U.S. Surgeon General's

(2001) report *Youth Violence*, and presented in abnormal psychology and criminology textbooks. But is it valid?

The reader is referred to two prior publications that articulate the main hypotheses derived from this taxonomic theory. The original paper proposing the two prototypes and their different etiologies ended with a section headed "Strategies for Research" which described predictions about epidemiology, age, social class, risk correlates, offense types, desistence from crime, abstainers from crime, and the longitudinal stability of antisocial behavior (Moffitt, 1993, pp. 694–696). The paper specified which findings would disconfirm the theory. A version published elsewhere specified disconfirmable hypotheses about sex and race (Moffitt, 1994). Ten years ago, when these hypotheses from the taxonomy were put forward, none of them had been tested, but since then several have been tested by us and by others. This chapter reviews the results of that research and points out where more empirical work is needed.

## A THUMBNAIL SKETCH OF THE TWO PROTOTYPES

In a nutshell, we suggested that life-course-persistent antisocial behavior originates early in life, when the difficult behavior of a high-risk young child is exacerbated by a high-risk social environment. According to the theory, the child's risk emerges from inherited or acquired neuropsychological variation, initially manifested as subtle cognitive deficits, difficult temperament, or hyperactivity. The environment's risk comprises factors such as inadequate parenting, disrupted family bonds, and poverty. The environmental risk domain expands beyond the family as the child ages, to include poor relations with people such as peers and teachers. Opportunities to learn prosocial skills are lost. Over the first two decades of development, transactions between the individual and the environment gradually construct a disordered personality with hallmark features of physical aggression and antisocial behavior persisting to midlife. The theory predicts that antisocial behavior will infiltrate multiple adult life domains: illegal activities, problems with employment, and victimization of intimate partners and children. This infiltration diminishes the possibility of reform.

In contrast, we suggested that adolescence-limited antisocial behavior emerges alongside puberty, when otherwise ordinary healthy youngsters experience psychological discomfort during the relatively role-less years between their biological maturation and their access to mature privileges and responsibilities, a period we called the "maturity gap." They experience dissatisfaction with their dependent status as a child, and impatience for what they anticipate are the privileges and rights of adulthood. While young people are in this "gap," it is virtually normative for them to find the delinquent style appealing and to mimic it as a way to demonstrate autonomy from parents, win affiliation with peers, and hasten social maturation. However, because their predelinquent development was normal, most adolescence-limited delinquents are able to desist from crime when they age into real adult roles, returning gradually to a more conventional lifestyle. This recovery may be delayed if the antisocial activities of adolescence-limited delinquents attract factors we called "snares," such as a criminal record, incarceration, addiction, or truncated education without credentials. Such snares can compromise the ability to make a successful transition to adulthood.

The literature contains other theoretical statements about early-onset antisocial behavior, but this one differs in that it offered not only an account of onset processes, but included an explanation of the processes leading to maintenance and desistence.

## LIFE-COURSE-PERSISTENT ORIGINS

### The Hypothesis That Life-Course-Persistent Antisocial Development Emerges from Early Neurodevelopmental and Family-Adversity Risk Factors

The original hypothesis about childhood risk specified that predictors of life-course-persistent antisocial behavior should include "health, gender, temperament, cognitive abilities, school achievement, personality traits, mental disorders (e.g., hyperactivity), family attachment bonds, child-rearing practices, parent and sibling deviance, and socioeconomic status, but not age" (Moffitt, 1993, p. 695).

Our tests of this hypothesis have been carried out in the Dunedin Multidisciplinary Health and Development Study, a 30-year longitudinal study of a birth cohort of 1,000 New Zealanders (Moffitt, Caspi, Rutter, & Silva, 2001). These tests have examined childhood predictors measured between ages 3 and 13, operationalizing the two prototypes of antisocial behavior using both categorical and continuous statistical approaches. These studies showed that the life-course-persistent path was differentially predicted by individual risk characteristics, including undercontrolled temperament measured by observers at age 3, neurological abnormalities and delayed motor development at age 3, low intellectual ability, reading difficulties, poor scores on neuropsychological tests of memory, hyperactivity, and slow heart rate (Jeglum-Bartusch, Lynam, Moffitt, & Silva, 1997; Moffitt, 1990; Moffitt & Caspi, 2001; Moffitt, Lynam, & Silva, 1994). The life-course-persistent path was also differentially predicted by parenting risk factors, including teenage single parents, mothers with poor mental health, mothers who were observed to be harsh or neglectful, as well as by experiences of harsh and inconsistent discipline, much family conflict, many changes of primary caretaker, low family socioeconomic status (SES), and rejection by peers in school. In contrast, study members on the adolescence-limited path, despite being involved in teen delinquency to the same extent as their counterparts on the life-course-persistent path, tended to have backgrounds that were normative or sometimes even better than the average Dunedin child's (Moffitt & Caspi, 2001).

These Dunedin findings about differential neurodevelopmental and family risk correlates for childhood-onset versus adolescent-onset offenders are generally in keeping with findings reported from other samples in eight countries. These studies operationalized the types using a variety of conceptual approaches and statistical methods (Aguilar, Sroufe, Egeland, & Carlson, 2000; Arseneault, Tremblay, Boulerice, & Saucier, 2002; Chung, Hill, Hawkins, Gilchrist, & Nagin, 2002; Dean, Brame, & Piquero, 1996; Donnellan, Ge, & Wenk, 2000; Fergusson, Horwood, & Nagin, 2000; Kjelsberg, 1999; Kratzer & Hodgins, 1999; Magnusson, af Klintberg, & Stattin, 1994; Maughan, Pickles, Rowe, Costello, & Angold, 2001; Mazerolle, Brame, Paternoster, Piquero, & Dean, 2000; Nagin et al., 1995; Patterson, Forgatch, Yoerger, & Stoolmiller, 1998; Piquero, 2001; Piquero & Brezina, 2001; Raine, Yaralian, Reynolds, Venables, & Mednick, 2002; Roeder, Lynch, & Nagin, 1999; Tibbetts & Piquero, 1999; Ruchkin, Koposov, Vermeiren, & Schwab-Stone, in press). However, at least one research team found mixed evidence for the taxonomy (cf. Brame, Bushway, & Paternoster, 1999; Paternoster & Brame, 1997).

Other studies, although not necessarily presented as a formal test of the two types, have reported findings consonant with our predictions about differential childhood risk. For example, children's hyperactivity interacts with poor parenting skill to predict antisocial behavior that has an early onset and escalates to delinquency (Patterson, De Garmo, & Knutson, 2000), an interaction that fits the hypothesized origins of the life-course-persistent path. Other studies have reported that measures of infant nervous system maldevelopment interact with poor parenting and social adversity to predict aggression that is chronic from childhood to adolescence (Arseneault et al., 2002) and early-onset violent crime (Raine, Brennan, & Mednick, 1994; Raine, Brennan, Mednick, & Mednick 1996), but not nonviolent crime (Raine, Brennan, & Mednick, 1997; Arseneault, Tremblay, Boulerice, Seguin, & Saucier, 2000). Also consistent with our prediction that infant nervous system maldevelopment contributes to long-term life-course-persistent antisocial outcomes, prenatal malnutrition has been found to predict adult antisocial personality disorder (Neugebauer, Hoek, & Susser, 1999).

Our differential risk prediction encountered a particular challenge from a longitudinal study of a low-SES Minneapolis sample (Aguilar et al., 2000). This research team observed that differences between their childhood-onset and adolescent-onset groups were not significant for neurocognitive and temperament measures taken prior to age 3, but that significant differences did emerge later in childhood. The authors inferred that childhood psychosocial adversity is sufficient to account for the origins of life-course-persistent antisocial behavior, which is similar to Patterson and Yoerger's (1997) thesis that unskilled parenting is sufficient to account for the early-onset antisocial type. Such exclusive socialization hypotheses are probably not defensible, in view of emerging evidence that the life-course-persistent pattern of antisocial behavior appears to have substantial heritable liability (DiLalla & Gottesman, 1989; Eley, Lichtenstein, & Moffitt, in press; Taylor, Iacono, & McGue, 2000), a finding we revisit below. The lack of significant early-childhood differences in the Minneapolis study may have arisen from methodological features of the study, including the unrepresentative and homogeneous nature of the sample (all high-risk, low-SES individuals), irregular sex composition of the groups (more females than males were antisocial), or weak psychometric qualities of the infant measures (poor predictive validity). Infant measures are known for their poor predictive validity (McCall & Carriger, 1993), and thus it is possible that the failure of the infant measures to predict the life-course-persistent path is part of such measures' more general failure to predict anything. Other studies have reported a significant relation between life-course-persistent-type offending and perinatal complications or low birth weight, problems known to be associated with neurocognitive and temperamental difficulties in infancy (Arseneault et al., 2000; Arseneault, Tremblay, et al., 2002; Kratzer & Hodgins, 1999; Tibbetts & Piquero, 1999; Raine, Brennan, & Mednick, 1994). These studies illustrate desirable features for testing neurodevelopmental risks from the beginning of infancy for persistent antisocial behavior: large representative samples, infant measures with proven predictive validity, and attention to interactions between neurodevelopmental and social adversity. Despite the potential shortcomings of the Aguilar et al. (2000) study for testing the origins of the life-course-persistent type, this study remains the only one that has reported objective measures of infants' temperament and neurocognitive status prior to age 3. As such, this study constitutes a challenge that must be taken seriously, and it warrants replication.

## What Research Is Needed?

Research already documents that life-course-persistent antisocial behavior has the predicted neurodevelopmental correlates in the perinatal and middle childhood periods, but clearly more research is needed to fill in the critical gap between birth and age 3. This might be accomplished by following up the antisocial outcomes of infants tested with newer neurocognitive measures having documented predictive validity, such as the infant attention–habituation paradigm (Sigman, Cohen, & Beckwith, 1997). Another feature of life-course-persistent theory that needs testing is the argument that antisocial behavior becomes persistent because a child's early difficult behavior provokes harsh treatment or rejection from parents, teachers, and peers, which in turn promotes more difficult child behavior. Adoption studies have shown an initial *child effect*, that is, children carrying a genetic liability to antisocial behavior provoke harsh parenting responses from their adoptive parents (Ge et al., 1996; O'Connor, Deater-Deckard, Fulker, Rutter, & Plomin, 1998). Such adoption studies could be followed up to ascertain whether this process beginning with a child effect ultimately leads to antisocial behavior that persists longer term.

## The Hypothesis That Genetic Etiological Processes Contribute More to Life-Course-Persistent Than to Adolescence-Limited Antisocial Development

DiLalla and Gottesman (1989) observed that adult crime seemed to be more heritable than adolescent juvenile delinquency. Our 1993 paper agreed with these authors that if the life-course-persistent type's causal factors are partly inherited, and if most antisocial adults are life-course-persistent but most antisocial adolescents are not, this could account for the observed greater heritability in adult than adolescent samples (Moffitt 1993, p. 694). As it turns out, the lack of heritability among juveniles in the DiLalla and Gottesman review probably resulted from low power and insensitive measurement; in 1989 the entire literature of behavior genetic studies of juvenile delinquency consisted of only 175 twin pairs, and the measure of antisocial behavior was conviction, a rare outcome for juveniles. Since then a large number of better designed behavioral genetic studies have proven that juvenile antisocial behavior is heritable. Among these, three groups of studies suggest that life-course-persistent antisocial behavior does have stronger heritable origins than adolescence-limited antisocial behavior.

The first of these groups of studies has taken a behavioral or phenotypic approach, identifying subtypes on the basis of the Aggression and Delinquency scales from the Child Behavior Checklist (CBCL; Achenbach, 1985). The Aggression scale is thought to be associated with the life-course-persistent prototype because it measures antisocial personality and physical violence and its scores are stable across development, whereas the Delinquency scale is associated with the adolescence-limited prototype because it measures rule breaking and its mean scores rise steeply during adolescence (Stanger, Achenbach, & Verhulst, 1997). In fact, both life-course-persistent and adolescence-limited young people engage in the behaviors on the Delinquency scale, but adolescence-limited young people are relatively more numerous and if they have less genetic risk, we would expect the Delinquency scale to yield low heritability estimates. Twin and adoption studies of these scales report higher heritability for aggression (around 60%) than delinquency (around 30–40%), while the shared environment is significant only for the Delinquency scale (also around 30–40%) (e.g., Deater-Deckard & Plomin, 1999; Edelbrock, Rende, Plomin, & Thompson, 1995; Eley, Lichtenstein, & Stevenson, 1999), although there is an exception to this pattern from a small sample (e.g. Schmitz, Fulker, & Mrazek, 1995).

The second group of studies has taken a developmental approach by defining life-course-persistent antisocial behavior in terms of preadolescent onset, or onset in adolescence with duration into adulthood, in contrast to adolescence-limited antisocial behavior seen only during the adolescent stage. The first of these studies demonstrated that antisocial behavior persisting from adolescence to adulthood was significantly more heritable than that reported only in adolescence (Lyons et al., 1995), a finding that has been replicated in a separate sample (Jacobson, Neale, Prescott, & Kendler, 2001). The second study examined onset of antisocial behavior before and during adolescence, and found early-onset antisocial behavior to be strongly familial and substantially heritable in contrast to adolescent-onset antisocial behavior, which was not very familial and was largely influenced by the shared environment (Taylor et al., 2000). A recent study explored genetic and environmental influences on aggression and delinquency in 1,000 Swedish twin pairs ages 8–9 years and again at ages 13–14 years (Eley et al., in press). Continuity from childhood to adolescence in the CBCL Aggression scale was largely mediated by genetic influences, whereas continuity in the Delinquency scale was mediated both by the shared environment and by genetic influences. This longitudinal study suggests that aggression is a stable heritable trait, whereas delinquency is more strongly influenced by the environment and shows less genetic stability over time.

The third group of studies are the four studies of large representative samples of very young twins. Arseneault et al. (in press) reported 82% heritability for antisocial behavior among 5-year-olds, Dionne, Tremblay, Boivin, Laplante, and Pérusse (2003) reported 58% heritability for aggression among 18-month-olds, van den Ord, Verhulst, and Boomsma (1996) reported 69% heritability for aggression among 3-year-olds, and van der Valk, Verhulst, Stroet, and Boomsma (1998) reported 50% heritability for externalizing behavior among 2- to 3-year-old boys and 75% heritability for girls. These high estimates for very young twins contrast with the lower estimate of no more than 40% heritability for adolescent and adult antisocial behavior from a recent meta-analysis (Rhee & Waldman, 2002).

Taken together, these three groups of studies suggest that the pattern of antisocial behavior that begins early in life and persists into adulthood is characterized by aggressive personality, includes physical aggression, and is associated with relatively higher heritability estimates than is late-onset, transient delinquency.

*What Research Is Needed?*

According to the taxonomic theory, the genetic component of variation in early-onset antisocial behavior ought to comprise not only the direct effects of genes, but also the effects of correlations between vulnerability genes and risky environments, and interactions between them as well. Research using measured genes and measured environments is needed to pick these elements apart. In addition, it would be useful to ascertain the genetic and environmental architecture of individual differences in trajectories of anti-social behavior over time. Such trajectories could be derived in longitudinal studies of twins by applying nonparametric mixture modeling tools to repeated measures of antisocial behavior (for demonstrations of these models, see Nagin et al., 1995, and Roeder et al., 1999). The theory would predict strong twin similarity for membership in a childhood-onset, life-course-persistent trajectory, but less twin similarity for membership in an adolescent-onset trajectory.

### Are Two Groups Enough?: Who Are the Low-Level Chronic Criminal Offenders?

The original theoretical taxonomy asserted that two prototypes, life-course-persistent and adolescence-limited offenders, account for the preponderance of the population's antisocial behavior, and thus warrant the preponderance of attention by theory and research. Researchers testing for the presence of the two types have since uncovered a third type that replicates across longitudinal studies. These offenders have been labeled "low-level chronics" because they have been found to offend persistently at a low rate from childhood to adolescence (Fergusson et al., 2000) or from adolescence to adulthood (D'Unger, Land, McCall, & Nagin, 1998; Nagin et al., 1995).

We identified a small group of Dunedin study males who had exhibited extreme, pervasive, and persistent antisocial behavior problems during childhood, but who surprisingly engaged in only low to moderate delinquency during adolescence, not extreme enough to meet criteria for membership in the life-course-persistent group (Moffitt, Caspi, Dickson, Silva, & Stanton, 1996). Like the life-course-persistent offenders, they had extremely undercontrolled temperaments as 3-year-olds (Moffitt et al., 1996); unpublished analyses showed that they also suffered family adversity in childhood and had low intelligence. This group was a surprise to the theory, because the theory argued that an early-onset chain of cumulative interactions between aggressive children and risky environments will perpetuate disordered behavior. On that basis, we had predicted that "false positive subjects, who meet criteria for a stable and pervasive antisocial childhood history and yet recover (eschew delinquency) after puberty, should be extremely rare" (Moffitt, 1993, p. 694). When we discovered this group, we optimistically labeled it the "recovery group" (Moffitt et al., 1996). However, our study of this group has revealed no protective factors. Since persuaded by other samples' findings about low-level chronics, we followed up the so-called recovery group at age 26. We found that recovery was clearly a misnomer, as their modal offending pattern over time fit a pattern referred to by criminologists as "intermittency," in which some offenders are not convicted for a period but then reappear in the courts (Laub & Sampson, 2001). This Dunedin group's long-term offending pattern closely resembles that of the "low-level chronic offenders" first identified in trajectory analyses of a British cohort (Nagin et al., 1995).

Anticipating true recoveries from serious childhood conduct disorder to be extremely rare, the taxonomic theory had argued that teens who engage in less delinquency than predicted might have off-putting personal characteristics that excluded them from the social peer groups in which most delinquency happens. Consistent with this prediction, the members of this low-level chronic group, unlike other cohort men, were often social isolates; their informants reported that they had difficulty making friends, none had married, few held jobs, and many had diagnoses of agoraphobia and/or social phobia. Almost all social phobics meet criteria for avoidant, dependent, and/or schizotypal personality disorders (Alnaes & Torgersen, 1988). We speculate that men in this group may suffer from these isolating personality disorders. As many as one-third of this group had diagnosable depression, their personality profile showed elevated neuroticism, and their informants rated them as the most depressed, anxious men in the cohort. This pattern in which formerly antisocial boys develop into depressed, anxious, socially isolated men resembles closely a finding from a British longitudinal study of males followed from ages 8 to 32. In that study also at-risk antisocial boys who became adult "false positives" (committing less crime than predicted) had few or no friends, held low-paying jobs, lived in dirty home conditions, and had been described in case records as withdrawn, highly strung, obsessional, nervous, or timid (Farrington, Gallagher, Morley, St. Ledger, & West, 1988).

Robins (1966) is often quoted as having said that one-half of all conduct problem boys do not grow up to have antisocial personalities. Such quotations are intended to imply that early conduct problems are fully malleable and need not be a cause for pessimism. However, less often quoted is Robins's (1966) observation that conduct problem boys who do not develop antisocial personalities generally suffer other forms of maladjustment as adults. Only 15% of Dunedin's 87 conduct problem boys (i.e., 47 in the life-course-persistent group and 40 in the low-level chronic group) truly recovered, escaping all adjustment problems by age 26. Taken together, findings from Dunedin and the studies by Farrington and Robins are consistent with our theory's original assertion that childhood-onset antisocial behavior is *virtually always* a prognosticator of poor adult adjustment.

## What Research Is Needed?

Several studies have detected low-level chronic offenders, but only two have been able to shed any light on their personal characteristics. The characteristics are suggestive of avoidant, dependent, schizotypal personality disorders and/or low intelligence, but these outcomes have not been directly measured in adulthood. It is important to know if this group has psychopathology to test the theory's assertion that serious childhood-onset antisocial behavior reliably signals a long-term process of maladjustment.


## ADOLESCENCE-LIMITED ORIGINS

### The Hypothesis That Adolescence-Limited Antisocial Behavior Is Influenced by the Maturity Gap and by Social Mimicry of Antisocial Models

The original theory asserted that "individual differences should play little or no role in the prediction of short-term adolescent offending careers. Instead, the strongest predictors of adolescence-limited offending should be peer delinquency, attitudes toward adolescence and adulthood reflecting the maturity gap [such as a desire for autonomy], cultural and historical contexts influencing adolescence, and age" (Moffitt, 1993, p. 695).

Most research on the taxonomy to date has focused on testing hypotheses about the etiology of life-course-persistent offenders. Unfortunately, adolescence-limited offenders have been relegated to the status of a contrast group and the original hypotheses about the distinct etiology of adolescent-onset offending have not captured the research imagination. This is unfortunate because adolescent-onset offenders are quite common (one-quarter of both males and females as defined in the Dunedin cohort) and their antisocial activities are not benign.

Aguilar et al. (2000) discovered that adolescent-onset delinquents experienced elevated internalizing symptoms and perceptions of stress at age 16, which may be consistent with the taxonomy's assertion that these adolescents experience psychological discomfort during the maturity gap. In a study of the Glueck's sample, adolescents' concerns about appearing immature increased their likelihood of delinquency (Zebrowitz, Andreoletti, Collins, Lee, & Blumenthal, 1998). Developmental research shows that when ordinary young people age into adolescence they begin to admire good students less and to admire aggressive, antisocial peers more (Bukowski, Sippola, & Newcomb, 2000; Luthar & McMahon, 1996). In adolescence, teens who place a high value on conforming to adults' rules become unpopular with peers (Allen, Weissberg, & Hawkins, 1989). Our Dunedin studies documented that the adolescence-limited path is more strongly associated with delinquent peers, as compared with the life-course-persistent path (Jeglum-Bartusch et al., 1997; Moffitt & Caspi, 2001). We also showed that an increase in young teens' awareness of peers' delinquency antedates and predicts onset of their own later delinquency (Caspi, Lynam, Moffitt, & Silva, 1993). Others have shown that delinquent peer influence directly promotes increases in the type of delinquency that begins in adolescence (Simons, Wu, Conger, & Lorenz, 1994; Vitaro, Tremblay, Kerr, Pagani, & Bukowski, 1997). (These same studies suggest that when antisocial behavior begins younger, the direction of influence runs the other way: the child's own early antisocial behavior promotes increases at adolescence in the number of delinquent peers who selectively affiliate with him.) One ethnographic study has illustrated how the maturity-gap explains *kortteliralli*, the street-racing alcoholic youth culture of Finland (Vaaranen, 2001).

The most direct test of the adolescence-limited etiological hypothesis was carried out in the Youth in Transition Survey of 2,000 males (Piquero & Brezina, 2001). This study was introduced to the literature with lines by rocker Alice Cooper that reflect the ennui of the maturity gap: "I'm in the middle without any plans, I'm a boy and I'm a man." The study tested the hypothesis that desires for autonomy promoted adolescent-onset offending. It found that, as predicted, the offenses committed by adolescence-limited delinquents were primarily rebellious (not physically aggressive), and that this rebellious offending was accounted for by the interaction between maturational timing and aspects of peer activities that were related to personal autonomy. However, one measure of youth autonomy in this study did not yield a significant finding.

It is important to acknowledge that alternative accounts of late-onset delinquency have been put forward. In particular, Patterson and Yoerger (1997) outlined a learning model in which decreases in parents' monitoring and supervision when their children enter adolescence cause adolescents to begin offending. We had argued that although parents' monitoring and supervision were certainly negatively correlated with adolescent-onset delinquency, the direction of cause and effect was unclear, and our adolescence-limited theory would say that this correlation arises because teens' desires to gain autonomy via delinquency motivate them to evade their parents' supervision (Moffitt, 1993, p. 693). A longitudinal study of 1,000 Swedish 14-year-olds and their parents suggested that our interpretation may be correct (Kerr & Stattin, 2000). Adolescents actively controlled their parents' access to information about their activities, and teens who took part in deviant behavior limited their parents' capacity to monitor them. The study showed that parents' efforts to supervise and monitor were not very effective in controlling their children's activities, and could even backfire if teens felt controlled.

*What Research Is Needed?*

Clearly, there is little research testing whether measures of the maturity gap and social mimicry can account for adolescence-limited delinquency, so any studies with this aim would add to our understanding. Short-term longitudinal studies of young teens might ask if a developmental increase in attitudes rejecting childhood and favoring autonomy is correlated with a growing interest in and approval of illicit activities. Moreover, there is the curious fact that life-course-persistent antisocials are rejected by their childhood peers but later become more popular with their adolescent peers. The theory of social mimicry predicted this shift, but more longitudinal research following individuals' changes in social standing is needed to understand it fully. Finally, we should consult historical and anthropological work to ascertain if times and cultures having low levels of delinquency are times and cultures having a clearly demarcated transition from childhood dependency to adulthood rights and responsibilities.

### The Hypothesis That Abstainers from Delinquency Are Rare Individuals Who Are Excluded from Normative Peer Group Activities in Adolescence

If, as the theory says, adolescence-limited delinquency is normative adaptational social behavior, then the existence of teens who abstain from delinquency requires an explanation. The original theory speculated that teens committing no antisocial behavior would be rare, and that they must have either structural barriers that prevent them from learning about delinquency, no maturity gap because of early access to adult roles, or personal characteristics unappealing to other teens that cause them to be excluded from teen social group activities (Moffitt, 1993, pp. 689, 695). In other words, if ordinary teens take up delinquent behavior, then teens who eschew delinquency must be extraordinary.

Consistent with the rarity prediction, the Dunedin cohort contained only a small group of males who avoided virtually any antisocial behavior during childhood and adolescence (Moffitt et al., 1996). These Dunedin abstainers described themselves at age 18 on personality measures as extremely overcontrolled, fearful, interpersonally timid, and socially inept, and they were latecomers to sexual relationships (i.e., virgins at age 18). Dunedin abstainers fit the profile Shedler and Block (1990) reported for youth who abstained from drug experimentation in a historical period when it was normative: overcontrolled, not curious, not active, not open to experience, socially isolated, and lacking social skills. Dunedin abstainers were unusually good students, fitting the profile of the compliant good student who during adolescence can become unpopular with peers (Allen et al., 1989; Bukowski et al., 2000). Dunedin's age-26 follow-up data confirm that these men have not become so-called late-onset offenders (Moffitt,

Caspi, Harrington, & Milne, 2002). Although their teenaged years had been troubling, their style became more successful in adulthood. As adults they retained their self-constrained personality, had virtually no crime or mental disorder, were likely to have settled into marriage, were delaying children (a desirable strategy for a generation needing prolonged education to succeed), were likely to be college-educated, held high-status jobs, and expressed optimism about their own futures.

### What Research Is Needed?

To our knowledge, the developmental histories of adolescents who abstain from delinquency have not been examined in other samples (apart from the 1990 paper by Shedler and Block), so our finding that abstainers are introverts as teens remains to be confirmed. Adolescent sociometric studies might ask if delinquent abstention is indeed correlated with unpopularity and social isolation. Further study of abstainers is critical for testing the hypothesis that adolescence-limiteds' delinquency is normative adaptational behavior by ordinary young people.

## OUTCOMES

### The Hypothesis That Life-Course-Persistent and Adolescence-Limited Delinquents Develop Different Personality Structures

The original theory hypothesized the following about the development of life-course-persistent offenders: "Over the years, an antisocial personality is slowly and insidiously constructed and accumulating consequences of the youngster's personality problems prune away options for change. A person–environment interaction process is needed to account for emerging antisocial behavior, but after some age, will the 'person' main effect alone predict adult outcome?" (Moffitt, 1993, p. 684).

Our Dunedin studies of adolescents' personality characteristics measured at age 18 showed that the life-course-persistent path was differentially associated with weak bonds to family and with the psychopathic personality traits of alienation, callousness, and impulsivity. In contrast, the adolescence-limited path at age 18 was differentially associated with a tendency to endorse unconventional values and with a personality trait called "social potency" (Moffitt et al., 1996). We assessed personality traits 10 years later at age 26, this time using not only self-reports but reports from informants who knew the Dunedin study members well (Moffitt et al., 2002). The self- and informant reports concurred that the life-course-persistent men had more negative emotionality (they were stress-reactive, alienated, and aggressive) and were less agreeable (less social closeness, more callous) compared to adolescence-limited men. Life-course-persistent men were no longer particularly impulsive, but the adolescence-limited men were still somewhat elevated on this scale at age 26. It appears from these repeated Dunedin assessments that the life-course-persistent pathway leads to a disordered antisocial personality structure resembling the psychopath: aggressive, alienated, and callous. Adolescence-limited men, in contrast, are unconventional, valuing spontaneity and excitement.

In another study, 4,000 California Youth Authority inmates were given the California Personality Inventory in the 1960s and then followed up into the 1980s (Donnellan, Ge, & Wenk, in press). Taxonomy comparison groups were defined as early starters versus later starters, and as chronic adult arrestees versus those arrested less often. The early-starter, chronic arrestees could be discriminated by extreme personality scale scores, in particular, low communality, little concern with impression, high irresponsibility, low control of emotions, low achievement motivation, low socialization, low tolerance (hostile, distrustful), and low well-being. These scales echo our Dunedin findings, with different instruments and informants, in which life-course-persistent offenders were disagreeable and high on negative emotionality.

### What Research Is Needed?

To our knowledge, the personality correlates of the taxonomy have only been examined in two samples, so the finding of differential personality structures remains to be confirmed by wider replication. The Dunedin finding that adolescence-limited offenders are unconventional excitement seekers raises the question of whether this approach-oriented personality style is present prospectively before they take up delinquency, and is an individual-difference risk factor for adolescent onset that was not anticipated by the theory. Childhood temperament studies that have measured the approach style might follow up their participants to ask if approach predicts adolescent-onset delinquency. Longitudinal research is also needed to determine if and when the antisocial personality style becomes "set," that is, able to predict adult antisocial outcomes alone, without any further environmental input.

### The Hypothesis That Life-Course-Persistent Development Is Differentially Associated in Adulthood with Serious Offending and Violence

The original theory predicted that life-course-persistent offenders, as compared to adolescence-limited offenders, would engage in a wider variety of offense types, including "more of the victim-oriented offenses, such as violence and fraud" (Moffitt, 1993, p. 695).

By the time the Dunedin cohort reached age 18, we reported that the life-course-persistent pathway was differentially associated with conviction for violent crimes (Jeglum-Bartusch et al., 1997; Moffitt et al., 1996), while the adolescence-limited pathway was differentially associated with nonviolent delinquent offenses (Jeglum-Bartusch et al., 1997). Moreover, we had shown that preadolescent antisocial behavior that was accompanied by neuropsychological deficits predicted greater persistence of crime and more violence up to age 18 (Moffitt et al., 1994).

Our follow-up at age 26 confirmed that life-course-persistent men as a group particularly differed from adolescence-limited men in the realm of violence, including violence against women and children. This finding was corroborated with large effect sizes by self-reports, informant reports, and official court conviction records (Moffitt et al., 2002). In a comparison of specific offenses, life-course-persistent men tended to specialize in serious offenses (carrying a hidden weapon, assault, robbery, violating court orders), whereas adolescence-limited men specialized in nonserious offenses (theft less than $5, public drunkenness, giving false information on application forms, pirating computer software). Life-course-persistent men accounted for five times their share of the cohort's violent convictions. Moreover, the life-course-persistent group's scores were elevated on self-reported and official conviction measures of abuse toward women, both physical abuse and controlling abuse (e.g., restricting her access to family, stalking her). Life-course-persistent men were also most likely to report that they had hit a child out of anger. Our finding that life-course-persistent offenders perpetrated more domestic violence was supported by the Christchurch Study's finding that people with childhood-onset antisocial behavior engaged in more partner violence than those with adolescent-onset antisocial behavior (Woodward, Fergusson, & Horwood, 2002).

In general, the empirical literature shows that the strongest long-term predictors of violence are the same predictors implicated by our theory of life-course-persistent offending: early-onset antisocial behavior, neurodevelopmental risk factors, and family risk factors (for a review, see Farrington, 1998). Moreover, research comparing violent crime versus general nonviolent delinquency has shown that violence is differentially predicted by birth complications (Raine et al., 1997), minor physical anomalies (Arseneault et al., 2000), difficult temperament (Henry, Caspi, Moffitt, & Silva, 1996), and cognitive deficits (Piquero, 2001), each of which are hypothetical risks for life-course-persistent development.

## What Research Is Needed?

The literature makes it clear that neurodevelopmental and family risks predict violence on a continuum, but only two studies have compared the adult violent outcomes of groups defined on the basis of early versus late delinquency onset. Moreover, research is needed to clarify why life-course-persistent offenders are more violent. Our theory implies that verbal cognitive deficits may limit their options for handling conflict, that they may have learned in their families that violence is an effective way to manage conflict, and that broken attachment bonds lead to alienation from their potential victims (Moffitt, 1994). But are any of these processes correct?

## The Hypothesis That Childhood-Onset Antisocial Behavior Will Persist into Middle Adulthood, Whereas Adolescent-Onset Antisocial Behavior Will Desist in Young Adulthood

We followed up the Dunedin cohort at age 26 (Moffitt et al., 2002), to test a hypothesis critical to the theory: that childhood-onset, but not adolescent-onset, antisocial behavior is associated in adulthood with antisocial personality and continued serious antisocial behavior that expands into maladjustment in work-life and victimization of partners and children (Moffitt, 1993, p. 695). Followed to age 26, the childhood-onset delinquents were the most elevated on psychopathic personality traits, mental health problems, substance dependence, number of children sired, domestic abuse, financial problems, work problems, and drug-related and violent crimes. The adolescent-onset delinquents at 26 were less extreme but also elevated on property offenses and financial problems. Interestingly, the adolescent-onset delinquents self-reported problems with mental health and substance dependence, but these difficulties were not corroborated by informants who knew them well. This discrepancy between self-reports and other sources was also found in a British longitudinal study in which offenders defined as adolescence-limited had desisted offending according to official police records, but continued into their 30s to self-report substance abuse and fighting (Nagin et al., 1995).

In a study of 4,000 California Youth Authority inmates followed into their 30s, significantly more early starters than later starters continued offending past age 21, past age 25, and past age 31; moreover, early onset and low cognitive ability were significant predictors of offending that continued into the 30s (Ge, Donnellan, & Wenk, 2001). Similarly, a large Swedish study reported less crime in adulthood among offenders who possessed positive personal characteristics resembling the characteristics of Dunedin adolescence-limited offenders (Stattin, Romelsjo, & Stenbacka, 1997).

The Rutgers Health and Human Development Project also followed its longitudinal sample into adulthood and reported a test of the taxonomy using nonparametric mixture modeling to detect trajectory groups (White, Bates, & Buyske, 2001). However, this paper's Figure 1, showing delinquency trajectories for the resulting groups, suggests that the group labeled "persistent" in this study was in reality adolescence-limited, because this group's trajectory showed very low levels of offending at ages 12 and 28, but a very pronounced adolescent offending peak at age 18. This sample may not have contained life-course-persistent members because it was re-cruited via random telephone dialing with an initial 17% rate of refusal to the phone call and afterwards a 52% completion rate for enrollment in data collection. Families with life-course-persistent risk characteristics are known to be difficult to engage as research participants. Given the strong possibility that groups were mislabeled in this study, it is unclear what to make of it, vis-à-vis the taxonomy.

## What Research Is Needed?

Overall, our theory's prediction that childhood-onset antisocial behavior persists longer into adulthood than adolescent-onset delinquency seems to be on fairly solid empirical footing. It has been known for decades that early onset of offending predicts a longer duration of crime career, and this association was recently affirmed by two careful reviews (Gendreau, Little, & Goggin, 1996; Krohn, Thornberry, Rivera, & LeBlanc, 2001). Nonethe-less, the adolescence-limited groups in the Dunedin and British studies con-tinued to self-report adjustment problems as adults, and we need research to understand what accounts for this. More important, longitudinal studies are needed that follow the life-course-persistent, low-level chronic, ab-stainer, and adolescence-limited groups to reveal the very-long-term impli-cations of their experiences in the first two decades of life. Here we put for-ward a new prediction, that the life-course-persistents' antisocial lifestyle, violence, socioeconomic stress, and hostile personality will place them at greatest risk in midlife for poor physical health, cardiovascular disease, and early mortality. Follow-up studies should measure such health outcomes.

# GENDER

### The Hypothesis That Most Female Antisocial Behavior Is the Adolescence-Limited Type

The original statement of the taxonomy asserted that the theory describes the behavior of females as well as it describes the behavior of males. The full text of the theory that included predictions about females was pub-lished as a book chapter that is not widely available (Moffitt, 1994). There-fore we quote the original statement, written in January 1991:

> The crime rate for females is lower than for males. In this developmental taxonomy, much of the gender difference in crime is attributed to sex differ-ences in the risk factors for life-course persistent antisocial behavior. Little girls are less likely than little boys to encounter all of the putative initial links in the causal chain for life-course persistent antisocial development. Research has shown that girls have lower rates than boys of symptoms of nervous system dysfunction, difficult temperament, late verbal and motor

milestones, hyperactivity, learning disabilities, reading failure, and child-hood conduct problems. Most girls lack the personal diathesis elements of the evocative, reactive, and proactive person/environment interactions that initiate and maintain life-course persistent antisocial behavior.

Adolescence-limited delinquency, on the other hand, is open to girls as well as to boys. According to the theory advanced here, girls, like boys, should begin delinquency soon after puberty, to the extent that they (1) have access to antisocial models, and (2) perceive the consequences of de-linquency as reinforcing. However, exclusion from gender-segregated male antisocial groups may cut off opportunities for girls to learn delin-quent behaviors. Girls are physically more vulnerable than boys to risk of personal victimization (e.g., pregnancy, or injury from dating violence) if they affiliate with life-course persistent antisocial males. Thus, lack of ac-cess to antisocial models and perceptions of serious personal risk may dampen the vigor of girls' delinquent involvement somewhat. Nonethe-less, girls should engage in adolescence-limited delinquency in significant numbers. (Moffitt, 1994, pp. 39–40)

The original theory thus proposed that (1) fewer females than males would become delinquent (and conduct-disordered) overall, and that (2) within delinquents the percentage who are life-course-persistent would be larger among males than among females. Following from this, (3) the ma-jority of delinquent females will be of the adolescence-limited type, and fur-ther, (4) their delinquency will have the same causes as adolescence-limited males' delinquency.

These predictions were borne out in the Dunedin cohort (Moffitt & Caspi, 2001; Moffitt et al., 2001). As predicted, the male:female difference was very large for the life-course-persistent form of antisocial behavior (10:1) but negligible for the adolescence-limited form (1.5:1). Childhood-onset females had high-risk neurodevelopmental and family backgrounds, but adolescent-onset females did not, which documented that females and males on the same trajectories share the same risk factors. We have de-scribed the elements of the adolescence-limited causal pathway among Dunedin females, showing that each girl's delinquency onset is linked to the timing of her own puberty (Moffitt et al., 2001), that delinquent peers are a necessary condition for onset of delinquency among adolescent girls (Caspi & Moffitt, 1991; Caspi et al., 1993), and that an intimate relationship with an offender promotes girls' antisocial behaviors (Moffitt et al., 2001).

Few empirical tests of this taxonomy have compared how females and males fit the two developmental trajectories, but it appears that our find-ings about females are broadly consistent with these previous studies. Fergusson et al. (2000), studying the Christchurch sample (n = 1,000), found that a single model described male and female trajectories of antiso-cial behavior, and the male-to-female ratio was 4:1 for early-onset versus only 2:1 for late-onset subjects. Kratzer and Hodgins (1999), studying a

Swedish cohort ($n$ = 13,000), found similar childhood risk factors for males and females in the life-course-persistent group, and the male-to-female ratio was 15:1 for early-onset versus only 4:1 for late-onset subjects. Mazerolle et al. (2000), studying a Philadelphia cohort ($n$ = 3,655), reported that early onset signaled persistent and diverse offending for males and females alike. A longitudinal study of 820 girls analyzed with a semiparametric mixture model found a stable, highly antisocial group, but this group contained only 1.4% of the girls (Cote, Zoccolillo, Tremblay, Nagin, & Vitaro, 2001). All studies concur that females are seldom childhood-onset or life-course-persistent-type (the exception is Aguilar et al., 2000, whose early-onset group had as many girls as boys). These accumulating findings suggest that the two theories of the origins of life-course-persistent and adolescence-limited offending are explanatory across the sexes and irrespective of sex. Because few females have the risk factors for life-course-persistent development, this theory explains the wide sex difference in serious, persistent, antisocial behavior. Because the risk factors for adolescence-limited offending are equal-opportunity ones, this theory explains the sex similarity for nonserious, transient delinquency during the teenage years (Moffitt et al., 2001).

## What Research Is Needed?

The dearth of gender comparisons originates from a pragmatic circumstance. An ideal test of this theory requires a large representative (nonclinical, nonadjudicated) sample followed longitudinally from childhood to adulthood with repeated measures of antisocial behavior. To date few such studies have included females. It would be useful to have a large sample including both life-course-persistent and adolescence-limited girls in sufficient numbers to test all components of our theory.

## RACE

### The Hypothesis That Both Life-Course Persistent and Adolescence-Limited Developmental Processes Are Exacerbated by Societal Race Prejudice

The original statement of the taxonomy asserted that the theory applies to ethnic minority populations as well as to whites. The discussion of race was published in a book chapter not widely available (Moffitt, 1994). Therefore we paraphrase the original statement:

> In the United States, the crime rate for black Americans is higher than the crime rate for whites. The race difference may be accounted for by a relatively higher prevalence of both life-course-persistent and adolescence-limited subtypes among contemporary African Americans. Life-course-

persistent antisocials might be anticipated at elevated rates among black Americans because the putative root causes of this type are elevated by institutionalized prejudice and by poverty. Among poor black families, prenatal care is less available, infant nutrition is poorer, and the incidence of exposure to toxic and infectious agents is greater, placing infants at risk for the nervous system problems that research has shown to interfere with prosocial child development. To the extent that family bonds have been loosened and poor black parents are under stress, and to the extent that poor black children attend disadvantaged schools, for poor black children the snowball of cumulative continuity may begin rolling earlier, and it may roll faster downhill. In addition, adolescence-limited crime is probably elevated among black youths as compared to white youths in contemporary America. If racially segregated communities provide greater exposure to life-course-persistent role models, then circumstances are ripe for black teens with no prior behavior problems to mimic delinquent ways in a search for status and respect. Moreover, black young people spend more years in the maturity gap, on average, than whites because ascendancy to valued adult roles and privileges comes later, if at all. Legitimate desirable jobs are closed to many young black men; they do not often shift from having "little to lose" to having a "stake in conformity" overnight by leaving schooling and entering a good job. Indeed, the biological maturity gap is perhaps best seen as an instigator of adolescent-onset delinquency for black youths, with an economic maturity gap maintaining offending into adulthood. (Moffitt, 1994, p. 39)

Our research with the Pittsburgh Youth Survey has documented that childhood risk factors associated with life-course-persistent offending (low IQ and impulsive undercontrol) are related to early-onset frequent delinquent offending and physical aggression among black and white males alike (Caspi et al., 1994; Lynam, Moffitt, & Stouthamer-Loeber, 1993; Lynam et al., 2000). However, these studies have not specifically divided Pittsburgh delinquents into childhood- versus adolescent-onset comparison groups (because the cohort of the Pittsburgh Study having IQ and personality data were not followed beyond age 13).

We know of only two studies that have directly compared life-course-persistent versus adolescent offender groups across races, and they seem to offer opposite findings. Donnelan et al. (2000) designated the taxonomy groups within 2,000 young adult California Youth Authority inmates. On a comprehensive set of measures of cognitive ability, life-course-persistent offenders scored below adolescence-limited offenders. However, this predicted finding of differential cognitive risk applied to adjudicated whites and Hispanics, but not to adjudicated African Americans. In contrast, a study of the Baltimore sample of the National Collaborative Perinatal Project examined race differences in the etiological process hypothesized to underly life-course-persistent antisocial behavior (Piquero, Moffitt, & Lawton, 2002). Results showed that several variables helped to explain differences between whites and blacks in the level of chronic offending. However, although black participants had higher mean levels of risk factors than whites, the developmental processes predicting chronic offending were the same across groups defined by race. Specifically, low birth weight in combination with adverse familial environments predicted chronic offending from adolescence to age 33 among whites and African Americans alike, although the effect size reached statistical significance among only African Americans, a pattern opposite to that reported by Donnelan et al. (2000). One further study is relevant. In the Providence sample of the National Collaborative Perinatal Project, Piquero and Buka (2002) found the expected higher prevalence of offenders among African Americans compared to whites. However, crime career patterns such as the concentration of crimes in a few offenders, and the significant prediction of adult crime from chronic juvenile delinquency, applied equally well to both races. This fits our theory's notion that causal developmental processes are the same across racial groups, but that African Americans end up with higher levels of crime because they begin the processes with higher levels of risk factors.

## What Research Is Needed?

The theory asserted that life-course-persistent and adolescence-limited processes should apply to both whites and ethnic minorities (neurodevelopmental and family risks should predict early onset across races, and the maturity gap and peer influences should predict late onset across races). Together these causal processes should be able to account for the elevated prevalence of delinquency among ethnic minorities, because minority group members experience higher levels of both sets of risk factors (see Rowe, Vazsonyi, & Flannery, 1994, for an explanation of how to test this). There is one caveat; if the maturity gap lasts longer for African American young men, this would make it difficult to distinguish the life-course-persistent versus adolescence-limited groups on the basis of chronic offending into adulthood, so researchers examining ethnic minorities should operationalize the groups using other features as well, such as early childhood onset, antisocial personality traits, and recidivistic violence.

## RESEARCH NEEDED ON OTHER HYPOTHESES

Before 1993 virtually no research compared delinquent subtypes defined on a developmental basis, but now this research strategy has become almost commonplace. Many research teams have assessed representative samples with prospective measures of antisocial behavior from childhood to adulthood, and this has enabled comparisons based on age of onset and persistence. Now that the requisite databases are available, other hypotheses derived from the original taxonomic theory need to be tested. We suggested that "snares" (e.g., a criminal record, incarceration, addiction, or truncated education without credentials) should explain variation in the age at desistence from crime during the adult age period, particularly among adolescent-limited offenders (Moffitt, 1993, p. 691). We asserted that the two groups would react differently to turning-point opportunities: life-course-persistent offenders would selectively get undesirable partners and jobs and would in turn expand their repertoire into domestic abuse and workplace crime, whereas adolescence-limited offenders would get good partners and jobs and would in turn desist from crime (Moffitt, 1993, p. 695). We speculated that adolescence-limited offenders must rely on peer support for crime, but life-course-persistent offenders should be willing to offend alone (Moffitt, 1993, p. 688). We suggested that childhood measures of antisocial behavior in longitudinal studies should be more highly correlated with adult measures than with adolescent measures (Moffitt, 1993, p. 695). To our knowledge, these hypotheses have not been systematically examined. Obviously, there is still a lot of work to do.

## ACKNOWLEDGMENT

Preparation of this chapter was supported by the U.S. National Institute of Mental Health (Grant Nos. MH45070, MH49414, and MH56344) and the British Medical Research Council.

## REFERENCES

Achenbach, T. M. (1985). *Assessment and taxonomy of child and adolescent psychopathology.* Newbury Park, CA: Sage.

Aguilar, B., Sroufe, L. A., Egeland, B., & Carlson, E. (2000). Distinguishing the early-onset-persistent and adolescent-onset antisocial behavior types: From birth to 16 years. *Development and Psychopathology, 12,* 109–132.

Allen, J. P., Weissberg, R. P., & Hawkins, J. A. (1989). The relation between values and social competence in early adolescence. *Developmental Psychology, 25,* 458–464.

Alnaes, R., & Torgersen, S. (1988). The relationship between DSM-III symptom disorders (Axis I) and personality disorders (Axis II) in an outpatient population. *Acta Psychiatrica Scandinavica, 78,* 485–492.

American Psychiatric Association. (1994). *Diagnostic and statistical manual of mental disorders* (4th ed.). Washington, DC: Author.

Arseneault, L., Moffitt, T. E., Caspi, A., Taylor, A., Rijsdijk, F., Jaffee, S., Ablow, J. C., & Measelle, J. R. (in press). Strong genetic effects on cross-situational antisocial behavior among 5-year-old children, according to mothers', teachers', examiner-observers', and twin's self-reports. *Journal of Child Psychology and Psychiatry.*

Arseneault, L., Tremblay, R. E., Boulerice, B., & Saucier, J.-F. (2002). Obstetric complications and adolescent violent behaviors: Testing two developmental pathways. *Child Development, 73,* 496–508.

Arseneault, L., Tremblay, R. E., Boulerice, B., Seguin, J. R., & Saucier, J.-F. (2000). Minor physical anomalies and family adversity as risk factors for adolescent violent delinquency. *American Journal of Psychiatry, 157*, 917–923.

Brame, R., Bushway, S., & Paternoster, R. (1999). On the use of panel research designs and random effects models to investigate static and dynamic theories of criminal offending. *Criminology, 37*, 599–642.

Brezina, T. (2000). Delinquent problem-solving: An interpretive framework for criminological theory and research. *Journal of Research in Crime and Delinquency, 37*, 3–30.

Bukowski, W. M., Sippola, L. K., & Newcomb, A. F. (2000). Variations in patterns of attraction to same- and other-sex peers during early adolescence. *Developmental Psychology, 36*, 147–154.

Caspi, A., Lynam, D., Moffitt, T. E., & Silva, P. A. (1993). Unraveling girls' delinquency: Biological, dispositional, and contextual contributions to adolescent misbehavior. *Developmental Psychology, 29*, 19–30.

Caspi, A., & Moffitt, T. E. (1991). Individual differences are accentuated during periods of social change: The sample case of girls at puberty. *Journal of Personality and Social Psychology, 61*, 157–168.

Caspi, A., & Moffitt, T. E. (1995). The continuity of maladaptive behavior: From description to explanation in the study of antisocial behavior. In D. Cicchetti & D. Cohen (Eds.), *Developmental psychopathology* (Vol. 2, pp. 472–511). New York: Wiley.

Caspi, A., Moffitt, T. E., Silva, P. A., Stouthamer-Loeber, M., Schmutte, P., & Krueger, R. (1994). Are some people crime-prone?: Replications of the personality–crime relation across nation, gender, race, and method. *Criminology, 32*, 301–333.

Chung, I., Hill, L. D., Hawkins, J. D., Gilchrist, K. G., & Nagin, D. (2002). Childhood predictors of offense trajectories. *Journal of Research in Crime and Delinquency, 39*, 60–90.

Cote, S., Zoccolillo, M., Tremblay, R. E., Nagin, D., & Vitaro, F. (2001). Predicting girls' conduct disorder in adolescence from childhood trajectories of disruptive behaviors. *Journal of the American Academy of Child and Adolescent Psychiatry, 40*, 678–684.

Dean, C. W., Brame, R., & Piquero, A. R. (1996). Criminal propensities, discrete groups of offenders, and persistence in crime. *Criminology, 34*, 547–574.

Deater-Deckard, K., & Plomin, R. (1999). An adoption study of the etiology of teacher and parent reports of externalizing behavior problems in middle childhood. *Child Development, 70*, 144–154.

DiLalla, L. F., & Gottesman, I. I. (1989). Heterogeneity of causes for delinquency and criminality: Lifespan perspectives. *Development and Psychopathology, 1*, 339–349.

Dionne, G., Tremblay, R., Boivin, M., Laplante, D., & Pérusse, D. (2003). Physical aggression and expressive vocabulary in 19–month-old twins. *Developmental Psychology, 39*(2), 261–273.

Donnellan, M. B., Ge, X., & Wenk, E. (2000). Cognitive abilities in adolescence-limited and life-course-persistent criminal offenders. *Journal of Abnormal Psychology, 109*, 396–402.

Donnellan, M. B., Ge, X., & Wenk, E. (in press). Personality characteristics of juvenile offenders: Differences in the CPI by age at first arrest and frequency of offending. *Personality and Individual Differences.*

D'Unger, A. V., Land, K. C., McCall, P. L., & Nagin, D. S. (1998). How many latent classes of delinquent/criminal careers? *American Journal of Sociology, 103*, 1593–1630.

Earls, F. (1987). Sex differences in psychiatric disorders: Origins and developmental influences. *Psychiatric Developments, 1*, 1–23.

Edelbrock, C., Rende, R., Plomin, R., & Thompson, L. A. (1995). A twin study of competence and problem behavior in childhood and early adolescence. *Journal of Child Psychology and Psychiatry, 36*, 775–785.

Eley, T. C., Lichtenstein, P., & Moffitt, T. E. (in press). A longitudinal analysis of the etiology of aggressive and non-aggressive antisocial behaviour. *Development and Psychopathology.*

Eley, T. C., Lichtenstein, P., & Stevenson, J. (1999). Sex differences in the etiology of aggressive and non-aggressive antisocial behavior: Results from two twin studies. *Child Development*, 70, 155–168.

Eme, R. F. (1992). Selective female affliction in the developmental disorders of childhood: A literature review. *Journal of Clinical Child Psychology*, 21, 354–364.

Farrington, D. P. (1998). Predictors, causes, and correlates of male youth violence. *Crime and Justice: An Annual Review of Research*, 24, 421–476.

Farrington, D. P., Gallagher, B., Morley, L., St. Ledger, R. J., & West, D. (1988). Are there any successful men from criminogenic backgrounds? *Psychiatry*, 51, 116–130.

Fergusson, D. M., Horwood, L. J., & Nagin, D. S. (2000). Offending trajectories in a New Zealand birth cohort. *Criminology*, 38, 525–552.

Ge, X., Conger, R. D., Cadoret, R. J., Neiderhauser, J. M., Yates, W., Troughton, E., & Stewart, M. A. (1996). The developmental interface between nature and nurture: A mutual influence model of child antisocial behavior and parent behaviors. *Developmental Psychology*, 32, 574–589.

Ge, X., Donnellan, M. B., & Wenk, E. (2001). The development of persistent criminal offending in males. *Criminal Justice and Behavior*, 28, 731–755.

Gendreau, P., Little, T., & Goggin, C. (1996). A meta-analysis of the predictors of adult offender recidivism: What works! *Criminology*, 34, 575–607.

Henry, B., Caspi, A., Moffitt, T. E., & Silva, P. A. (1996). Temperamental and familial predictors of violent and non-violent criminal convictions: From age 3 to age 18. *Developmental Psychology*, 32, 614–623.

Howell, J. C., & Hawkins, J. D. (1998). Prevention of youth violence. *Crime and Justice: A Review of Research*, 24, 263–316.

Jacobson, K. C., Neale, M. C., Prescott, C. A., & Kendler, K. S. (2001, July). *Behavioural genetic confirmation of a life-course perspective on antisocial behavior*. Presentation at the annual meeting of the Behaviour Genetics Association, Cambridge, UK.

Jeglum-Bartusch, D., Lynam, D., Moffitt, T. E., & Silva, P. A. (1997). Is age important?: Testing general versus developmental theories of antisocial behavior. *Criminology*, 35, 13–47.

Kerr, M., & Stattin, H. (2000). What parents know, how they know it, and several forms of adolescent adjustment: Further support for reinterpretation of monitoring. *Developmental Psychology*, 36, 366–380.

Kjelsberg, E. (1999). Adolescent-limited versus life-course-persistent criminal behaviour in adolescent psychiatric inpatients. *European Child and Adolescent Psychiatry*, 8, 276–282.

Kratzer, L., & Hodgins, S. (1999). A typology of offenders: A test of Moffitt's theory among males and females from childhood to age 30. *Criminal Behaviour and Mental Health*, 9, 57–73.

Krohn, M. D., Thornberry, T. P., Rivera, C., & LeBlanc, M. (2001). Later delinquency careers of very young offenders. In R. Loeber & D. P. Farrington (Eds.), *Child delinquents* (pp. 67–94). Thousand Oaks, CA: Sage.

Lahey, B. B., Waldman, I. D., & McBurnett, K. (1999). The development of antisocial behavior: An integrative causal model. *Journal of Child Psychology and Psychiatry*, 40, 669–682.

Laub, J. H., & Sampson, R. J. (2001). Understanding desistence from crime. *Crime and Justice: An Annual Review of Research*, 28, 1–69.

Laucht, M. (2001). Antisoziales Verhalten im jugendalter: Entstehungsbedingungen und Verlaufsformen. *Zeitschrift fur Kinder-Jugendpsychiatry*, 29, 297–311.

Luthar, S. S., & McMahon, T. J. (1996). Peer reputation among inner-city adolescents: Structure and correlates. *Journal of Research on Adolescence*, 6, 581–603.

Lynam, D. R., Caspi, A., Moffitt, T. E., Wikström, P. O., Loeber, R., & Novak, S. P. (2000). The interaction between impulsivity and neighborhood context on offending: The effects of impulsivity are stronger in poorer neighborhoods. *Journal of Abnormal Psychology*, 109, 563–574.

Lynam, D., Moffitt, T. E., & Stouthamer-Loeber, M. (1993). Explaining the relation between IQ and delinquency: Class, race, test motivation, school failure, or self-control? *Journal of Abnormal Psychology*, 102, 187–196.

Lyons, M. J., True, W. R., Eisen, S. A., Goldberg, J., Meyer, J. M., Faraone, S. V., Eaves, L. J., & Tsuang, M. T. (1995). Differential heritability of adult and juvenile antisocial traits. *Archives of General Psychiatry*, *53*, 906–915.

Magnusson, D., af Klintberg, B., & Stattin, H. (1994). Juvenile and persistent offenders: Behavioral and physiological characteristics. In R. D. Kettelinus & M. Lamb (Eds.), *Adolescent problem behaviors* (pp. 81–91). Hillsdale, NJ: Erlbaum.

Maughan, B., Pickles, A., Rowe, R., Costello, E. J., & Angold, A. (2001). Developmental trajectories of aggressive and non-aggressive conduct problems. *Journal of Quantitative Criminology*, *16*, 199–222.

Mazerolle, P., Brame, R., Paternoster, R., Piquero, A., & Dean, C. (2000). Onset age, persistence, and offending versatility: Comparisons across gender. *Criminology*, *38*, 1143–1172.

McCall, R. B., & Carriger, M. S. (1993). A meta-analysis of infant habituation and recognition memory performance as predictors of later IQ. *Child Development*, *64*, 57–79.

Moffitt, T. E. (1990). Juvenile delinquency and attention-deficit disorder: Developmental trajectories from age three to fifteen. *Child Development*, *61*, 893–910.

Moffitt, T. E. (1993). "Life-course-persistent" and "adolescence-limited" antisocial behavior: A developmental taxonomy. *Psychological Review*, *100*, 674–701.

Moffitt, T. E. (1994). Natural histories of delinquency. In E. Weitekamp & H. J. Kerner (Eds.), *Cross-national longitudinal research on human development and criminal behavior* (pp. 3–61). Dordrecht, The Netherlands: Kluwer Academic Press.

Moffitt, T. E. (1997). Adolescence-limited and life-course-persistent offending: A complementary pair of developmental theories. In T. Thornberry (Ed.), *Advances in criminological theory: Developmental theories of crime and delinquency* (pp. 11–54). London: Transaction Press.

Moffitt, T. E., & Caspi, A. (2001). Childhood predictors differentiate life-course persistent and adolescence-limited pathways, among males and females. *Development and Psychopathology*, *13*, 355–375.

Moffitt, T. E., Caspi, A., Dickson, N., Silva, P. A., & Stanton, W. (1996). Childhood-onset versus adolescent-onset antisocial conduct in males: Natural history from age 3 to 18. *Development and Psychopathology*, *8*, 399–424.

Moffitt, T. E., Caspi, A., Harrington, H., & Milne, B. (2002). Males on the life-course persistent and adolescence-limited antisocial pathways: Follow-up at age 26. *Development and Psychopathology*, *14*, 179–206.

Moffitt, T. E., Caspi, A., Rutter, M., & Silva, P. A. (2001). *Sex differences in antisocial behaviour: Conduct disorder, delinquency, and violence in the Dunedin Longitudinal Study*. Cambridge, UK: Cambridge University Press.

Moffitt, T. E., Lynam, D., & Silva, P. A. (1994). Neuropsychological tests predict persistent male delinquency. *Criminology*, *32*, 101–124.

Nagin, D. S., Farrington, D. P., & Moffitt, T. E. (1995). Life-course trajectories of different types of offenders. *Criminology*, *33*, 111–139.

National Institute of Mental Health. (2000). *Child and adolescence violence research* (NIH Publication No. 00–4706). Bethesda, MD: National Institute of Health.

Neugebauer, R., Hoek, H. W., & Susser, E. (1999). Prenatal exposure to wartime famine and development of antisocial personality disorder in early adulthood. *Journal of the American Medical Association*, *282*, 455–462.

O'Connor, T. G., Deater-Deckard, K., Fulker, D., Rutter, M., & Plomin, R. (1998). Genotype–environment correlations in later childhood and early adolescence: Antisocial behavioral problems and coercive parenting. *Developmental Psychology*, *34*, 970–981.

Osgood, D. W. (1998). Interdisciplinary integration: Building criminology by stealing from our friends. *The Criminologist*, *23*, 1–4, 41.

Paternoster, R., & Brame, R. (1997). Multiple routes to delinquency?: A test of developmental and general theories of crime. *Criminology*, *35*, 49–84.

Patterson, G. R., DeGarmo, D. S., & Knutson, N. (2000). Hyperactive and antisocial behaviors:

Comorbid or two points in the same process? *Development and Psychopathology, 12*, 91–106.

Patterson, G. R., Forgatch, M. S., Yoerger, K. L., & Stoolmiller, M. (1998). Variables that initiate and maintain an early-onset trajectory for juvenile offending. *Development and Psychopathology, 10*, 531–548.

Patterson, G. R., & Yoerger, K. (1997). A developmental model for later-onset delinquency. In R. Deinstbeir & D. W. Osgood (Eds.), *Motivation and delinquency* (pp. 119–177). Lincoln: University of Nebraska Press.

Piquero, A. R. (2001). Testing Moffitt's neuropsychological variation hypothesis for the prediction of life-course persistent offending. *Psychology, Crime and Law, 7*, 193–216.

Piquero, A. R., & Brezina, T. (2001). Testing Moffitt's account of adolescence-limited delinquency. *Criminology, 39*, 353–370.

Piquero, A. R., & Buka, S. (2002). Linking juvenile and adult patterns of criminal activity in the Providence Cohort of the National Collaborative Perinatal Project. *Journal of Criminal Justice, 30*, 259–272.

Piquero, A. R., Moffitt, T. E., & Lawton, B. (in press). Race and crime: The contribution of individual, familial, and neighborhood level risk factors to life-course-persistent offending. In D. Hawkins & K. Kempf-Leonard (Eds.), *Race, crime, and the juvenile justice system*. Chicago: University of Chicago Press.

Raine, A., Brennan, P., & Mednick, S. A. (1994). Birth complications combined with early maternal rejection at age 1 year predispose to violent crime at age 18 years. *Archives of General Psychiatry, 51*, 984–988.

Raine, A., Brennan, P., & Mednick, S. A. (1997). Interaction between birth complications and early maternal rejection in predisposing individuals to adult violence: Specificity to serious, early-onset violence. *American Journal of Psychiatry, 154*, 1265–1271.

Raine, A., Brennan, P., Mednick, B., & Mednick, S. A. (1994). High rates of violence, crime, academic problems, and behavioral problems in males with both early neuromotor deficits and unstable family environments. *Archives of General Psychiatry, 53*, 544–549.

Raine, A., Yaralian, P. S., Reynolds, C., Venables, P. H., & Mednick, S. A. (2002). Spatial but not verbal cognitive deficits at age 3 years in persistently antisocial individuals. *Development and Psychopathology, 14*, 25–44.

Rhee, S. H., & Waldman, I. D. (2002). Genetic and environmental influences on antisocial behavior: A meta-analysis. *Psychological Bulletin, 128*, 490–529.

Robins, L. N. (1966). *Deviant children grown up*. Baltimore: Williams & Wilkins.

Roeder, K., Lynch, K. G., & Nagin, D. S. (1999). Modeling uncertainty in latent class membership: A case study in criminology. *Journal of the American Statistical Association, 94*, 766–776.

Rowe, D. C., Vazsonyi, A. T., & Flannery, D. J. (1994). No more than skin deep: Ethnic and racial similarity in developmental process. *Psychological Review, 101*, 396–413.

Ruchkin, V. V., Koposov, R. A., Vermeiren, R., & Schwab-Stone, M. (in press). Psychopathology and the age of onset of conduct problems in juvenile delinquents. *Journal of Clinical Psychiatry*.

Schmitz, S., Fulker, D. W., & Mrazek, D. A. (1995). Problem behavior in early and middle childhood: An initial behavior genetic analysis. *Journal of Child Psychology and Psychiatry, 36*, 1443–1458.

Scott, E. S., & Grisso, T. (1997). The evolution of adolescence: A developmental perspective on juvenile justice reform. *Journal of Criminal Law and Criminology, 88*, 137–189.

Shedler, J., & Block, J. (1990). Adolescent drug use and psychological health. *American Psychologist, 45*, 612–630.

Sigman, M., Cohen, S. E., & Beckwith, L. (1997). Why does infant attention predict adolescent intelligence? *Infant Behavior and Development, 20*, 133–140.

Silverthorn, P., & Frick, P. J. (1999). Developmental pathways to antisocial behavior: The delayed-onset pathway in girls. *Development and Psychopathology, 11*, 101–126.

Simons, R. L., Wu, C. I., Conger, R., & Lorenz, F. O. (1994). Two routes to delinquency: Differences between early and late starters in the impact of parenting and deviant peers. *Criminology, 32*, 247–275.

Stanger, C., Achenbach, T., & Verhulst, F. C. (1997). Accelerated longitudinal comparisons of aggressive versus delinquent syndromes. *Development and Psychopathology, 9*, 43–58.

Stattin, H., Romelsjo, A., & Stenbacka, M. (1997). Personal resources as modifiers of the risk for future criminality. *British Journal of Criminology, 37*, 198–223.

Taylor, J., Iacono, W. G., & McGue, M. (2000). Evidence for a genetic etiology for early-onset delinquency. *Journal of Abnormal Psychology, 109*, 634–643.

Tibbetts, S., & Piquero, A. (1999). The influence of gender, low birth weight and disadvantaged environment on predicting early onset of offending: A test of Moffitt's interactional hypothesis. *Criminology, 37*, 843–878.

U.S. Surgeon General. (2001). *Youth violence: A report of the surgeon general. http://www.surgeongeneral.gov/library/youthviolence/.*

Vaaranen, H. (2001). The blue-collar boys at leisure: An ethnography on cruising club boys' drinking, driving, and passing time in cars in Helsinki. *Mannsforsking, 1*, 48–57.

van den Oord, E. J. C. G., Verhulst, F. C., & Boomsma, D. I. (1996). A genetic study of maternal and paternal ratings of problem behaviors in 3–year-old twins. *Journal of Abnormal Psychology, 105*, 349–357.

van der Valk, J. C., Verhulst, F. C., Stroet, T. M., & Boomsma, D. I. (1998). Quantitive genetic analysis of internalising and externalising problems in a large sample of 3-year-old twins. *Twin Research, 1*, 25–33.

Vitaro, F., Tremblay, R. E., Kerr, M., Pagani, L., & Bukowski, W. M. (1997). Disruptiveness, friends' characteristics, and delinquency in early adolescence: A test of two competing models of development. *Child Development, 68*, 676–689.

White, H. R., Bates, M. E., & Buyske, S. (2001). Adolescence-limited versus persistent delinquency: Extending Moffitt's hypothesis into adulthood. *Journal of Abnormal Psychology, 110*, 600–609.

Woodward, L. J., Fergusson, D. M., & Horwood, L. J. (2002). Romantic relationships of young people with early and late onset antisocial behavior problems. *Journal of Abnormal Child Psychology, 30*, 231–243.

Zebrowitz, L. A., Andreoletti, C., Collins, M., Lee, S. H., & Blumenthal, J. (1998). Bright, bad, babyfaced boys: Appearance stereotypes do not always yield self-fulfilling prophecy effects. *Journal of Personality and Social Psychology, 75*, 1300–1320.

Zucker, R. A., Ellis, D. A., Fitzgerald, H. E., Bingham, C. R., & Sanford, K. (1996). Other evidence for at least two alcoholisms: II. Life-course variation in antisociality and heterogeneity of alcoholic outcome. *Development and Psychopathology, 8*, 831–848.

# 4

# A Developmental Propensity Model of the Origins of Conduct Problems during Childhood and Adolescence

BENJAMIN B. LAHEY
IRWIN D. WALDMAN

In this chapter, we present an overview of a causal model of the origins of conduct problems during childhood and adolescence. We use the term *conduct problems* to refer to behaviors that violate important behavioral norms or laws. In this sense, both juvenile crimes and DSM-IV symptoms of conduct disorder (CD) are conduct problems. The diagnosis of CD is viewed as the extreme end of the continuum of conduct problems, with the point of demarcation between CD and "normal behavior" reflecting a convention rather than a dichotomy in nature (Lahey et al., 1994). Thus, the present model is applicable to both CD and juvenile delinquency. The milder behavior problems that define DSM-IV oppositional defiant disorder (ODD) are not considered to be conduct problems in this chapter, but we discuss their association with conduct problems.

The dependent variable for the model is the youth's developmental trajectory of conduct problems. In the general terminology of longitudinal data analysis, trajectories are defined by the youth's *intercept* (i.e., essentially the level of conduct problems at the youngest age at which conduct problems are measured) and *slope* (i.e., increasing or decreasing trends over time). In this chapter, we focus on school-age children, from the age of school entry through age 17 years. We believe that it will be possible to extend the present model back in time, however, to encompass the earliest phases of the development of conduct problems.

In this chapter, we state hypotheses that are based on data, but we often go beyond current data. In all cases these hypotheses are advanced in the context of suggested studies that would expose them to risk of refutation. The present model should be considered to be preliminary, partly because key analyses of data from our recent studies from which the hypotheses were induced have not been through peer review.

## ONTOGENY OF CONDUCT PROBLEMS

A necessary first step in determining the causes of conduct problems is to describe their ontogeny. Several seminal papers (Farrington, 1991; Loeber, 1988; Moffitt, 1993; Patterson, Reid, & Dishion, 1992) suggest that there are multiple developmental pathways for conduct problems. Moffitt (1993) proposed a "developmental taxonomy" in which two groups of antisocial youth were distinguished based on their ages of onset and trajectories of conduct problems. She posited that these groups of antisocial youth differ enough to require different causal explanations. We believe that Moffitt is fundamentally correct in postulating that youth with the earliest and the latest ages of onset of conduct problems tend to be antisocial for different reasons, but our model differs from her model in two ways. First, we believe that differences in conduct problems based on their age of onset fall along a continuum of ages of onset, rather than reflecting a true developmental taxonomy. Second, we posit that the same set of causal factors influence conduct problems that emerge at all ages, but the strength and pattern of these causal influences vary along the continuum of the age of onset of conduct problems.

### Individual Differences in the Ontogeny of Conduct Problems

In the general population, minor aggression (mostly bullying and fighting), lying, and hurting animals are common at school entry, but their prevalence declines with increasing age through adolescence. We refer to these as *developmentally early* conduct problems. In contrast, the prevalence of many nonaggressive conduct problems (e.g., stealing, running away from home, truancy, breaking and entering) and serious forms of aggression (e.g., mugging, use of a weapon, and forced sex) increases from middle childhood through adolescence. We term these *developmentally late* conduct problems.

At school entry, there is a broad range of involvement in developmentally early conduct problems (intercepts), with a small group of children already exhibiting high levels that impair the child's social and academic functioning. Another small group of children exhibits no conduct problems at school entry, whereas most children fall between these extremes of this continuum. Over the course of development, youth change from their initial level of conduct problems (intercepts) in every possible direction (slopes).

In general, however, trajectories of conduct problems from school entry through late adolescence are predicted reasonably well by individual differences in the level of developmentally early conduct problems at school entry (Lahey & Loeber, 1994). Children with the highest initial levels of developmentally early conduct problems at school entry are more likely to show persistent or worsening problems over time and are less likely to desist (Brame, Nagin, & Tremblay, 2001; Nagin & Tremblay, 1999). Similarly, children with higher levels of developmentally early conduct problems at school entry both begin to engage in developmentally late conduct problems at younger ages and show steeper slopes, reaching higher levels of developmentally late conduct problems during adolescence than children with lower levels of conduct problems at school entry (Brame et al., 2001; Sampson & Laub, 1992). Children who are high in developmentally early conduct problems at school entry generally do not advance to serious forms of violence during adolescence and adulthood unless they exhibit precocious development of developmentally late conduct problems during childhood or early adolescence (Haemaelaeinen & Pulkkinen, 1996). As a result, adolescents who engage in high levels of serious adolescent delinquency rarely "come out of nowhere." Few very well-behaved young children engage in substantial levels of delinquency during adolescence, and when they do, they mostly (but not exclusively) engage in nonaggressive behaviors (e.g., theft and truancy) and usually do not engage in violent behaviors (Brame et al., 2001).

## Meaning of Age of Onset

Tremblay (Tremblay et al., 1996, 1999; Tremblay, 2000) convincingly argued for a reconceptualization of the term *age of onset*. He used population-based data to demonstrate that many toddlers hit, kick, intentionally break things, take other children's toys, state untruths, and resist the authority of adults from the time they can walk and talk (Tremblay et al., 1999). Although not all toddlers engage in such behaviors—for example, only about 40% of Canadian 24-month-olds "sometimes" or "often" hit, kick, or bite (Tremblay et al., 1996)—they are certainly common enough to be viewed as normative. Over the course of development, the prevalence of these behaviors declines greatly, suggesting to Tremblay that most children "unlearn" them as a result of socialization.

Although we believe that Tremblay's (2000) view is essentially correct, it can be reconciled with traditional approaches of the age of onset of conduct problems. Typically, age of onset is measured by asking respondents (usually parents) to report the age at which a specific conduct problem first occurred. We believe that respondents answer such questions for developmentally early behaviors by reporting the age at which they first viewed the behavior as atypical. A prevalent behavior (e.g., taking toys from others during play) might come to be viewed as atypical either because the immature behavior changed through maturation and social learning into a more serious behavior (e.g., taking a toy when the owner was not looking) or because a behavior (e.g., hitting) persisted unchanged to an age when it was no longer viewed as normative. Moreover, not all conduct problems fit the ontogenic pattern described by Tremblay. For developmentally late behaviors, the report of age of onset actually reflects the first occurrence of the behavior (e.g., breaking and entering). Thus, we believe the concept of age of onset has meaning if it is viewed from the perspective of how the informant answers such questions.

## Improvement in Childhood Conduct Problems

Nearly half of all children who engage in high levels of conduct problems show considerable improvement by early adolescence (Fergusson, Lynskey, & Horwood, 1996; Moffitt, Caspi, Dickson, Silva, & Stanton, 1996; Nagin & Tremblay, 1999). The dominance of developmental models since Moffitt's (1993) influential paper, which focuses on the onset of conduct problems, may have unintentionally contributed to a neglect of children whose behavior improves over time. A number of studies suggest that children with early conduct problems who improve over time have less extreme levels of conduct problems in childhood, have higher intelligence scores, have fewer delinquent friends, come from families with higher socioeconomic status (SES), have mothers who did not give birth as teenagers, and have parents who are less antisocial and have fewer mental health problems (Fergusson et al., 1996; Lahey, Loeber, Burke, & Rathouz, 2002; Nagin & Tremblay, 2001). As we will see, the inverse of these factors is also associated with the onset of conduct problems, suggesting that risks for initiating and persisting in conduct problems often overlap.

## CHILD CHARACTERISTICS THAT INCREASE THE LIKELIHOOD OF CONDUCT PROBLEMS

Gottfredson and Hirschi (1990) proposed that variations in antisocial behavior can be explained by individual differences in *antisocial propensity*. Although situational influences on conduct problems can be strong, a large body of evidence suggests that the origins of conduct problems cannot be understood without taking individual differences in persons into account. Antisocial propensity is inferred from individual differences in conduct problems, but to avoid circularity it must be defined and measured in independent terms. Thus, Gottfredson and Hirschi (1990) and Farrington (1991, 1995) have provided similar lists of hypothesized components of individual differences in antisocial propensity, including lower intelligence and higher levels of daring, impulsivity, activity level, and physical strength. The present model builds on this conceptual foundation.

In our model, central roles are ascribed both to characteristics of children associated with their propensity to exhibit conduct problems and to transactions with the environment that increase or decrease the likelihood that such antisocial propensity will be manifested in the youth's behavior. Thus, we distinguish two questions about the causes of conduct problems: (1) what are the causes of the child characteristics that constitute antisocial propensity, and (2) what are the causal factors that determine which children will make the developmental transition from antisocial *propensity* to antisocial *behavior*?

We posit that multiple child factors contribute to antisocial propensity. These factors influence conduct problems that emerge at all ages, from early childhood through late adolescence, but their influence varies with the age of onset of conduct problems. This is primarily because the strength of the various causal influences on conduct problems influences the age of onset of conduct problems. For youth with earlier ages of onsets of conduct problems, we posit that atypical temperament and low cognitive ability play significant roles, working through transactions with the social environment to increase the level of conduct problems over time. The age of onset of conduct problems increases as the components of antisocial propensity (cognitive abilities and temperament) play progressively less important roles, with peer influence and other social factors playing more important roles. Thus, following the lead of Moffitt (1993), we posit differences in causal influences on earlier and later onset conduct problems, but we view these as reflecting a continuum of differences in age of onset. In the remainder of this section, we present specific hypotheses about the nature of these predisposing child characteristics.

## Three Hypothesized Dimensions of Temperament Relevant to Conduct Problems

Like others, we use the term *temperament* to refer to substantially heritable and relatively persistent individual differences in global aspects of socioemotional responding that emerge early in childhood and constitute the foundation for many personality traits later in life (Buss & Plomin, 1975, 1984; Caspi, 1998). Because we seek to explain the origins of psychopathology partly in terms of individual differences in temperament, it is essential to distinguish between temperament and psychopathology. We recognize, however, that the conceptual boundary between temperament and psychopathology is fuzzy. In both cases, they are latent constructs inferred from the child's behavior. We use the term *temperament* to refer to global aspects of socioemotional behavior and the term *psychopathology* to refer to more specific behaviors with serious consequences for the youth's adaptive functioning, but this distinction is not always clear-cut. Unlike most temperament and personality researchers, however, we have taken care to avoid overlap in the items that define our hypothesized dimensions of temperament and psychopathology. For example, although it may make sense for models of personality to include terms like "anxious," "aggressive," and "depressed" in the scales of the trait of negative emotionality, such items cannot be included in studies relating temperament to psychopathology as it would raise the possibility that any correlation between negative emotionality and psychopathology is based only on these overlapping items.

The three dimensions of temperament described next are based on two steps in our effort to define the aspects of temperament that are most relevant to the development of conduct problems. First, we conducted a review of the existing literature on early temperament-like child characteristics associated with increased risk for conduct problems. That is, rather than attempting to construct a new general model of temperament, our purpose is to identify aspects of temperament that may function as developmental antecedents to conduct problems. Our first description of the aspects of temperament that are relevant to conduct problems (Lahey, Waldman, & McBurnett, 1999) included the construct of *oppositional temperament*, which was defined by the symptoms of oppositional defiant disorder. In this version, we have replaced the construct of oppositional temperament with the broader construct of "negative emotionality."

After compiling a broad list of temperamental attributes that had been found to be correlated with child conduct problems, our second step was to create an investigational scale composed of these items. A parent rating scale was created that is suitable for children ages 4–17 years, consisting of items thought to tap the three hypothesized dimensions of socioemotional responding. A parallel form of the same scale was created for youth self-reports by 9- to 17-year-olds. We conducted a study of a population-based sample enriched with clinic attendees of 1,382 children and adolescents ranging in age from 4 to 17. Exploratory factor analyses and construct validity analyses of part of that sample have been reported (Lahey, Applegate, & Waldman, 2001), but have not yet been published in peer-review journals. This exploratory factor analysis yielded three factors that were consistent with the three aspects of temperament described below. Analyses of these data supported the change from our earlier model (Lahey, Waldman, et al., 1999), as oppositional defiant behavior was found to be correlated with all three temperament dimension in the present model and not just with negative emotionality (Lahey et al., 2001). We are in the process of conducting additional studies to test the hypothesis that the three dimensions of temperament described next are independent from one another and are concurrently and predictively related to conduct problems.

*Negative Emotionality*

Most trait models of personality include a dimension defined by experiencing negative emotions frequently, intensely, and with little provocation (see reviews by Bouchard & Loehlin, 2001; Zuckerman, Kuhlman, Joireman, Teta, & Kraft, 1993). This dimension is often referred to as *neuroticism* (Digman & Inouye, 1986; Eysenck, 1947; Goldberg, 1993; McCrae & Costa, 1987), but we will use the term *negative emotionality* (Watson, Clark, & Tellegen, 1988). Among adults, negative emotionality is positively correlated with a wide range of mental health problems, including antisocial behavior (Addad & Leslau, 1990; Berman & Paisey, 1984; Eysenck & Eysenck, 1970, 1977; Eysenck & McGurk, 1980; Gershuny & Sher, 1998; Goma-I.-Freixnet, 1995; Krueger, 1999; Moffitt, Caspi, Rutter, & Silva, 2001; Rahman, 1992; Roberts, & Kendler, 1999).

The existing literature on the relation between negative emotionality and child conduct problems is less consistent, however. A number of studies have found significant concurrent or prospective associations of negative emotionality with child conduct problems (Eisenberg et al., 1996; Gabrys, 1983; Gjone & Stevenson, 1997; Rowe & Flannery, 1994). On the other hand, a number of studies have not found negative emotionality to be significantly correlated with delinquent behavior/conduct problems (Fonseca & Yule, 1995; Furnham & Thompson, 1991; Heaven, 1996; John, Caspi, Robins, Moffitt, & Stouthamer-Loeber, 1994; Powell & Stewart, 1983; Rushton & Chrisjohn, 1981; Shapland & Rushton, 1975; Tranah, Harnett, & Yule, 1998). This lack of consistency may reflect differences in the operationalization of negative emotionality across studies or may indicate that the relation between negative emotionality and child conduct problems is complex.

*Daring*

Farrington and West (1993) found that children rated by parents as "daring" in childhood were considerably more likely to be chronic criminal offenders during adolescence and adulthood. Farrington and West's (1993) construct of *daring* may be related to some aspects of sensation seeking (Zuckerman, 1996) and novelty seeking (Cloninger, 1987), both of which have been found to be positively correlated with conduct problems in diverse samples (Arnett, 1996; Daderman, 1999; Daderman, Wirsen, & Hallman, 2001; Goma-I.-Freixnet, 1995; Greene, Krcmar, Walters, Rubin, & Hale, 2000; Luengo, Otero, Carrillo-de-la-Pena, & Miron, 1994; Newcomb & McGee, 1991; Schmeck & Poustka, 2001; Simo & Perez, 1991; Wasson, 1980). Thus, some items used to characterize our dimension of daring were based on our earlier studies of sensation seeking in children (Russo et al., 1993).

Farrington and West's (1993) construct of daring also may be inversely related to Kagan's construct of *behavioral inhibition*. Kagan and colleagues (Garcia-Coll, Kagan, & Reznick, 1987; Kagan, Reznick, & Snidman, 1988; Kagan, Reznick, Snidman, Gibbons, & Johnson, 1988) used laboratory observations to classify toddlers as "behaviorally inhibited" or "disinhibited." Young children in Kagan et al.'s studies were exposed to a variety of novel situations, including an unfamiliar adult and a lighted robot that emerged from behind a curtain and spoke to the children. Observers monitored the children's fretfulness, latency to approach persons and objects, and latency to vocalize. At the extremes of the distribution of inhibition scores, there was significant stability over time. A number of studies show that toddlers classified as disinhibited readily approached unfamiliar stimuli and were quick to vocalize. As preschoolers, disinhibited children spontaneously vocalized and readily followed the examiner's requests to "misbehave": to scribble in a book, spill juice on the floor, and throw a ball at the examiner's face. Highly inhibited children behaved in much the opposite manner. Most importantly, from our perspective, disinhibition was later found to predict conduct problems during later childhood and early adolescence in several samples (Biederman et al., 2001; Hirshfeld et al., 1992; Hirshfeld-Becker et al., 2002; Kerr, Tremblay, Pagani-Kurtz, & Vitaro, 1997; Raine, Reynolds, Venables, Mednick, & Farrington, 1998; Schwartz, Snidman, & Kagan, 1996).

Cloninger (1987) also identified a dimension of temperament, termed *harm avoidance*, which may also describe some aspects of the inverse pole of daring. Persons high in harm avoidance are cautious, apprehensive, and inhibited in the face of novel or dangerous situations. Two longitudinal population-based studies have found that children with higher harm avoidance scores were less likely to engage in significant antisocial behavior in adolescence and young adulthood (Sigvardsson, Bohman, & Cloninger, 1987; Tremblay, Pihl, Vitaro, & Dobkin, 1994).

## Prosociality

From preschool through adolescence, youth who engage in more conduct problems show less sympathy and concern for others (Cohen & Strayer, 1996; Eisenberg, Fabes, & Murphy, 1996; Frick, O'Brien, Wootton, & McBurnett, 1994; Hastings, Zahn-Waxler, Robinson, Usher, & Bridges, 2000; Hughes, White, Sharpen, & Dunn, 2000; Luengo et al., 1994; Miller & Eisenberg, 1988). Goodman (2001) developed a prosocial behavior scale that is composed of items that are seemingly related to sympathy, including sharing, helping, kindness, consideration for others, and volunteering. In a representative British sample of 10,438 children and adolescents ranging in age from 5 to 15 (Meltzer, Gatward, Goodman, & Ford, 2000), the correlation between this prosocial behavior scale and conduct problems (lying, fighting, stealing, disobedience, temper tantrums) was −.42 for parent reports, −.57 for teacher reports, and −.31 for youth self-reports (R. Goodman, personal communication, 2001). Even more impressively, Haemaelaeinen and Pulkkinen (1996) obtained peer ratings on a similar prosocial behavior scale at age 8 years and found that it predicted criminal offenses by age 27 years after controlling for early conduct problems and school failure.

Based on these findings, and the theoretical foundations provided by Eisenberg and Mussen (1991), Hoffman (1982), and Zahn-Waxler, Robinson, and Emde (1992), we propose the construct of *prosociality* to refer to a dimension of temperament characterized by dispositional sympathy for others. Because our exploratory factor analysis suggested that guilt over misdeeds and respect for rules were also part of this factor, we suggest that these are linked to the prosociality dimension. This is important, as many studies have found that children who engage in high levels of conduct problems exhibit little guilt over their misdeeds (e.g., Frick et al., 1994; Loeber, Farrington, Stouthamer-Loeber, & Van Kammen, 1998).

### Comment on Extraversion

Many structural theories of personality specify a broad dimension of *extraversion* that is characterized by positive emotionality, high energy, and sociability (Digman & Inouye, 1986; Eysenck, 1947; Goldberg, 1993; McCrae & Costa, 1987). In their meta-analysis, Miller and Lynam (2001) found that the correlation of antisocial behavior with extraversion is usually positive, but is sometimes negative. We did not specify a dimension of temperament that corresponds to extraversion in the present model, but will explore it in future studies.

### Relation to Existing Structural Models of Personality and Temperament

It is important to consider the possible relations of our three hypothesized dimensions of temperament to the major models of personality and temperament. The three-factor and five-models models of personality (Costa & McCrae, 1995; Eysenck, 1947; Goldberg & Rosolack, 1994) and widely used child temperament scales (Buss & Plomin, 1975, 1984; Presley & Martin, 1994; Rothbart, Ahadi, Hershey, & Fisher, 2001) all identify a dimension of negative emotionality with content similar to our construct. Thus, it seems likely that our dimension of negative emotionality is similar to the corresponding dimension in other personality and temperament models.

We believe that our dimensions of daring and prosociality will ultimately be found to be related to Eysenck's (1947) broad construct of psychoticism and to the five-factor dimensions of concientiousness and agreeableness (Costa & McCrae, 1995; Digman & Inouye, 1986; John et al., 1994). Of the three dimensions in Eysenck's model, psychoticism is most strongly and consistently associated with antisocial behavior, particularly with physical aggression (Berman & Paisey, 1984; Goma-I.-Freixnet, 1995; Miller & Lynam, 2001). Similarly, a number of studies of adult ratings of children and adolescents have found that the five-factor dimensions of agreeableness and conscientiousness are inversely correlated with self-reports of delinquent behavior and adult ratings of behavior problems and school adjustment (e.g., Digman & Inouye, 1986; Graziano, 1994; John et al., 1994). This suggests that psychoticism, agreeableness, and conscientiousness are pertinent to our goal of identifying the dimensions of temperament that are most related to conduct problems. How are these constructs related to our hypothesized dimensions of temperament?

The items in Eysenck's dimension of *psychoticism* refer to the lack of emotional closeness, empathy, and conventional behavior that is characteristic of individuals who exhibit psychosis. Costa and McCrae (1995) have argued that agreeableness and conscientiousness reflect distinct dimensions that are conflated in Eysenck's dimension of psychoticism. Indeed, many studies have shown that psychoticism is inversely correlated at substantial levels with both agreeableness and conscientiousness in the five-factor model of personality (e.g., Costa & McCrae, 1995; Goldberg & Rosolack, 1994). In discussing the inverse correlation of psychoticism with antisocial behavior, Costa and McCrae (1995) have hypothesized that agreeableness and conscientiousness are each inversely related to antisocial behavior for different reasons: "Agreeable people tend to be courteous and law abiding because they are mindful of the rights and feelings of others, and because they trust that laws and customs are designed for the common good. Conscientious people also tend to be polite and law abiding, not necessarily because they are prosocial in disposition, but because their conduct is guided by rules" (p. 316).

Thus, it is important to consider the possible relations between the current model and the five-factor dimensions of agreeableness and conscientiousness. Graziano and Eisenberg (1997) suggested that the five-factor model construct of agreeableness incorporates the key elements of Eisenberg and Mussen's (1991) construct of dispositional sympathy, which includes many of the elements of our dimension of prosociality. Furthermore, the items used to operationalize the five-factor dimension of agreeableness (e.g., sympathetic, generous, kind, cooperative, and trusting) suggest that agreeableness is similar to our prosociality dimension in content. Thus, it is possible that our dimension of prosociality incorporates many central elements of the five-factor dimension of agreeableness.

In contrast, the item content of the conscientiousness dimension in the

NEO (Costa & McCrae, 1987), which is the personality scale that was developed to measure five-factor model traits in adults, does not overlap with our hypothesized dimension of daring. It is interesting, however, that when the authors of the NEO conducted an exploratory factor analysis of a scale developed to measure Eysenck's three-factor model, they extracted five factors that they interpreted as corresponding to their five-factor model (Costa & McCrae, 1995). Because the Eysenck scale used a different set of items, the five factors that Costa and McCrae extracted had different item content than the NEO scales. The scale that Costa and McCrae identified as conscientiousness in this study was composed of the items of risk taking, impulsive, sensation seeking, and irresponsible. The first three of these items appear to be similar to our dimension of daring. Thus, it is possible that our dimension of daring bears some empirical relation to the five-factor dimension of conscientiousness, even if the item content of this dimension in the NEO scale is different.

## Temperament Profiles and Antisocial Propensity

Each of the three hypothesized dimensions of temperament in our model is believed to index a separate aspect of propensity to antisocial behavior. It is not yet clear if they contribute to the likelihood of conduct problems interactively, but the risk for antisocial behavior can only be assessed comprehensively by taking all three dimensions into account. Specifically, we hypothesize that children who are high in negative emotionality, low in prosociality, and high in daring will have the greatest propensity to conduct problems. In contrast, youth with the "antitype" of this high-risk profile (i.e., youth who are low in negative emotionality, high in prosociality, and low in daring) will be very unlikely to engage in conduct problems at any time during childhood or adolescence. We hypothesize that this low-risk antisocial propensity profile *protects* such youth from social pressures to engage in antisocial behavior throughout childhood and adolescence.

Our hypothesis that conduct problems are related to a profile of temperaments is not original; only the details are new. Thirty years ago, Eysenck (1964, 1996) hypothesized that individuals who are high in the dimensions of neuroticism, psychoticism, and extraversion are more likely to commit crimes. Similarly, using Cloninger's (1987) model of personality, Tremblay et al. (1994) demonstrated the importance of temperament profiles by showing that children rated as being high in novelty seeking, low in harm avoidance, and low in reward dependence exhibited greater conduct problems during early adolescence than youth with any other temperament profile. In addition, Caspi et al. (1994), Krueger et al. (1994), and Moffitt and colleagues (Moffit et al., 1996; Moffit, Caspi, Harrington, & Milne, 2002) administered Tellegen's (1982) personality questionnaire to a longitudinal sample during adolescence and found the profile of higher negative emotionality and lower "constraint" to be associated with greater antisocial behavior in adolescence and adulthood. Tellegen's construct of constraint appears to reflect both higher prosociality and lower daring in the present model (both of which we view as "constraining" the expression of negative emotionality in conduct problems). Thus, because our model is quite similar to earlier trait theories, any value of the present model must derive from the details of its hypotheses. In particular, the present model posits somewhat different dimensions of temperament that are operationalized using measures that do not overlap with psychopathology, includes cognitive-verbal deficits ignored in most temperament/personality models, places antisocial propensity in developmental context, integrates the temperament model with a social learning model, and uses the concepts of contemporary behavior genetics to frame our hypotheses regarding both environmental and genetic influences.

A number of papers have addressed the relation between child temperament/personality and conduct problems by defining dichotomous types of personality instead of dimensions. In several samples of children and adolescents across countries, Block's (1961) personality Q-sort was used to empirically induce three personality types in a sample of adolescent males (Asendorpf, Borkenau, Ostendorf, & Van Aken, 2001; Asendorpf & van Aken, 1999; Hart, Hofmann, Edelstein, & Keller, 1997; Robins, Johns, Caspi, Moffitt, & Stouthamer-Loeber, 1996). Youth were classified as "resilient," "overcontrolled," or "undercontrolled," with the latter having characteristics similar to our high-risk temperament profile and exhibiting substantially more conduct problems than other personality types in all studies. These studies are potentially important in describing a group of youth who are at very high risk for conduct problems. Unfortunately, Block's Q-sort includes many items that refer to symptoms of externalizing and internalizing psychopathology, raising concerns that the correlation with conduct problems is based partly or wholly on overlapping items in the measure of personality and conduct problems.

Although we loosely speak of our high-risk temperament profile as referring to a group of youth in this chapter, we are not hypothesizing that they constitute a taxonomic type like the "undercontrolled type." Rather, we believe that variation along all three continuous dimensions of temperament is important in the prediction of conduct problems. This means two things: First, we hypothesize that youth with deviant scores on only one or two of the dimensions of temperament will be at increased risk for later conduct problems (i.e., increased risk is not limited to youth who exhibit all elements of the "profile"). Second, among youth who exhibit the high-risk profile, we hypothesize that youth whose scores on the three temperament dimensions deviate more from the norm will be at greater risk for conduct problems.

*Development of Temperament*

We believe that the three dimensions of temperament described in the present chapter can be measured reliably beginning in preschool, and perhaps earlier. For example, observational measures of prosociality and negative emotionality used with 4-year-olds (e.g., Hughes et al., 2000) and observational measures of behavioral disinhibition (which we refer to as "daring") used with toddlers (Kagan et al., 1988) have been found to be related to conduct problems. Additional work is needed to determine the earliest ages at which each dimension of temperament can be measured and how these dimensions change over the course of development. For example, are there individual differences in the behavior of 1-year-olds that reliably predict prosociality later in life?

A chapter that addresses the role of temperament in the origins of conduct problems cannot fail to address the construct of "difficult temperament." There is evidence that children who are rated as having difficult temperament during infancy and toddlerhood are at increased risk for stable, aggressive conduct problems (Kingston & Prior, 1995; Olson, Bates, Sandy, & Lanthier, 2000; Sanson & Prior, 1999). The empirical relationship between difficult temperament in the first year of life and the present model, if any, remains to be described. We hypothesize, however, that ratings of infant difficultness will predict the high-risk profile of temperament. That is, we predict that infants rated as difficult will tend to be high in negative emotionality, low in prosociality, and high in daring during later childhood. If this hypothesis is supported, it would link two literatures regarding the developmental antecedents of conduct problems.

## Cognitive Abilities and Antisocial Propensity

In addition to the three dimensions of temperament, we hypothesize that lower cognitive ability and slow language development increase risk for conduct problems. Many studies suggest that cognitive ability scores, particularly verbal abilities, are inversely related to individual differences in conduct problems (Elkins, Iacono, Doyle, & McGue, 1997; Ge, Donnellan, & Wenk, 2000; Kratzer & Hodgins, 1999; Lynam, Moffitt, & Stouthamer-Loeber, 1993; Moffitt & Silva, 1988; Stattin & Klackenberg-Larsson, 1993). This correlation does not appear to be explainable in terms of differences in SES, greater ability of more intelligent youth to avoid detection of their antisocial behaviors, or differences in test motivation (Lynam et al., 1993; Moffitt & Silva, 1988). The specific cognitive deficits associated with conduct problems have been referred to variously using the partially overlapping terms of "intelligence," "neuropsychological dysfunction," and "executive functioning." At this time it is not yet clear if one construct is more defensible than others. Emerging evidence suggests that a cluster of executive function and language abilities is associated with early-onset conduct problems, even controlling for general intelligence (Giancola, Martin, Tarter, Pelham, & Moss, 1996; Seguin, Boulerice, Harden, Tremblay, & Pihl, 1999), but further research is needed on this important topic.

It is important to note that lower verbal intelligence is correlated with slower language development in early childhood (Sparks, Ganschow, & Thomas, 1996). An association between early deficits in language development and conduct problems is well documented by both cross-sectional and prospective studies of children from the general population (Stattin & Klackenberg-Larsson, 1993) and children with language disorders and other verbal deficits (Baker & Cantwell, 1987; Beitchman et al., 2001; Cohen et al., 1998; Dery, Toupin, Pauze, Mercier, & Fortin, 1999; Pennington & Ozonoff, 1996).

It should be noted that although we have preliminary evidence that the three dimensions of temperament are essentially orthogonal (only weakly intercorrelated), it is not yet clear that cognitive-linguistic deficits are fully independent of the three dimensions of temperament. Indeed, there are two reasons for thinking that intelligence and temperament may not be orthogonal. First, in three studies, youth classified as "undercontrolled," which shares many characteristics with our high-risk temperament profile, had lower intelligence scores, on average (Asendorpf et al., 2001; Hart et al., 1997; Robins et al., 1996), suggesting that our temperament dimensions may also be linked to lower intelligence. Second, Nigg and Huang-Pollock (Chapter 8, in this volume) and Blair (2002) in his developmental neurobiological model both suggest that cognitive-linguistic abilities and negative emotionality are causally intertwined. As further evidence is gathered, therefore, it may well be necessary to modify our model to include causal links between cognitive-linguistic ability and one or more of the dimensions of temperament.

## GENETIC AND ENVIRONMENTAL INFLUENCES

We first review current findings on genetic and environmental influences on conduct problems and the temperamental and cognitive elements of antisocial predisposition. Then we propose specific hypotheses regarding the mechanisms of these influences. As we detail later in this chapter, we examine genetic influences in the context of a social learning model of the origins of conduct problems. We believe that the critically important role of social learning in the origins of conduct problems can only be fully understood when taking the complex interplay of genetic and environmental influences into account.

## Genetic and Environmental Influences on the Dimensions of Antisocial Propensity

There is strong and consistent evidence that Eysenck's dimensions of neuroticism, extraversion, and psychoticism have substantial genetic influences and significant environmental influences (Eysenck, 1990; Lake, Eaves, Maes, Heath, & Martin, 2000; Macaskill, Hopper, White, & Hill, 1994; Pedersen, Plomin, McClearn, & Friberg, 1988). Similarly, studies using the construct of negative emotionality have found evidence of substantial heritability during adulthood (McGue, Bacon, & Lykken, 1993; Tellegen et al., 1988). Studies of adults' empathic concern about the welfare of others have similarly found substantial heritability (Matthews, Batson, Horn, & Rosenman, 1981; Rushton, Fulker, Neale, Nias, & Eysenck, 1986).

Furthermore, negative emotionality is substantially heritable in toddlers, school-age children, and adolescents (Cyphers, Phillips, Fulker, & Mrazek, 1990; Emde et al., 1992; Gjone & Stevenson, 1997; Goldsmith, Buss, & Lemery, 1997; Phillips & Matheny, 1997; Saudino, Plomin, & DeFries, 1996). Similarly, twin studies of infants, children, and adults consistently suggest that empathy/prosocial behavior is moderately heritable (Davis, Luce, & Kraus, 1994; Emde et al., 1992; Rushton et al., 1986; Zahn-Waxler et al., 1992). Behavioral disinhibition and extraversion are also substantially heritable in toddlers and children (Cyphers et al., 1990; DiLalla, Kagan, & Reznick, 1994; Emde et al., 1992; Goldsmith et al., 1997; Phillips & Matheny, 1997; Robinson, Kagan, Reznick, & Corley, 1992).

There are, of course, also significant environmental influences on each of the three dimensions of temperament. The nature of these environmental influences is largely unknown, but several theorists have hypothesized that empathy, for example, can be influenced through socializing interactions with parents (Eisenberg, Fabes, & Murphy, 1996; Eisenberg & Mussen, 1991; Grusec, 1991). If the present model is correct in positing that temperament plays an important role in the origins of conduct problems, then understanding environmental influences on temperament in enough detail to develop preventive interventions must be a high priority. Keenan and Shaw (Chapter 6, this volume) provide an important perspective on this key issue. Genetic influences on cognitive ability and the development of language skills are also well documented (Plomin & Petrill, 1997), even during the toddler years (Eley, Dale, & Bishop, 2001; Emde et al., 1992; Petrill et al., 1997).

## Genetic and Environmental Influences on Conduct Problems

There is abundant evidence from twin and adoption studies that child and adolescent conduct problems are influenced by both genetic and environmental factors (Deater-Deckard & Plomin, 1999; Edelbrock, Rende, Plomin, & Thompson, 1995; Eley, Lichtenstein, & Stevenson, 1999; Ge et al., 1996; Gjone & Stevenson, 1997; Mason & Frick, 1994; Meyer et al., 2000; Miles & Carey, 1997; O'Connor, Neiderhiser, Reiss, Hetherington, & Plomin, 1998; Rhee & Waldman, 2002; Rodgers, Muster, & Rowe, 2001; Rowe, 1983; Rowe, Almeida, & Jacobson, 1999; Rutter, 1997; Rutter et al., 1997; Schmitz, Fulker, & Mrazek, 1995; van den Oord, Boomsma, & Verhulst, 1994). These include both genetic influences on the onset of conduct problems and on their persistence over time (Robinson et al., 1992; Saudino et al., 1996). Later in this chapter, we present specific hypotheses regarding the mechanisms of genetic influences on conduct problems.

## CONDUCT PROBLEMS AND THEIR CO-OCCURRENCE WITH OTHER PROBLEMS

Youth with childhood conduct problems are more likely to meet diagnostic criteria for attention-deficit/hyperactivity disorder (ADHD) and ODD during childhood than youth with later ages of onset of conduct problems (Hinshaw, Lahey, & Hart, 1993; Lahey et al., 1998; Loeber, Green, Keenan, & Lahey, 1995; Moffitt, 1990; Moffitt et al., 1996). There is also increasing evidence that children with early-onset conduct problems and co-occurring ADHD and ODD are more likely to exhibit aggression, to show persistent or worsening conduct problems over time, and to exhibit psychopathic characteristics later in life (Henry, Caspi, Moffitt, & Silva, 1996; Lynam, 1998).

We hypothesize that early-onset conduct problems, ADHD, and ODD often co-occur because they reflect essentially the *same* underlying temperamental and cognitive propensities. That is, the high-risk profile of temperament and cognitive deficits is not specifically associated with conduct problems, but is a risk profile for all disruptive behavior disorders. Why, then, do many children exhibit only one or two of these three disorders? We hypothesize two reasons:

1. Differences in the child's transactions with the social environment will determine which children will exhibit which combination of ADHD, ODD, and CD behaviors. We expand on this key hypothesis later in the chapter.

2. We also expect variations in the *degree* of variation in each dimension of propensity to be a factor in determining the pattern of disruptive behaviors that each child exhibits. Most children who exhibit only ADHD or only ODD are hypothesized to have only moderately atypical propensity profiles, whereas we expect most children with co-occurring early-onset conduct problems, ADHD, and ODD to have extremely atypi-

cal propensity profiles. There is evidence that supports the hypothesis that children with co-occurring conduct problems, ADHD, and ODD have the highest levels of antisocial propensity. In the Australian Temperament Project, children with comorbid conduct problems and ADHD at age 8 years were more likely to receive high ratings on negative emotionality/irritability from infancy onward than children with only conduct problems, only ADHD, or neither disorder (Sanson & Prior, 1999). In addition, Waschbusch (2002) conducted a meta-analysis of 12 studies of over 6,000 girls and boys and found that verbal intelligence scores were related to conduct problems, but, confirming earlier qualitative reviews (Henry & Moffitt, 1997; Hinshaw, 1992; Hogan, 1999), children with both conduct problems and ADHD tended to have lower verbal intelligence scores than children with only conduct problems, only ADHD, or neither disorder. Indeed, children who exhibited only conduct problems and not ADHD did not differ from controls in verbal intelligence.

## Paradoxical Relation between Anxiety and Conduct Problems

Four well-established findings about conduct problems and anxiety have long seemed contradictory, but can perhaps be explained by the present model. First, anxiety disorders co-occur with conduct problems at greater than chance rates in childhood, adolescence, and adulthood (Loeber & Keenan, 1994; Zoccolillo, 1992). Second, children with conduct problems who are socially withdrawn are at increased risk for persistent and serious conduct problems (Blumstein, Farrington, & Moitra, 1985; Kerr et al., 1997; Serbin, Moskowitz, Schwartzman, & Ledingham, 1991). Third, shyness or anxiety in childhood in the absence of early conduct problems is associated with a *decreased* risk of later conduct problems (Graham & Rutter, 1973; Kohlberg, Ricks, & Snarey, 1984; Mitchell & Rosa, 1981; Sanson, Pedlow, Cann, Prior, & Oberklaid, 1996). Fourth, delinquents with higher levels of anxiety show lower rates of recidivism (Quay & Love, 1977).

Thus, anxiety and shyness sometimes appear to *foster* conduct problems and sometimes seem to *protect against* conduct problems. In terms of the present model, we hypothesize that shyness or anxiety that reflects low daring (i.e., timidity and shyness) will protect against the development of conduct problems. To the extent that anxiety reflects negative emotionality, however, anxiety will be positively correlated with conduct problems (because negative emotionality is positively correlated with conduct problems). In addition, when children are considered to be socially withdrawn or shy because they are low in prosociality (i.e., they do not care about other children), their social withdrawal will be positively correlated with conduct problems because prosociality is inversely related to conduct problems.

This hypothesis is consistent with the recent findings of a follow-up at age 26 years of the Dunedin Longitudinal Study (Moffitt et al., 2002). Personality measures administered in adolescence showed that males who abstained from antisocial behavior from childhood into adulthood could be said to be anxious in the sense of be low in daring, but were prosocial and low in negative emotionality. Boys showing life-course-persistent conduct problems exhibited the opposite pattern. What is needed, of course, is a prospective test of this hypothesis using measures of temperament administered in childhood rather than in adolescence.

## Genotype–Environment Interactions and Correlations

Like others, we believe that the environment plays a profoundly important role in the development of conduct problems. In order to fully understand environmental influences and harness their power in prevention and treatment, however, the role of the environment must be studied in the context of its interplay with genetic influences. In particular, we believe that genetic and environmental influences on conduct problems work partly through both genotype–environment interactions and genotype–environment correlations (Rutter, 1997; Rutter et al., 1997).

### Genotype–Environment Interactions

Specifically, we hypothesize two types of genotype–environment interactions:

1. There is evidence that genetic influences on conduct problems can be muted by favorable social learning environments. In particular, a number of adoption studies indicate that conduct problems in the adopted-away offspring of antisocial parents are less common when they are raised by well-adjusted adoptive parents than by adoptive parents with problems like their biological parents (Bohman, 1996; Cadoret, Yates, Troughton, Woodward, & Stewart, 1995).

2. Different individuals respond in different ways to the social factors that encourage conduct problems. For example, some youth who are poorly supervised and live in neighborhoods in which there are many delinquent role models will engage in serious delinquent acts with these peers, but most will not. We posit that genetic influences increase or decrease the likelihood that youth will respond to the social press to engage in delinquent behavior. Recently, Caspi et al. (2002) have provided striking evidence that maltreated children who have a particular allele of the gene that encodes monoamine oxidase A, which is an enzyme that inactivates a number of neurotransmitters, are more likely to engage in antisocial behavior than maltreated children without this allele. We expect that many such gene–environment interactions will need to be examined to understand the role of both genes and the environment.

Although previous studies of genotype–environment interaction have examined differences in the magnitude of genetic and environmental influences as a function of naturally occurring variation in environments, it would be possible to increase the power for examining such interactions by creating experimenter-manipulated environments. That is, future twin studies of genotype–environment interaction for conduct problems could employ designs that incorporate random assignment to environmental manipulations (e.g., early parent training) to explore genotype–environment interactions. It is possible that such studies would find greater evidence of genotype–environment interactions on conduct problems than naturalistic studies by increasing the range of variation in trait-relevant social environments.

### Genotype–Environment Correlations

Passive, evocative, and active genotype–environment correlations are also thought to be involved in the development of conduct problems (Plomin, DeFries, & Loehlin, 1977; Rutter, 1997; Rutter et al., 1997). That is, genetic and environmental influences on the origins of conduct problems are not independent, but are correlated.

The hypothesis of *passive genotype–environment correlations* means that the antisocial propensity that the child brings to the family, and the causally significant aspects of the family environment in which the child is raised, share the same genetic influences. Children with the greatest antisocial propensity tend to have absent antisocial fathers and to be raised by younger antisocial mothers with mental health problems (Klerman, 1993; Lahey et al., 1988; Lahey, Russo, Walker, & Piacentini, 1989; Nagin, Pogarsky, & Farrington, 1997; Wahler & Hann, 1987; Wakschlag et al., 2000). We hypothesize that this is partly because the same genes influence the behavior of both parents and their children. Because antisocial families are poorly prepared to provide the kinds of skilled childrearing that could prevent the development of conduct problem, this genotype–environment correlation helps propel the developmental progression from antisocial propensity to conduct problems.

*Evocative genotype–environment* correlations reflect the effects of the child's genetically influenced temperament and cognitive characteristics on the social environment, and the effects, in turn, of the social environment on the development of conduct problems. Consistent with the social learning model (Patterson, 1982; Reid & Patterson, 1989), we hypothesize that parenting plays the key role in the developmental transformation of antisocial predisposition into conduct problems. Cognitively and temperamentally predisposed children are less likely to develop conduct problems if they are raised in adaptive social environments. Unfortunately, the child's predisposing characteristics are hypothesized to evoke exactly the kinds of coercive, harsh, nonresponsive, inconsistent, and negative parenting behaviors that transform antisocial propensity into conduct problems (Anderson, Lytton, & Romney, 1986; Ge et al., 1996; Loeber & Tengs, 1986; Patterson, 1982; Sanson & Prior, 1999).

*Active genotype–environment correlations* mean that, partly because of genetic influences, some children are more likely than others to seek out social environments that foster the development of conduct problems. For example, children who are on a developmental pathway to adolescent conduct problems preferentially associate with delinquent peers who foster their delinquent behavior. There is evidence that association with delinquent peers is partly genetically influenced (Rowe & Osgood, 1984).

## INTERPLAY OF CHILD AND ENVIRONMENTAL FACTORS

How do individual differences in antisocial propensity cause conduct problems? The answer lies in the crucially important interplay between child characteristics (propensity) and the social environment (Keenan & Shaw, 1995). Consider, for example, two aspects of the interplay of negative emotionality with the social environment. First, by definition, toddlers who are high in negative emotionality become highly upset when they are frustrated or annoyed (e.g., by other children playing with a toy they want, by teachers instructing them to change activities, or by being bumped by another child). Their largely unlearned, intense, and nonspecific affective responses during toddlerhood provide a fertile behavioral basis for oppositional behavior. Indeed, little is required from the social environmental to shape such global affective reactions into oppositional behaviors (defiance, tantrums, etc.). In addition, such children respond in intensely negative ways to frustrating disciplinary restrictions, raising the likelihood of the increasingly aversive parent–child exchanges that Patterson (1982) refers to as the "coercion cycle." Second, as Tremblay (2000) demonstrated, it is common (but far from universal) for toddlers to be aggressive: to hit, kick, and bite. We posit that toddlers who are high in negative emotionality are both (1) more likely to be aggressive, and (2) to be aggressive in affect-laden ways that have serious consequences for self and others. For example, we hypothesize that toddlers who are high in negative emotionality tend to be aggressive in emotionally intense ways that are reinforced by their dominating other children (and sometimes adults).

Prosociality and daring are thought to influence the development of conduct problems in similar ways. For example, consider a social exchange in which a preschool child hits another child in an argument over a toy. For a child who is low in prosociality, the victim's crying and acquiescence might reinforce the aggression, but this same reaction might be punishing to a child who is high in prosociality. Similarly, a peer's suggestion that they leave the school building without permission might seem exciting and desirable to a child who is high on daring, but too risky to a child who is low on daring. In many such ways, the three dimensions of temperament that children bring to their social environments both shape the environment and influence his or her reaction to it.

Although the mechanisms of the inverse association between cognitive ability and conduct problems are not yet clear, we suspect that there are multiple ways in which deficient cognitive and verbal skills contribute to the development of conduct problems. For example, in early childhood, individual differences in intelligence are manifested partly as differences in the development of communication skills (Stattin & Klackenberg-Larsson, 1993). Following Keenan and Shaw (1997), we posit that toddlers with better communication skills are easier to socialize. This is because they comprehend parental instructions better, can communicate their wishes better, and hence are less likely to become frustrated during interactions with their parents.

Two recent studies suggest important ways in which cognitive deficits might interact with negative emotionality to adversely affect the social environment. In the words of Hughes, Cutting, and Dunn (2001), preschool children with high levels of behavior problems "act nasty" when frustrated in rigged competitive tasks more often than other children. In everyday life, it is likely that below-average cognitive abilities increase the likelihood of actual failure in school tasks, games, and sports. Thus, if children with less well developed cognitive skills and early conduct problems often fail, and react emotionally when they fail, they may be children that their well-behaved peers would reject (Maszk, Eisenberg, & Guthrie, 1999) and children that teachers find difficult to discipline in constructive ways.

During primary school, children who are low in cognitive abilities and exhibit conduct problems are at increased risk for grade retention. Using longitudinal data, Pagani, Tremblay, Vitaro, Boulerice, and McDuff (2001) found that grade retention did not improve academic performance but increased future conduct problems, particularly in boys. This might happen because grade retention places the aggressive child in an environment with younger and weaker classmates who are more likely to reinforce his or her antisocial behavior by cowering and complying. This study has important implications both for theories of the origins and maintenance of conduct problems and for public policy, as recent moves toward greater grade retention in the United States could foster the development of conduct problems.

## SPECIFYING AND EVALUATING THE MODEL

In this section, we lay out the major specific hypotheses of the current model and suggest critical empirical tests needed to evaluate the validity of the present model.

## Key Hypotheses Regarding the Origins of Conduct Problems

Many hypotheses regarding the origins of conduct problems are embedded in the text above. In this section, we offer a number of hypotheses that deserve particular attention and suggest studies needed to provide the most stringent tests of these hypotheses.

### Mediation of Genetic Influences

There is growing evidence that the genetic influences on childhood conduct problems, ODD, and ADHD overlap to a considerable degree (Coolidge, Thede, & Young, 2000; Eaves et al., 2000; Thapar, Harrington, & McGuffin, 2001; Waldman, Rhee, Levy, & Hay, 2001). We hypothesize an explanation for this overlap in genetic influences that is based on our model of predisposing child characteristics. This hypothesis is the cornerstone of our model, as we believe it provides a necessary blueprint for understanding genetic and environmental influences on conduct problems.

In our model, genetic influences do not have a direct impact on conduct problems. Broad dimensions of human behavior have direct genetic influences, but specific complex behaviors, such as stealing and vandalism, do not. Genetic influences on conduct problems are hypothesized to be *indirect*, through the four broad dimensions of antisocial propensity. Specifically, we hypothesize that the temperamental and cognitive-verbal components of antisocial propensity (1) each have unique genetic influences, and (2) these components of propensity mediate the genetic influences on conduct problems (Lahey, Waldman, et al., 1999). Genetic influences are hypothesized to affect the environments in which conduct problems are learned partly due to the effects of child characteristics (temperament and cognitive ability) on the environment (active and evocative genotype–environment correlations), but also through passive genotype–environment correlations.

Four recent studies provide evidence relevant to our genetic mediation hypothesis. Schmitz et al. (1999) obtained maternal ratings of the negative emotionality of twins at the ages of 14, 20, 24, and 36 months and ratings on the Child Behavior Checklist (CBCL) at 48 months. Negative emotionality measured at all ages predicted CBCL Externalizing scores (composite of oppositional, aggressive, and nonaggressive conduct problems) at age 4 years. Consistent with our mediation hypothesis, 96% of the correlation between early negative emotionality and later conduct problems was explained by genetic influences common to both variables. In a well-conceived study, Lemery, Essex, and Smider (in press) developed "purified" measures of temperament and child behavior and emotional problems by eliminating overlapping items. In 270 pairs of twins, temperament measured at age 5 predicted behavior problems at age 7. More importantly, genetic influences on age 7 conduct problems were substantial and were entirely mediated by age 5 temperament measures. Although their dimensions of temperament differed from our own, two of the dimensions of temperament that Lemery et al. identified through exploratory factor analyses (negative affectivity and surgency) resemble our hypothesized dimensions of negative emotionality and daring enough to lend plausibility to our mediation hypothesis.

Over a much longer age span, Gjone and Stevenson (1997) also conducted multivariate behavior genetic analyses of a sample of 759 twin pairs who were 5–15 years old in the first assessment. Parent ratings of negative emotionality in the first assessment predicted both CBCL Aggression and Delinquency ratings 2 years later. Negative emotionality and Aggression scores shared common genetic influences, but neither common genetic nor shared environmental influences explained the prospective association between temperament and CBCL Delinquency scores. Although our model would have predicted some shared causal influences on negative emotionality and CBCL Delinquency scores, this finding is consistent with our hypothesis that developmentally early conduct problems, which constitute most of the Aggression scale items, and which are found mostly among youth with earlier ages of onset, have stronger genetic influences that the items on the Delinquency scale (which are also common among youth with later ages of onset).

There also is suggestive evidence that executive functioning shares a substantial proportion of its genetic influences with childhood conduct problems, ODD, and ADHD (Coolidge et al., 2000). This is consistent with our hypothesis that genetic influences on childhood conduct problems (and co-occurring ADHD and ODD) are mediated partly by deficits in verbal–executive aspects of cognitive ability.

At the molecular level, the nature of genetic influences on conduct problems is undoubtedly complex, but our model may facilitate their identification. As reviewed above, there is evidence that the genetic influences on conduct problems are shared with ADHD, ODD, and perhaps other mental disorders. Our model suggests that each of the components of antisocial propensity is influenced by a distinct sets of genes, which indirectly influence the development of conduct problems through the four components of antisocial propensity. If this hypothesis is correct, it may be easier to identify the smaller and more independent sets of genes that influence each of the four dimensions of antisocial propensity than to search for the multiple sets of overlapping genes that indirectly influence conduct problems and other types of mental health problems.

## Sex Differences in Conduct Problems

From about 4 years of age, boys are more likely than girls to engage in conduct problems (Keenan & Shaw, 1997; Lahey, Schwab-Stone, et al., 2000;

Moffitt et al., 2001; Tremblay et al., 1996). Because the magnitude of these sex differences is considerable, any successful explanation of sex differences will greatly inform general models of the origins of conduct problems. We hypothesize that the causes of conduct problems are the same for girls and boys, with sex differences in conduct problems arising mostly from sex differences in the *levels* of the components of antisocial propensity (Rhee & Waldman, 2002; Rowe, Vazsonyi, & Flannery, 1995). For example, boys lag behind girls on average in the development of language communication during the crucial toddler years (Sanson, Smart, Prior, & Oberklaid, 1993). Keenan and Shaw (1997) suggested that girls are easier to socialize for this reason and that the resulting differences in socialization help create sex differences in conduct problems. To take a second example, girls show higher levels of empathy and guilt than males from toddlerhood through adolescence (Keenan, Loeber, & Green, 1999; Keenan & Shaw, 1997; Zahn-Waxler et al., 1992). We posit that prosociality plays the same role in the development of conduct problems in girls and boys, but from an early age boys are less prosocial. This difference may reflect inherent sex differences in prosociality, early sex differences in socialization that create differences in prosociality, or both.

There is some evidence, however, that there could be more fundamental sex differences in genetic and environmental influences on conduct problems. Two studies suggest that genetic and environmental influences are similar for girls and boys on developmentally early conduct problems, but are more distinct on developmentally late conduct problems (Eley et al., 1999; Silberg et al., 1996). This could reflect sex differences in the magnitude of genetic influences, but it raises the possibility of unique causal influences on girls' conduct problems that are not included in the present model, such as genetic influences on pubertal timing. This seems plausible as some evidence suggests that early-maturing girls show an earlier and higher peak in conduct problems (Moffitt et al., 2001) and pubertal timing has strong genetic influences in girls (Pickles et al., 1998). There are many possible explanations for the potential sex difference in environmental influences on developmentally late conduct problems. First, they may reflect differences in the ways in which parents and teachers socialize girls and boys (Keenan & Shaw, 1997). Second, they may result from sex differences in the interaction between pubertal development and peer influences (Caspi, Lynam, Moffitt, & Silva, 1993). Third, girls may be more sensitive to some kinds of social influences than boys, with one potential difference of this type being greater sensitivity to family discord among girls than boys (Keenan et al., 1999).

There are three additional ways in which there could be fundamental sex differences in the causes of conduct problems. There is a substantial difference between girls and boys in the extent of co-occurrence of conduct problems with depression, substance abuse, and other disorders (Keenan et al., 1999), raising the possibility that conduct problems in girls may share more etiological influences with these other disorders than do boys. In addition, evidence from Gjone and Stevenson (1997) suggests that the association between negative emotionality and conduct problems may be stronger for boys than girls. Finally, although much remains to be learned (Keenan et al., 1999; Moffit et al., 2001), some studies suggest that girls who engage in conduct problems have similar characteristics regardless of their age of onset of conduct problems, whereas the characteristics of boys with earlier versus later ages of onset differ considerably (Kratzer & Hodgins, 1999; Silverthorn & Frick, 1999; Silverthorn, Frick, & Reynolds, 2001). Thus, there are many possible reasons why sex differences in conduct problems could reflect fundamental sex differences in the causal matrix. All of these possibilities deserve study, but a sensible first step would be to test the hypothesis that sex differences in conduct problems can be fully explained by sex differences in mean levels of the components of antisocial propensity. Moffit et al. (2001) provided important evidence of this possibility using a population-based sample of youth. When two dimensions of personality (negative emotionality and constraint) that were measured during adolescence were added to a regression model of sex differences in delinquent behavior, sex differences in personality accounted for nearly all of the sex differences.

### Demographics and Conduct Problems

An inverse relation between SES and conduct problems has been found in many population-based studies (Lahey, Miller, Gordon, & Riley, 1999). An important goal of any general model of conduct problems is to explain why this is the case, and also to explain why the great majority of children from low-SES families do *not* engage in serious conduct problems. We hypothesize that the multiple environmental factors associated with lower SES influence the developmental transition from antisocial propensity to conduct problems. These SES-linked environmental factors include living in high-crime neighborhoods, attending schools with delinquent peers, and the family's lack of economic resources—which affect access to daycare, afterschool care, mental health services, and the like (Harnish, Dodge, & Valente, 1995; Kilgore, Snyder, & Lentz, 2000). We hypothesize that these environmental circumstances foster the social learning of conduct problems (Caspi, Taylor, Moffitt, & Plomin, 2000). On the other hand, part of the correlation of lower SES with conduct problems reflects selection effects. There is evidence of downward socioeconomic mobility (or staying at the low SES of their family of origin) among parents who are antisocial and/or have mental health and substance abuse problems (Dohrenwend & Dohrenwend, 1974; Miech et al., 1999). In some instances, then, characteristics of persons lead them to live in adverse socioeconomic circumstances (selection effects) and these circumstances, in turn, influence their children (casual effects).

Why do most children living in low-SES circumstances not engage in serious antisocial behavior? Consistent with our general model, we hypothesize that children who are not temperamentally and cognitively predisposed to develop conduct problems will be less influenced by the environmental factors associated with lower SES than predisposed children. Because there are genetic influences on antisocial propensity, this means that the environmental influences associated with SES influence the child partly through genotype–environment interactions.

There is also evidence that women who give birth at younger ages are more likely to have children who engage in conduct problems (e.g., Levine, Pollack, & Comfort, 2001; Nagin et al., 1997). Following Jaffee, Caspi, Moffitt, and Silva (2001), we hypothesize that this reflects both person factors that select certain women into early childbearing and environmental influences on their offspring associated with early childbearing. These hypotheses regarding sociodemographic influences could be put to the strongest test in genetically informative, multigenerational designs, such as a study of the offspring of twin mothers.

## Race–Ethnic Differences in Conduct Problems

After controlling for SES and neighborhood factors, there is little or no difference in the prevalence of most conduct problems among African American, Hispanic, and non-Hispanic white youth (Bird et al., 2001; Loeber et al., 1998). There appear to be race–ethnic differences in some specific crimes, however, such as drug selling and assault with a deadly weapon (Blum et al., 2000). We hypothesize that these differences are mostly attributable to a marked difference in the tendency of youth in different race–ethnic groups to join antisocial gangs. Evidence is sparse for girls, but there is clear evidence that the boys who join gangs had high and escalating levels of aggressive and nonaggressive conduct problems prior to joining their first gang (Esbensen, Huizinga, & Weiher, 1993; Lahey, Gordon, Loeber, Stouthamer-Loeber, & Farrington, 1999). Over the past 100 years, the race–ethnic groups that have been most likely to join antisocial gangs have changed, with Irish immigrants being the mostly likely to join gangs around the turn of the 20th century, for example. At this time in history, misbehaving non-Hispanic white boys are much less likely to join gangs than misbehaving African American and Hispanic boys (Lahey, Gordon, et al., 1999). There is also clear evidence from longitudinal studies that during their period of gang membership, gang members show marked increases in the frequency of drug-related and violent offenses (so that they account for 10 times more assaults and drug sales than nongang members), which declines after their period of gang membership ends (Esbensen et al., 1993;

Thornberry, Krohn, Lizotte, & Chard-Wierschem, 1993). We posit that the powerful social influence of gang membership accounts for much of race–ethnic differences in serious adolescent antisocial behavior. The outlook for gang influence is guardedly optimistic, as there has been a 13% decline in the number of law enforcement jurisdictions in the United States with known gangs from 1996 to 2000 and a 5% decline in the number of gang members from 1999 to 2000. Still, there were an estimated 772,500 gang members in the United States during 2000 (Office of Juvenile Justice and Delinquency Prevention, 2002). In addition, there are findings that suggest other possible race–ethnic differences in the nature of social influences on conduct problems (such as parenting styles) that must be pursued in future studies (e.g., Deater-Deckard, Dodge, Bates, & Pettit, 1996; Donnellan, Ge, & Wenk, 2001). Given the profound importance of culture, it would not be surprising to find differences in causal influences on conduct problems, but such differences have not yet been convincingly demonstrated.

## Playing (and Refuting) the Devil's Advocate

The greatest threat to the validity of the present model of the origins of conduct problems (and other models that ascribe a role to temperament or personality constructs) is that the correlations on which they are based could be circular. Consider a parent who has been asked to complete two rating scales about her daughter, one composed of items referring to conduct problems and the other composed of items that assess her temperament. After rating the child's antisocial behavior, the parent is asked if her daughter "gets upset easily," "cares about the feelings of others," and "likes things that may be dangerous." The mother may answer these questions by thinking of her daughter's frequent fighting. Even if there is evidence to the contrary in the girl's behavior, the salience of her fighting may lead the mother to *infer* that her daughter is easily upset, unconcerned about others, and likes dangerous situations. A youth completing self-report instruments might complete them in the same circular way.

It is essential to move beyond this potential circularity in testing the present causal model. Several research strategies seem appropriate for this purpose:

1. It is important for some studies to use measures of temperament that are not completed by the same individuals who report on the child's conduct problems. A number of such studies have already been completed, however, which lend credibility to the model. For example, Kagan's (1992) laboratory measure of behavioral disinhibition, which is based on observations by independent observers, is associated with the development of conduct problems (Biederman et al., 2000; Schwartz et al., 1996). Similarly, observational measures have shown that preschoolers with conduct problems engage in less prosocial behavior and display more negative emo-

tion during play with a friend (Hughes et al., 2000) and react more emotionally to failure in a competitive task (Hughes et al., 2001). Eisenberg et al. (1996) used gaze aversion while watching a film of a distressed child and Zhou et al. (2002) used ratings of facial expressions while viewing slides depicting the positive or negative emotions of others as measures of empathy. Similarly, Hastings et al. (2000) used feigned accidents to the child's mother to observe the child's empathic response, with some aspects of empathy being correlated with conduct problems in both studies. Fortunately, structured tests of cognitive and language skills by examiners are relatively free of confounds if the examiners are unaware of child's behavior problems (but individual differences in behavior during assessments could bias the test results).

2. Because of the low cost and convenience of rating scales, particularly in large-scale population-based studies, it is essential to validate temperament rating scales against observational and laboratory measures.

3. The similarities of the current model of temperament to structural personality theories suggest another important way to validate measures of temperament and to understand their meaning. Eyseck's (1947) model, for example, has stimulated many studies of biological differences in individuals with varying scores on his dimensions of personality. For example, using functional magnetic resonance imaging, Canli et al. (2001) found striking correlations in the $r = .70–.85$ range between neuroticism scores and activity in frontal and limbic structures in response to negatively valenced stimuli. Similarly strong correlations were found between extraversion scores and brain activity in response to positively valenced stimuli. Such studies using measures of the our hypothesized dimensions of temperament would do much to validate the measures and further understanding of the individual differences in brain functioning associated with temperament. Other well-developed research programs on the neurobiology of personality and emotion (Davidson, Putnam, & Larson, 2000; Depue & Collins, 1999) and on individual differences in conditioning and reward sensitivity also provide highly promising avenues for validating the model (Beyts, Frcka, Martin, & Levey, 1983; Daugherty, Quay, & Ramos, 1993; Newman, Widom, & Stewart, 1985).

4. Prospective studies beginning early in childhood that test predictions about the future development of conduct problems will be essential to testing the model in the most informative manner. If, for example, preschool children with the high-risk propensity profile fail to show marked increases in conduct problems during later childhood and adolescence, the model would be disconfirmed.

5. The validity of the present model can also be evaluated by testing specific model-driven hypotheses, such as the hypothesis that the temperamental and cognitive-linguistic components of propensity mediate genetic influences on conduct problems.

## Studies Needed to Expose the Current Model to Risk of Refutation

The many specific hypotheses advanced in this chapter relate the social environment and individual differences in child characteristics (the components of antisocial propensity, sex, and race–ethnicity) to individual differences in the development of conduct problems. These hypotheses can be best tested in representative population-based samples that can map the relation of child characteristics and social environments onto individual differences in the development of conduct problems. Representative samples are needed to avoid sampling biases that create false correlations. These samples would need to contain sufficient numbers of children who engage in significant levels of conduct problems to provide adequate statistical power. This would require either large sample sizes or the oversampling of high-risk subgroups, such as lower SES families. Alternatively, well-reasoned comparisons of selected groups, such as clinic attendees and matched controls could be useful, but any use of nonrepresentative samples raises risks of artifacts due to biased sampling and population stratification. The hypotheses of independent genetic influences on the components of propensity and their mediation of genetic influences on conduct problems could be tested in genetically informative population-based samples, such as samples of twins or other siblings, with longitudinal studies providing the greatest information of both the timing of influences and the nature of influences on the persistence of conduct problems. Such scientifically strong studies are expensive and time-consuming, but, in the long run, they provide the quickest and most cost-effective way to advance knowledge of the causes of this troubling personal and social problem.

### ACKNOWLEDGMENT

The writing of this chapter was supported in part by Grant Nos. R01-MH42529, R01-MH53554, R01-MH51091, and K01-MH01818 from the National Institute of Mental Health.

### REFERENCES

Addad, M., & Leslau, A. (1990). Immoral judgment, extraversion, neuroticism, and criminal behaviour. *International Journal of Offender Therapy and Comparative Criminology, 34*, 1–13.

Anderson, K. E., Lytton, H., & Romney, D. M. (1986). Mothers' interactions with normal and conduct-disordered boys: Who affects whom? *Developmental Psychology, 22*, 604–609.

Arnett, J. J. (1996). Sensation seeking, aggressiveness, and adolescent reckless behavior. *Personality and Individual Differences, 20*, 693–702.

Asendorpf, J. B., Borkenau, P., Ostendorf, F., & van Aken, M. A. G. (2001). Carving personality description at its joints: Confirmation of three replicable personality prototypes for both children and adults. *European Journal of Personality, 15,* 169–198.

Asendorpf, J. B., & van Aken, M. A. (1999). Resilient, overcontrolled, and undercontrolled personality prototypes in childhood: Replicability, predictive power, and the trait–type issue. *Journal of Personality and Social Psychology, 77,* 815–832.

Baker, L., & Cantwell, D. P. (1987). A prospective psychiatric follow-up of children with speech/ language disorders. *Journal of the American Academy of Child and Adolescent Psychiatry, 26,* 546–553.

Beitchman, J. H., Wilson, B., Johnson, C. J., Atkinson, L., Young, A., Adlaf, E., Escobar, M., & Douglas, L. (2001). Fourteen-year follow-up of speech/language-impaired and control children: Psychiatric outcome. *Journal of the American Academy of Child and Adolescent Psychiatry, 40,* 75–82.

Berman, T., & Paisey, T. (1984). Personality in assaultive and non-assaultive juvenile male offenders. *Psychological Reports, 54,* 527–530.

Beyts, J., Frcka, G., Martin, I., & Levey, A. B. (1983). The influence of psychoticism and extraversion on classical eyelid conditioning using a paraorbital shock UCS. *Personality and Individual Differences, 4*(3), 275–283.

Biederman, J., Hirshfeld-Becker, D. R., Rosenbaum, J. F., Herot, C., Friedman, D., Snidman, N., Kagan, J., & Faraone, S. V. (2001). Further evidence of association between behavioral inhibition and social anxiety in children. *American Journal of Psychiatry, 158,* 1673–1679.

Bird, H. R., Canino, G. J., Davies, M., Zhang, H., Ramirez, R., & Lahey, B. B. (2001). Prevalence and correlates of antisocial behaviors among three ethnic groups. *Journal of Abnormal Child Psychology, 29,* 465–478.

Blair, C. (2002). School readiness: Integrating cognition and emotion in a neurobiological conceptualization of children's functioning at school entry. *American Psychologist, 57,* 111–127.

Block, J. (1961). *The Q-sort method in personality assessment and psychiatric research.* Springfield, IL: Thomas.

Blum, R., W., Beuhring, T., Shew, M. L., Bearinger, L. H., Sieving, R. E., & Resnick, M. D. (2000). The effects of race/ethnicity, income, and family structure on adolescent risk behaviors. *American Journal of Public Health, 90,* 1879–1884.

Blumstein, A., Farrington, D. P., & Moitra, S. (1985). Delinquency careers: Innocents, desisters, and persisters. In M. Tonry & N. Morris (Eds.), *Crime and justice.* Chicago: University of Chicago Press.

Bohman, M. (1996). Predispoistions to criminality: Swedish adoption studies in retrospect. In G. R. Bock & J. A. Goode (Eds.), *Genetics of criminal and antisocial behavior.* Chichester, UK: Wiley.

Bouchard, T. J., & Loehlin, J. C. (2001). Genes, evolution, and personality. *Behavior Genetics, 31,* 243–273.

Brame, B., Nagin, D. S., & Tremblay, R. E. (2001). Developmental trajectories of physical aggression from school entry to late adolescence. *Journal of Child Psychology and Psychiatry, 42,* 503–512.

Buss, A. H., & Plomin, R. (1975). *A temperament theory of personality development.* New York: Wiley-Interscience.

Buss, A. H., & Plomin, R. (1984). *Temperament: Early developing personality traits.* Hillsdale, NJ: Erlbaum.

Cadoret, R. J., Yates, W. R., Troughton, E., Woodward, G., & Stewart, M. A. (1995). Genetic–environmental interaction in the genesis of aggressivity and conduct disorders. *Archives of General Psychiatry, 52,* 916–924.

Canli, T., Zhao, Z., Desmond, J. E., Kang, E., Gross, J., & Gabrieli, J. D. E. (2001). An fMRI study of personality influences on brain reactivity to emotional stimuli. *Behavioral Neuroscience, 115,* 33–42.

Caspi, A. (1998). Personality development across the life course. In N. Eisenberg (Ed.), *Handbook of child psychology* (5th ed., Vol. 3, pp. 311–388). New York: Wiley.

Caspi, A., Lynam, D., Moffitt, T. E., & Silva, P. A. (1993). Unraveling girls' delinquency: Biological, dispositional, and contextual contributions to adolescent misbehavior. *Developmental Psychology, 29,* 19–30.

Caspi, A., McClay, J., Moffitt, T., Mill, J., Martin, J., Craig, I. W., Taylor, A., & Poulton, R. (2002). Role of genotype in the cycle of violence in maltreated children. *Science, 297,* 851–854.

Caspi, A., Moffitt, T. E., Silva, P. A., Stouthamer-Loeber, M., Schmutte, P. S., & Krueger, R. (1994). Are some people crime-prone?: Replications of the personality–crime relation across nation, gender, race and method. *Criminology, 32,* 301–333.

Caspi, A., & Roberts, B. W. (2001). Personality development across the life course: The argument for change and continuity. *Psychological Inquiry, 12,* 49–66.

Caspi, A., Taylor, A., Moffitt, T. E., & Plomin, R. (2000). Neighborhood deprivation affects children's mental health: Environmental risks idenitified in a genetic design. *Psychological Science, 11,* 338–342.

Cloninger, C. R. (1987). A systematic method for clinical description and classification of personality variants: A proposal. *Archives of General Psychiatry, 44,* 573–588.

Cohen, D. C., & Strayer, J. (1996). Empathy in conduct-disordered and comparison youth. *Developmental Psychology, 32,* 988–998.

Cohen, N. J., Menna, R., Vallance, D. D., Barwick, M. A., Im, N., & Horodezky, N. B. (1998). Language, social cognitive processing, and behavioral characteristics of psychiatrically disturbed children with previously identified and unsuspected language impairments. *Journal of Child Psychology and Psychiatry, 39,* 853–864.

Coolidge, F. L., Thede, L. L., & Young, S. E. (2000). Heritability and the comorbidity of attention deficit hyperactivity disorder with behavioral disorders and executive function deficits: A preliminary investigation. *Developmental Neuropsychology, 17,* 273–287.

Costa, P. T., & McCrae, R. R. (1987). *NEO.* Odessa, FL: Psychological Assessment Resources.

Costa, P. T., & McCrae, R. R. (1995). Primary traits of Eysenck's P-E-N system: Three and five-factor solutions. *Journal of Personality and Social Psychology, 69,* 308–317.

Cyphers, L. H., Phillips, K., Fulker, D. W., & Mrazek, D. A. (1990). Twin temperament during the transition from infancy to early childhood. *Journal of the American Academy of Child and Adolescent Psychiatry, 29,* 392–397.

Daderman, A. M. (1999). Differences between severely conduct-disordered juvenile males and normal juvenile males: The study of personality traits. *Personality and Individual Differences, 26,* 827–845.

Daderman, A. M., Wirsen, M. A., & Hallman, J. (2001). Different personality patterns in non-socialized (juvenile delinquents) and socialized (air force pilot recruits) sensation seekers. *European Journal of Personality, 15,* 239–252.

Daugherty, T. K., Quay, H. C., & Ramos, L. (1993). Response perseveration, inhibitory control, and central dopaminergic activity in childhood behavior disorders. *Journal of Genetic Psychology, 154,* 177–188.

Davidson, R. J., Putnam, K. M., & Larson, C. L. (2000). Dysfunction in the neural circuitry of emotion regulation—A possible prelude to violence. *Science, 289,* 591–594.

Davis, M. H., Luce, C., & Kraus, S. J. (1994). The heritability of characteristics associated with dispositional empathy. *Journal of Personality, 62,* 369–391.

Deater-Deckard, K., Dodge, K. A., Bates, J. E., & Pettit, G. S. (1996). Physical discipline among African American and European American mothers: Links to children's externalizing behaviors. *Developmental Psychology, 32,* 1065–1072.

Deater-Deckard, K., & Plomin, R. (1999). An adoption study of the etiology of teacher reports of externalizing problems in middle childhood. *Child Development, 70,* 144–154.

Depue, R. A., & Collins, P. F. (1999). Neurobiology of the structure of personality: Dopamine facilitation of incentive motivation and extraversion. *Behavioral and Brain Sciences, 22,* 491–569.

Dery, M., Toupin, J., Pauze, R., Mercier, H., & Fortin, L. (1999). Neuropsychological characteristics of adolescents with conduct disorder: Association with attention-deficit-hyperactivity and aggression. *Journal of Abnormal Child Psychology, 27*, 225–236.

Digman, J. M., & Inouye, J. (1986). Further specification of the five robust factors of personality. *Journal of Personality and Social Psychology, 50*, 116–123.

DiLalla, L. F., Kagan, J., & Reznick, J. S. (1994). Genetic etiology of behavioral inhibition among 2-year-old children. *Infant Behavior and Development, 17*, 405–412.

Dohrenwend, B. P., & Dohrenwend, B. S. (1974). Social and cultural influences on psychopathology. *Annual Review of Psychology, 25*, 417–452.

Donnellan, M. B., Ge, X., & Wenk, E. (2000). Cognitive abilities in adolescent-limited and life-course-persistent criminal offenders. *Journal of Abnormal Psychology, 109*, 396–402.

Eaves, L., Rutter, M., Silberg, J. L., Shillady, L., Maes, H., & Pickles, A. (2000). Genetic and environmental causes of covariation in interview assessments of disruptive behavior in child and adolescent twins. *Behavior Genetics, 30*, 321–334.

Edelbrock, C., Rende, R., Plomin, R., & Thompson, L. E. (1995). A twin study of competence and problem behavior in childhood and early adolescence. *Journal of Child Psychology and Psychiatry, 36*, 775–785.

Eisenberg, N., Fabes, R. A., Guthrie, I. K., Murphy, B. C., Maszk, P., Homlgren, R., & Suh, K. (1996). The relations of regulation and emotionality to problem behavior in elementary school children. *Development and Psychopathology, 8*, 141–162.

Eisenberg, N., Fabes, R. A., & Murphy, B. C. (1996). Parents' reactions to children's negative emotions: Relations to children's social competence and comforting behavior. *Child Development, 67*, 2227–2247.

Eisenberg, N., & Mussen, P. H. (1991). *The roots of prosocial behavior in children.* New York: Cambridge University Press.

Eley, T. C., Dale, P., & Bishop, D. (2001). Longitudinal analysis of the genetic and environmental influences on components of cognitive delay in preschoolers. *Journal of Educational Psychology, 93*, 698–707.

Eley, T. C., Lichtenstein, P., & Stevenson, J. (1999). Sex differences in the etiology of aggressive and nonaggressive antisocial behavior: Results from two twin studies. *Child Development, 70*, 155–168.

Elkins, I., Iacono, W., Doyle, A., & McGue, M. (1997). Characteristics associated with the persistence of antisocial behavior: Results from recent longitudinal research. *Aggression and Violent Behavior, 2*, 101–124.

Emde, R. N., Plomin, R., Robinson, J. A., Corley, R., DeFries, J., Fulker, D. W., Reznick, J. S., Campos, J., Kagan, J., & Zahn-Waxler, C. (1992). Temperament, emotion, and cognition at fourteen months: The MacArthur Longitudinal Twin Study. *Child Development, 63*, 1437–1455.

Eron, L. D., & Huesmann, L. R. (1984). The relation of prosocial behavior to the development of aggression and psychopathology. *Aggressive Behavior, 10*, 201–211.

Esbensen, F.-A., Huizinga, D., & Weiher, A. W. (1993). Gang and non-gang youth: Differences in explanatory factors. *Journal of Contemporary Criminal Justice, 9*, 94–116.

Eysenck, H. J. (1947). *Dimensions of personality.* New York: Praeger.

Eysenck, H. J. (1964). *Crime and personality.* New York: Houghton Mifflin.

Eysenck, H. J. (1990). Genetic and environmental contributions to individual differences: The three major dimensions of personality. *Journal of Personality, 58*, 245–261.

Eysenck, H. J. (1996). Psychology and crime: Where do we stand? *Psychology, Crime, and Law, 2*, 143–152.

Eysenck, S. G., & Eysenck, H. J. (1970). Crime and personality: An empirical study of the three-factor theory. *British Journal of Criminology, 10*, 225–239.

Eysenck, S. B., & Eysenck, H. J. (1977). Personality differences between prisoners and controls. *Psychological Reports, 40*, 1023–1028.

Eysenck, S. B., & McGurk, B. J. (1980). Impulsiveness and venturesomeness in a detention center population. *Psychological Reports, 47*, 1299–1306.

Farrington, D. P. (1991). Antisocial personality from childhood to adulthood. *Psychologist, 4,* 389–394.

Farrington, D. P. (1995). The development of offending and antisocial behaviour from childhood: Key findings from the Cambridge Study in Delinquent Development. *Journal of Child Psychology and Psychiatry, 6,* 929–964.

Farrington, D. P., & West, D. J. (1993). Criminal, penal and life histories of chronic offenders: Risk and protective factors and early identification. *Criminal Behaviour and Mental Health, 3,* 492–523.

Fergusson, D. M., Lynskey, M. T., & Horwood, L. J. (1996). Factors associated with continuity and change in disruptive behavior patters between childhood and adolescence. *Journal of Abnormal Child Psychology, 24,* 533–553.

Fonseca, A. C., & Yule, W. (1995). Personality and antisocial behavior in children and adolescents: An enquiry into Eysenck's and Gray's theories. *Journal of Abnormal Child Psychology, 23,* 767–781.

Frick, P. J., O'Brien, B. S., Wootton, J. M., & McBurnett, K. (1994). Psychopathy and conduct problems in children. *Journal of Abnormal Psychology, 103,* 700–707.

Furnham, A., & Thompson, J. (1991). Personality and self-reported delinquency. *Personality and Individual Differences, 12,* 585–593.

Gabrys, J. B. (1983). Contrasts in social behavior and personality of children. *Psychological Reports, 52,* 171–178.

Garcia-Coll, C., Kagan, J., & Reznick, J. S. (1984). Behavioral inhibition in young children. *Child Development, 55,* 1005–1019.

Ge, X., Conger, R. D., Cadoret, R. J., Neiderhiser, J. M., Yates, W., Troughton, E., & Stewart, M. A. (1996). The developmental interface between nature and nurture: A mutual influence model of child antisocial behavior and parent behaviors. *Developmental Psychology, 32,* 574–589.

Ge, X., Donnellan, M. B., & Wenk, E. (2001). The development of persistent criminal offending in males. *Criminal Justice and Behavior, 26,* 731–755.

Gershuny, B. S., & Sher, K. J. (1998). The relation between personality and anxiety: Findings from a 3-year prospective study. *Journal of Abnormal Psychology, 107,* 252–262.

Giancola, P. R., Martin, C. S., Tarter, R. E., Pelham, W. E., & Moss, H. B. (1996). Executive cognitive functioning and aggressive behavior in preadolescent boys at high risk for substance abuse/dependence. *Journal of Studies on Alcohol, 57,* 352–359.

Gjone, H., & Stevenson, J. (1997). A longitudinal twin study of temperament and behavior problems: Common genetic or environmental influences? *Journal of the American Academy of Child and Adolescent Psychiatry, 36,* 1448–1456.

Goldberg, L. R. (1993). The structure of phenotypic personality traits. *American Psychologist, 48,* 26–34.

Goldberg, L. R., & Rosolack, T. K. (1994). The big five factor structure as an integrative framework: An empirical comparison with Eysenck's P–E–N model. In C. F. Halverson, G. A. Kohnstamm, & R. P. Martin (Eds.), *The developing structure of temperament and personality from infancy to adulthood* (pp. 7–35). Hillsdale, NJ: Erlbaum.

Goldsmith, H. H., Buss, K. A., & Lemery, K. S. (1997). Toddler and childhood temperament: Expanded content, stronger genetic evidence, new evidence for the importance of environment. *Developmental Psychology, 33,* 891–905.

Goma-I.-Freixnet, M. (1995). Prosocial and antisocial aspects of personality. *Personality and Individual Differences, 19,* 125–134.

Goodman, R. (2001). Psychometric properties of the Strengths and Difficulties Questionnaire. *Journal of the American Academy of Child and Adolescent Psychiatry, 40,* 1337–1345.

Gottfredson, M. R., & Hirschi, T. (1990). *A general theory of crime.* Stanford, CA: Stanford University Press.

Graham P., & Rutter, M. (1973). Psychiatric disorders in the young adolescent: A follow-up study. *Proceedings of the Royal Society of Medicine, 66,* 1226–1229.

Graziano, W. G. (1994). The development of agreeableness as a dimension of personality. In C. F. Halverson, G. A. Kohnstamm, & R. P. Martin (Eds.), *The developing structure of temperament and personality from infancy to adulthood* (pp. 339–354) Hillsdale, NJ: Erlbaum.

Graziano, W. G., & Eisenberg, N. (1997). Agreeableness: A dimension of personality. In R. Higan, J. Johnson, & S. Briggs (Eds.), *Handbook of personality psychology* (pp. 795–824). San Diego, CA: Academic Press.

Greene, K., Krcmar, M., Walters, L. H., Rubin, D. L., & Hale, J. L. (2000). Targeting adolescent risk-taking behaviors: The contribution of egocentrism and sensation-seeking. *Journal of Adolescence, 23,* 439–461.

Grusec, J. E. (1991). Socializing concern for others in the home. *Developmental Psychology, 27,* 338–342.

Haemaelaeinen, M., & Pulkkinen, L. (1996). Problem behavior as a precursor of male criminality. *Development and Psychopathology, 8,* 443–455.

Harnish, J. D., Dodge, K. A., & Valente, E. (1995). Mother–child interaction quality as a partial mediator of the roles of maternal depressive symptomatology and socioeconomic status in the development of child conduct problems. *Child Development, 66,* 739–753.

Hart, D., Hofmann, V., Edelstein, W., & Keller, M. (1997). The relation of childhood personality types to adolescent behavior and development: A longitudinal study of Icelandic children. *Developmental Psychology, 33,* 195–205.

Hastings, P. D., Zahn-Waxler, C., Robinson, J., Usher, B., & Bridges, D. (2000). The development of concern for others in children with behavior problems. *Developmental Psychology, 36,* 531–546.

Heaven, P. C. L. (1996). Personality and self-reported delinquency: A longitudinal analysis. *Journal of Child Psychology and Psychiatry, 37,* 747–751.

Henry, B., Caspi, A., Moffitt, T. E., & Silva, P. A. (1996). Temperamental and familial predictors of violent and nonviolent criminal convictions: Age 3 to age 18. *Developmental Psychology, 32,* 614–623.

Hirshfeld, D. R., Rosenbaum, J. F., Biederman, J., Bolduc, E. A., Faraone, S. V., Snidman, N., Reznick, J. S., & Kagan, J. (1992). Stable behavioral inhibition and its association with anxiety disorder. *Journal of the American Academy of Child and Adolescent Psychiatry, 31,* 103–111.

Hirshfeld-Becker, D. R., Biederman, J., Faraone, S. V., Violette, H., Wrightsman, J., & Rosenbaum, J. F. (2002). Temperamental correlates of disruptive behavior disorders in young children: Preliminary findings. *Biological Psychiatry, 51,* 563–574.

Hinshaw, S. P., Lahey, B. B., & Hart, E. L. (1993). Issues of taxonomy and comorbidity in the development of conduct disorder. *Development and Psychopathology, 5,* 31–50.

Hoffman, M. L. (1982). Development of prosocial motivation: Empathy and guilt. In N. Eisenberg (Ed.), *The development of prosocial behavior* (pp. 281–313). New York: Academic Press.

Hogan, A. (1999). Cognitive functioning in children with oppositional defiant disorder and conduct disorder. In H. C. Quay & A. E. Hogan (Eds.), *Handbook of disruptive behavior disorders* (pp. 317–335). New York: Kluwer Academic/Plenum.

Hughes, C., Cutting, A. L., & Dunn, J. (2001). Acting nasty in the face of failure?: Longitudinal observations of "hard-to-manage" children playing a rigged competitive game with a friend. *Journal of Abnormal Child Psychology, 29,* 403–416.

Hughes, C., White, A., Sharpen, J., & Dunn, J. (2000). Antisocial, angry, and unsympathetic: "Hard-to-manage" preschoolers' peer problems and possible cognitive influences. *Journal of Child Psychology and Psychiatry, 41,* 169–179.

Jaffee, S., Caspi, A., Moffitt, T. E., & Silva, P. A. (2001). Why are children born to teen mothers at risk for adverse outcomes in young adulthood?: Results from a 20-year longitudinal study. *Development and Psychopathology, 13,* 377–397.

John, O. P., Caspi, A., Robins, R. W., Moffitt, T. E., & Stouthamer-Loeber, M. (1994). The "little five": Exploring the nomological network of the five-factor model of personality in adolescent boys. *Child Development, 65*, 160–178.

Kagan, J. (1992). Stable behavioral inhibition and its association with anxiety disorder. *Journal of the American Academy of Child and Adolescent Psychiatry, 31*, 103–111.

Kagan, J., Reznick, J. S., & Snidman, N. (1988). Biological bases of childhood shyness. *Science, 240*, 167–171.

Kagan, J., Reznick, J. S., Snidman, N., Gibbons, J., & Johnson, M. O. (1988). Childhood derivatives of inhibition and lack of inhibition to the unfamiliar. *Child Development, 59*, 1580–1589.

Keenan, K., Loeber, R., & Green, S. (1999). Conduct disorder in girls: A review of the literature. *Clinical Child and Family Psychology Review, 2*, 3–19.

Keenan, K., & Shaw, D. (1995). The development of coercive family processes: The interaction between aversive toddler behavior and parenting factors. In. J. McCord (Ed.), *Coercion and punishment in long-term perspectives* (pp. 165–180). New York: Cambridge University Press.

Keenan, K., & Shaw, D. (1997). Developmental and social influences on young girls' early problem behavior. *Psychological Bulletin, 121*, 95–113.

Kerr, M., Tremblay, R. E., Pagani-Kurtz, L., & Vitaro, F. (1997). Boy's behavioral inhibition and the risk of later delinquency. *Archives of General Psychiatry, 54*, 809–816.

Kilgore, K., Snyder, J., & Lentz, C. (2000). The contribution of parental discipline, parental monitoring, and school risk to early-onset conduct problems in African American boys and girls. *Developmental Psychology, 36*, 835–845.

Kingston, L., & Prior, M. (1995). The development of patterns of stable, transient, and school-age onset aggressive behavior in young children. *Journal of the American Academy of Child and Adolescent Psychiatry, 34*, 348–358.

Klerman, L. V. (1993). The relationship between adolescent parenthood and inadequate parenting. *Children and Youth Services Review, 15*, 309–320.

Kohlberg, L., Ricks, D., & Snarey, J. (1984). Childhood development as a predictor of adaptation in adulthood. *Genetic Psychology Monographs, 110*, 91–172.

Kratzer, L., & Hodgins, S. (1999). A typology of offenders: A test of Moffitt's theory among males and females from childhood to age 30. *Criminal Behaviour and Mental Health, 9*, 57–73.

Krueger, R. F. (1999). Personality traits in late adolescence predict mental disorders in early adulthood: A prospective-epidemiologic study. *Journal of Personality, 67*, 39–65.

Krueger, R. F., Schmutte, P. S., Caspi, A., Moffitt, T. E., Campbell, K., & Silva, P. A. (1994). Personality traits are linked to crime among males and females: Evidence from a birth cohort. *Journal of Abnormal Psychology, 103*, 328–338.

Lahey, B. B., Applegate, B., Barkley, R. A., Garfinkel, B., McBurnett, K., Kerdyk, L., Greenhill, L., Hynd, G. W., Frick, P. J., Newcorn, J., Biederman, J., Ollendick, T., Hart, E. L., Perez, D., Waldman, I., & Shaffer, D. (1994). DSM-IV field trials for oppositional defiant disorder and conduct disorder in children and adolescents. *American Journal of Psychiatry, 151*, 1163–1171.

Lahey, B. B., Applegate, B., & Waldman, I. D. (2001). *Three dimensions of personality/temperament related to child and adolescent psychopathology*. Presentation to the International Society for Research on Child and Adolescent Psychopathology, Vancouver, British Columbia, Canada.

Lahey, B. B., Gordon, R. A., Loeber, R., Stouthamer-Loeber, M., & Farrington, D. P. (1999). Boys who join gangs: A prospective study of predictors of first gang entry. *Journal of Abnormal Child Psychology, 27*, 261–276.

Lahey, B. B., & Loeber, R. (1994). Framework for a developmental model of oppositional defiant disorder and conduct disorder. In D. K. Routh (Ed.). *Disruptive behavior disorders in childhood*. New York: Plenum Press.

Lahey, B. B., Loeber, R., Burke, J., & Rathouz, P. J. (2002). Adolescent outcomes of childhood conduct disorder among clinic-referred boys: Predictors of improvement. *Journal of Abnormal Child Psychology, 30*, 333–348.

Lahey, B. B., Loeber, R., Quay, H. C., Applegate, B., Shaffer, D., Waldman, I., Hart, E. L., McBurnett, K., Frick, P. J., Jensen, P., Dulcan, M., Canino, G., & Bird, H. (1998). Validity of DSM-IV subtypes of conduct disorder based on age of onset. *Journal of the American Academy of Child and Adolescent Psychiatry, 37*, 435–442.

Lahey, B. B., McBurnett, K., & Loeber, R. (2000). Are attention-deficit hyperactivity disorder and oppositional defiant disorder developmental precursors to conduct disorder? In A. Sameroff, M. Lewis, & S. Miller (Eds.), *Handbook of developmental psychopathology* (2nd ed., pp. 431–446). New York: Plenum Press.

Lahey, B. B., Miller, T. L., Gordon, R. A., & Riley, A. (1999). Developmental epidemiology of the disruptive behavior disorders. In H. Quay & A. Hogan (Eds.), *Handbook of the disruptive behavior disorders.* San Antonio, TX: Academic Press.

Lahey, B. B., Piacentini, J. C., McBurnett, K., Stone, P. A., Hartdagen, S., & Hynd, G. W. (1988). Psychopathology in the parents of children with conduct disorder and hyperactivity. *Journal of the American Academy of Child and Adolescent Psychiatry, 27*, 163–170.

Lahey, B. B., Russo, M. F., Walker, J. L., & Piacentini, J. C. (1989). Personality characteristics of the mothers of children with disruptive behavior disorders. *Journal of Consulting and Clinical Psychology, 57*, 512–515.

Lahey, B. B., Schwab-Stone, M., Goodman, S. H., Waldman, I. D., Canino, G., Rathouz, P. J., Miller, T. L., Dennis, K. D., Bird, H., & Jensen, P. S. (2000). Age and gender differences in oppositional behavior and conduct problems: A cross-sectional household study of middle childhood and adolescence. *Journal of Abnormal Psychology, 109*, 488–503.

Lahey, B. B., Waldman, I. D., & McBurnett, K. (1999). The development of antisocial behavior: An integrative causal model. *Journal of Child Psychology and Psychiatry, 40*, 669–682.

Lake, R. I. E., Eaves, L. J., Maes, H. H. M., Heath, A. C., & Martin, N. G. (2000). Further evidence against the environmental transmission of individual differences in neuroticism from a collaborative study of 45,850 twins and relatives on two continents. *Behavior Genetics, 30*, 223–233.

Lemery, K. S., Essex, M. J., & Smider, N. A. (in press). Revealing the relationship between temperament and behavior problems by eliminating measurement confounding: Expert ratings and factor analysis. *Child Development.*

Levine, J. A., Pollack, H., & Comfort, M. E. (2001). Academic and behavioral outcomes among the children of young mothers. *Journal of Marriage and the Family, 63*, 355–369.

Loeber, R. (1982). The stability of antisocial and delinquent behavior: A review. *Child Development, 53*, 1431–1446.

Loeber, R. (1988). Natural histories of conduct problems, delinquency, and associated substance abuse: Evidence for developmental progressions. In B. B. Lahey & A. E. Kazdin (Eds.), *Advances in clinical child psychology* (Vol. 11). New York: Plenum Press.

Loeber, R., Farrington, D. P., Stouthamer-Loeber, M., & Van Kammen, W. (1998). *Antisocial behavior and mental health problems: Explanatory factors in childhood and adolescence.* Mahwah, NJ: Erlbaum.

Loeber, R., Green, S. M., Keenan, K., & Lahey, B. B. (1995). Which boys will fare worse?: Early predictors of the onset of conduct disorder in a six-year longitudinal study. *Journal of the American Academy of Child and Adolescent Psychiatry, 34*, 499–509.

Loeber, R., & Keenan, K. (1994). Interaction between conduct disorder and its comorbid conditions: Effects of age and gender. *Clinical Psychology Review, 14*, 497–523.

Loeber, R., & Tengs, T. (1986). The analysis of coercive chains between children, mothers, and siblings. *Journal of Family Violence, 1*, 51–70.

Luengo, M. A., Otero, J. M., Carrillo-de-la-Pena, M. T., & Miron, L. (1994). Dimensions of antisocial behaviour in juvenile delinquency: A study of personality variables. *Psychology Crime and Law, 1*, 27–37.

Lynam, D. R. (1998). Early identification of the fledgling psychopath: Locating the psycho-pathic child in the current nomenclature. *Journal of Abnormal Psychology, 107,* 566–575.

Lynam, D., Moffitt, T., & Stouthamer-Loeber, M. (1993). Explaining the relation between IQ and delinquency: Class, race, test motivation, school failure or self-control? *Journal of Abnormal Psychology, 102,* 187–196.

Macaskill, G. T., Hopper, J. L., White, V., & Hill, D. J. (1994). Genetic and environmental variation in Eysenck Personality Questionnaire scales measured on Australian adolescent twins. *Behavior Genetics, 24,* 481–491.

Mason, D. A., & Frick, P. J. (1994). The heritability of antisocial behavior: A meta-analysis of twin and adoption studies. *Journal of Psychopathology and Behavioral Assessment, 16,* 301–322.

Maszk, P., Eisenberg, N., & Guthrie, I. K. (1999). Relations of children's social status to their emotionality and regulation: A short-term longitudinal study. *Merrill-Palmer Quarterly, 45,* 468–492.

Matthews, K. A., Batson, C. D., Horn, J., & Rosenman, R. H. (1981). "Principles in his nature which interest him in the fortune of others . . . ": The heritability of empathic concern for others. *Journal of Personality, 49,* 237–247.

McGue, M., Bacon, S., & Lykken, D. T. (1993). Personality stability and change in early adult-hood: A behavioral genetic analysis. *Developmental Psychology, 29,* 96–109.

McRae, R. R., & Costa, P. T. (1987). Validation of the five-factor model of personality across instruments and observers. *Journal of Personality and Social Psychology, 52,* 81–90.

Meltzer, H., Gatward, R., Goodman, R., & Ford, T. (2000). *Mental health of children and adolescents in Great Britain.* London: Her Majesty's Stationery Office.

Meyer, J. M., Rutter, M., Silberg, J. L., Maes, H. H., Simonoff, E., Shillady, L. L., Pickles, A., Hewitt, J. K., & Eaves, L. J. (2000). Familial aggregation for conduct disorder symptomatology: The role of genes, marital discord and family adaptability. *Psychological Medicine, 30,* 759–774.

Miech, R. A., Caspi, A., Moffitt, T. E., Wright, B. R. E., & Silva, P. A. (1999). Low socioeconomic status and mental disorders: A longitudinal study of selection and causation during young adulthood. *American Journal of Sociology, 104,* 1096–1131.

Miles, D. R., & Carey, G. (1997). Genetic and environmental architecture of human aggression. *Journal of Personality and Social Psychology, 72,* 207–217.

Miller, J. D., & Lynam, D. R. (2001). Structural models of personality and their relation to antisocial behavior: A meta-analytic review. *Criminology, 39,* 765–792.

Miller, P. A., & Eisenberg, N. (1988). The relation of empathy to aggressive and externalizing/antisocial behavior. *Psychological Bulletin, 103,* 324–344.

Mitchell, S., & Rosa, P. (1981). Boyhood behaviour problems as precursors of criminality: A fifteen year study. *Journal of Child Psychology and Psychiatry, 22,* 19–33.

Moffitt, T. E. (1990). Juvenile delinquency and attention deficit disorder: Boys' developmental trajectories from age 3 to 15. *Child Development, 61,* 893–910.

Moffitt, T. E. (1993). Adolescence-limited and life-course-persistent antisocial behavior: A developmental taxonomy. *Psychological Review, 100,* 674–701.

Moffitt, T. E., Caspi, A., Dickson, N., Silva, P., & Stanton, W. (1996). Childhood-onset versus adolescent-onset antisocial conduct problems in males: Natural history from ages 3 to 18 years. *Development and Psychopathology, 8,* 399–424.

Moffitt, T. E., Caspi, A., Harrington, H., & Milne, B. J. (2002). Males on the life-course-persistent and adolescence-limited antisocial pathways: Follow-up at age 26 years. *Development and Psychopathology, 14,* 179–207.

Moffitt, T. E., Caspi, A., Rutter, M., & Silva, P. A. (2001). *Sex differences in antisocial behaviour.* Cambridge, UK: Cambridge University Press.

Moffitt, T. E., & Silva, P. A. (1988). IQ and delinquency: A direct test of the differential detection hypothesis. *Journal of Abnormal Psychology, 97,* 330–333.

Nagin, D. S., Pogarsky, G., & Farrington, D. P. (1997). Adolescent mothers and the criminal behavior of their children. *Law and Society Review*, *31*, 137–162.

Nagin D., & Tremblay, R. E. (1999). Trajectories of boys' physical aggression, opposition, and hyperactivity on the path to physically violent and non-violent delinquency. *Child Development*, *70*, 1181–1196.

Nagin, D. S., & Tremblay, R. E. (2001). Parental and early childhood predictors of persistent physical aggression in boys from kindergarten to high school. *Archives of General Psychiatry*, *58*, 389–394.

Newcomb, M. D., & McGee, L. (1991). Influence of sensation seeking on general deviance and specific problem behaviors from adolescence to young adulthood. *Journal of Personality and Social Psychology*, *61*, 614–628.

Newman, J. P., Widom, C. S., & Stewart, N. (1985). Passive avoidance in syndromes of disinhibition: Psychopathy and extraversion. *Journal of Personality and Social Psychology*, *48*, 1316–1327.

O'Connor, T. G., Neiderhiser, J. M., Reiss, D., Hetherington, E. M., & Plomin, R. (1998). Genetic contributions to continuity, change, and co-occurrence of antisocial and depressive symptoms in adolescence. *Journal of Child Psychology and Psychiatry*, *39*, 323–336.

Office of Juvenile Justice and Delinquency Prevention. (2002). *National youth gang survey trends from 1996 to 2000*. Washington, DC: Author.

Olson, S. L., Bates, J. E., Sandy, J. M., & Lanthier, R. (2000). Early developmental precursors of externalizing behavior in middle childhood and adolescence. *Journal of Abnormal Child Psychology*, *28*, 119–133.

Pagani, L., Tremblay, R. E., Vitaro, F., Boulerice, B., & McDuff, P. (2001). Effects of grade retention on academic performance and behavioral development. *Development and Psychopathology*, *13*, 297–315.

Patterson, G. R. (1982). *Coercive family interactions*. Eugene, OR: Castalia.

Patterson, G. R., Reid, J. B., & Dishion, T. J. (1992). *Antisocial boys*. Eugene, OR: Castalia.

Pedersen, N. L., Plomin, R., McClearn, G. E., & Friberg, L. (1988). Neuroticism, extraversion, and related traits in adult twins reared apart and reared together. *Journal of Personality and Social Psychology*, *55*, 950–957.

Pennington, B. F., & Ozonoff, S. (1996). Executive functions and developmental psychopathology. *Journal of Child Psychology and Psychiatry*, *37*, 51–87.

Petrill, S. A., Saudino, K., Cherny, S. S., Emde, R. N., Hewitt, J. K., Fulker, D. W., & Plomin, R. (1997). Exploring the genetic etiology of low general cognitive ability from 14 to 36 months. *Developmental Psychology*, *33*, 544–548.

Phillips, K., & Matheny, A. P. (1997). Evidence for genetic influence on both cross-situation and situation-specific components of behavior. *Journal of Personality and Social Psychology*, *73*, 129–138.

Pickles, A., Pickering, K., Simonoff, E., Silberg, J., Meyer, J., & Maes, H. (1998). Genetic "clocks" and "soft" events: A twin model for pubertal development and other recalled sequences of developmental milestones, transitions, or ages at onset. *Behavior Genetics*, *28*, 243–253.

Plomin, R., DeFries, J. C., & Loehlin, J. C. (1977). Genotype–environment interaction and correlation in the analysis of human behavior. *Psychological Bulletin*, *84*, 309–322.

Plomin, R., & Petrill, S. A. (1997). Genetics and intelligence: What's new? *Intelligence*, *24*, 53–77.

Powell, G. E., & Stewart, R. A. (1983). The relationship of personality to antisocial and neurotic behaviours as observed by teachers. *Personality and Individual Differences*, *4*, 97–100.

Presley, R., & Martin, R. P. (1994). Toward a structure of preschool temperament: Factor structure of the Temperament Assessment Battery for Children. *Journal of Personality*, *62*, 415–448.

Quay, H. C., & Love, C. T. (1977). The effect of a juvenile diversion program on rearrests. *Criminal Justice and Behavior*, *4*, 377–396.

Rahman, A. (1992). Psychological factors in criminality. *Personality and Individual Differences*, *13*, 483–485.

Raine, A., Reynolds, C., Venables, P. H., Mednick, S. A., & Farrington, D. P. (1998). Fearlessness, stimulation-seeking, and large body size at age 3 years as early predispositions to childhood aggression at age 11 years. *Archives of General Psychiatry*, *55*, 745–751.

Reid, J. B., & Patterson, G. R. (1989). The development of antisocial behavior patterns in childhood and adolescence. *European Journal of Personality*, *3*, 107–119.

Rhee, S. H., & Waldman, I. D. (2002). Genetic and environmental influences on antisocial behavior: A meta-analysis of twin and adoption studies. *Psychological Bulletin*, *128*, 490–529.

Roberts, S., & Kendler, K. S. (1999). Neuroticism and self-esteem as indices of the vulnerability to major depression in women. *Psychological Medicine*, *29*, 1101–1109.

Robins, R. W., Johns, O. P., Caspi, A., Moffitt, T. E., & Stouthamer-Loeber, M. (1996). Resilient, overcontrolled, and undercontrolled boys: Three replicable personality types. *Journal of Personality and Social Psychology*, *70*, 157–171.

Robinson, J. L., Kagan, J., Reznick, J. S., & Corley, R. (1992). The heritability of inhibited and unihibited behavior: A twin study. *Developmental Psychology*, *28*, 1030–1037.

Rodgers, J. L., Muster, M., & Rowe, D. C. (2001). Genetic and environmental influences on delinquency: DF analysis of NLSY kinship data. *Journal of Quantitative Criminology*, *17*, 145–168.

Rothbart, M. K., Ahadi, S. A., Hershey, K. L., & Fisher, P. (2001). Investigations of temperament at three to seven years: The Children's Behavior Questionnaire. *Child Development*, *72*, 1394–1408.

Rowe, D. C. (1983). Biometrical genetic models of self-reported delinquent behavior: A twin study. *Behavior Genetics*, *13*, 473–489.

Rowe, D. C., Almeida, D. M., & Jacobson, K. C. (1999). School context and genetic influences on aggression in adolescence. *Psychological Science*, *10*, 277–280.

Rowe, D. C., & Flannery, D. J. (1994). An examination of environmental and trait influences on adolescent delinquency. *Journal of Research in Crime and Delinquency*, *31*, 374–389.

Rowe, D. C., & Osgood, D. W. (1984). Heredity and sociology theories of delinquency: A reconsideration. *American Sociological Review*, *49*, 526–540.

Rowe, D. C., Vazsonyi, A. T., & Flannery, D. J. (1995). Sex differences in crime: Do means and within-sex variation have similar causes? *Journal of Research in Crime and Delinquency*, *32*, 84–100.

Rushton, J. P., & Chrisjohn, R. D. (1981). Extraversion, neuroticism, psychoticism and self-reported delinquency: Evidence from eight separate samples. *Personality and Individual Differences*, *2*, 11–20.

Rushton, J. P., Fulker, D. W., Neale, M. C., Nias, D. K., & Eysenck, H. J. (1986). Altruism and aggression: The heritability of individual differences. *Journal of Personality and Social Psychology*, *50*, 1192–1198.

Russo, M. F., Stokes, G. S., Lahey, B. B., Christ, M. A. G., McBurnett, K., Loeber, R., Southamer-Loeber, M., & Green, S. M. (1993). A sensation seeking scale for children: Further refinement and psychometric development. *Journal of Psychopathology and Behavior Assessment*, *15*, 69–86.

Rutter, M. L. (1997). Nature–nurture integration: The example of antisocial behavior. *American Psychologist*, *52*, 390–398.

Rutter, M., Dunn, J., Plomin, R., Siminoff, E., Pickles, A., Maughan, B., Ormel, J., Meyer, J., & Eaves, L. (1997). Integrating nature and nurture: Implications of person–environment correlations and interactions for developmental psychopathology. *Development and Psychopathology*, *9*, 335–364.

Sampson, R. J., & Laub, J. H. (1992). Crime and deviance. *Annual Review of Sociology*, *18*, 63–84.

Sanson, A., Pedlow, R., Cann, W., Prior, M., & Oberklaid, F. (1996). Shyness ratings: Stability and correlates in early childhood. *International Journal of Behavioral Development, 19,* 705–724.

Sanson, A., & Prior, M. (1999). Temperament and behavioral precursors to oppositional defiant disorder and conduct disorder. In H. Quay & A. Hogan (Eds.), *Handbook of the disruptive behavior disorders* (pp. 397–417). New York: Kluwer Academic/Plenum.

Sanson, A., Smart, D., Prior, M., & Oberklaid, F. (1993). Precursors of hyperactivity and aggression. *Journal of the American Academy of Child and Adolescent Psychiatry, 32,* 1207–1216.

Saudino, K. J., Plomin, R., & DeFries, J. C. (1996). Tester-rated temperament at 14, 20 and 24 months: Environmental change and genetic continuity. *British Journal of Developmental Psychology, 14,* 129–144.

Schmeck, K., & Poustka, F. (2001). Temperament and disruptive behavior disorders. *Psychopathology, 4,* 159–163.

Schmitz, S., Fulker, D. W., & Mrazek, D. A. (1995). Problem behavior in early and middle childhood: An initial behavior genetic analysis. *Journal of Child Psychology and Psychiatry, 36,* 1443–1458.

Schmitz, S., Fulker, D. W., Plomin, R., Zahn-Waxler, C., Emde, R. N., & DeFries, J. C. (1999). Temperament and problem behavior during early childhood. *International Journal of Behavioral Development, 23,* 333–355.

Schwartz, C. E., Snidman, N., & Kagan, J. (1996). Early childhood temperament as a determinant of externalizing behavior in adolescence. *Developmental Psychopathology, 8,* 527–537.

Seguin, J. R., Boulerice, B., Harden, P. W., Tremblay, R. E., & Pihl, R. O. (1999). Executive functions and physical aggression after controlling for attention deficit hyperactivity disorder, general memory and IQ. *Journal of Child Psychology and Psychiatry, 40,* 1197–1208.

Serbin, L. A., Moskowitz, D. S., Schwartzman, A. E., & Ledingham, J. E. (1991). Aggressive, withdrawn, and aggressive/withdrawn children in adolescence: Into the next generation. In D. J. Pepler & K. H. Rubin (Eds.), *The development and treatment of childhood aggression.* Hillsdale, NJ: Erlbaum.

Shapland, J., & Rushton, J. P. (1975). Crime and personality: Further evidence. *Bulletin of the British Psychological Society, 28,* 66–67.

Sigvardsson, S., Bohman, M., & Cloninger, C. R. (1987). Structure and stability of childhood personality: Prediction of later social adjustment. *Journal of Child Psychology and Psychiatry, 28,* 929–946.

Silberg, J. L., Rutter, M., Meyer, J., Maes, H., Hewitt, J., Siminoff, E., Pickles, A., Loeber, R., & Eaves, L. (1996). Genetic and environmental influences on the covariation between hyperactivity and conduct disturbance in juvenile twins. *Journal of Child Psychology and Psychiatry, 37,* 803–816.

Silverthorn, P., & Frick, P. J. (1999). Developmental pathways to antisocial behavior: The delayed-onset pathway in girls. *Development and Psychopathology, 11,* 101–126.

Silverthorn, P., Frick, P. J., & Reynolds, R. (2001). Timing of onset and correlates of severe conduct problems in adjudicated girls and boys. *Journal of Psychopathology and Behavioral Assessment, 23,* 171–181.

Simo, S., & Perez, J. (1991). Sensation seeking and antisocial behaviour in a junior student sample. *Personality and Individual Differences, 12,* 965–966.

Sparks, R., Ganschow, L., & Thomas, A. (1996). Role of intelligence tests in speech/language referrals. *Perceptual and Motor Skills, 83,* 195–204.

Stattin, H., & Klackenberg-Larsson, I. (1993). Early language and intelligence development and their relationship to future criminal behavior. *Journal of Abnormal Psychology, 102,* 369–378.

Tellegen, A. (1982). *Brief manual for the Multidimensional Personality Questionnaire.* Minneapolis: University of Minnesota.

Tellegen, A., Lykken, D. T., Bouchard, T. J., Wilcox, K. J., Segal, N. L., & Rich, S. (1988). Personality similarity in twins reared apart and together. *Journal of Personality and Social Psychology, 54*, 1031–1039.

Thapar, A., Harrington, R., & McGuffin, P. (2001). Examining the comorbidity of ADHD-related behaviours and conduct problems using a twin study design. *British Jounal of Psychiatry, 179*, 224–229.

Thornberry, T. P., Krohn, M. D., Lizotte, A. J., & Chard-Wierschem, D. (1993). The role of juvenile gangs in facilitating delinquent behavior. *Journal of Research in Crime and Delinquency, 30*, 55–87.

Tranah, T., Harnett, P., & Yule, W. (1998). Conduct disorder and personality. *Personality and Individual Differences, 24*, 741–745.

Tremblay, R. E. (2000). The development of aggressive behaviour during childhood: What have we learned in the past century? *International Journal of Behavioral Development, 24*, 129–141.

Tremblay, R. E., Boulerice, B., Harden, P. W., McDuff, P., Perusse, D., Pihl, R. O., & Zoccolillo, M. (1996). Do children in Canada become more aggressive as they approach adolescence? In M. Cappe & I. Fellegi (Eds.), *Growing up in Canada*. Ottawa, Ontario: Statistics Canada.

Tremblay, R. E., Japel, C., Perusse, D., McDuff, P., Boivin, M., Zoccolillo, M., & Montplaisir, J. (1999). The search for the age of "onset" of physical aggression: Rousseau and Bandura revisited. *Criminal Behaviour and Mental Health, 9*, 8–23.

Tremblay, R. E., Pihl, R. O., Vitaro, F., & Dobkin, P. L. (1994). Predicting early onset of male antisocial behavior from preschool behavior. *Archives of General Psychiatry, 51*, 732–739.

van den Oord, E. J., Boomsma, D. I., & Verhulst, F. C. (1994). A study of problem behaviors in 10- to 15-year old biologically related and unrelated international adoptees. *Behavior Genetics, 24*, 193–205.

Wahler, R. G., & Hann, D. M. (1987). An interbehavioral approach to clinical child psychology: Toward an understanding of troubled families. In D. H. Ruben & D. J. Delpratto (Eds.), *New ideas in therapy: Introduction to an interdisciplinary approach*. New York: Greenwood Press.

Wakschlag, L. S., Gordon, R. A., Lahey, B. B., Loeber, R., Green, S. M., & Leventhal, B. L. (2000). Maternal age at first birth and boys' risk for conduct disorder. *Journal of Research on Adolescence, 10*, 417–441.

Waldman, I. D. (1996). Aggressive children's hostile perceptual and response biases: The role of attention and impulsivity. *Child Development, 67*, 1015–1033.

Waldman, I. D., Rhee, S. H., Levy, F., & Hay, D. A. (2001). Genetic and environmental influences on the covariation among symptoms of attention deficit hyperactivity disorder, oppositional defiant disorder, and conduct disorder. In D. A. Hay & F. Levy (Eds.), *Attention, genes, and ADHD*. Hillsdale, NJ: Erlbaum.

Waschbusch, D. A. (2002). A meta-analytic examination of comorbid hyperactive-impulsive-attention problems and conduct problems. *Psychological Bulletin, 128*, 118–150.

Wasson, A. S. (1980). Stimulus-seeking, perceived school environment and school misbehavior. *Adolescence, 15*, 603–608.

Watson, D., Clark, L. A., & Tellegen, A. (1988). Development and validation of brief measures of positive and negative affect: The PANAS scales. *Journal of Personality and Social Psychology, 54*, 1063–1070.

Zahn-Waxler, C., Robinson, J. L., & Emde, R. N. (1992). The development of empathy in twins. *Developmental Psychology, 28*, 1038–1047.

Zhou, Q., Eisenberg, N., Losoya, S. H., Fabes, R. A., Reiser, M., Guthrie, I. K., Murphy, B. C., Cumberland, A. J., & Shepard, S. (2002). The relations of parental warmth and positive expressiveness to children's empathy-related responding and social functioning: A longitudinal study. *Child Development, 73*, 893–915.

Zoccolillo, M. (1992). Co-occurrence of conduct disorder and its adult outcomes with depressive and anxiety disorders: A review. *Journal of the American Academy of Child and Adolescent Psychiatry, 31*, 547–556.

Zuckerman, M. (1996). The psychobiological model for impulsive unsocialized sensation seeking: A comparative approach. *Neuropsychobiology, 34*, 125–129.

Zuckerman, M., Kuhlman, D. M., Joireman, J., Teta, P., & Kraft, M. (1993). A comparison of three structural models for personality: The big three, the big five, and the alternative five. *Journal of Personality and Social Psychology, 65*, 757–768.

$\boxed{5}$

# Social Mechanisms of Community Influences on Crime and Pathways in Criminality

PER-OLOF H. WIKSTRÖM
ROBERT J. SAMPSON

The correlation between community contextual characteristics and levels of criminal offending has long been documented in criminological research. However, the causal mechanisms that link contextual features of communities to acts of offending are poorly understood. To improve our understanding of the influence of community characteristics on crime we need to (1) better theorize the mechanisms that link community contextual characteristics to acts of crime and individual pathways in criminality, (2) advance methods and improve measurements of the community context and its characteristics (ecometrics), and (3) focus our efforts on exploring cross-level interactions—that is, the interactions between individuals and contexts in producing acts of crime and shaping individual pathways in criminality. This chapter aims to contribute to theories of crime causation by advancing criminological approaches to these three realms.

## STATE OF THE FIELD

The role of the community context for offending has (re-)emerged as a key topic within criminology. Indeed, the need to better understand the causal mechanisms by which community contextual characteristics influence crime and pathways in crime, especially the role of concentrated neighborhood disadvantage, has come to occupy a prominent place in academic as well as policy discussions (e.g., Sampson, Morenoff, & Gannon-Rowley, 2002; Wilson, 1987). It may be argued that to advance our knowledge about the causes of crime we particularly need to better address questions about the potential interaction between individual and community characteristics in producing acts of crime and pathways in criminality (e.g., Wikström, 1998; Wikström & Loeber, 2000). A special problem in advancing knowledge about community contextual influences is that, in comparison with psychometrics, what has been called "ecometrics," that is, the measurement of ecological settings, is highly underdeveloped (see Raudenbush & Sampson, 1999). Overall, we believe that the field of criminology is characterized by the following major limitations to knowledge on the community-level causes of crime.

1. *Studies of developmental pathways have neglected the influence of the wider social context.* Research on criminal careers and individual development documents some distinctive developmental patterns in onset, duration, variation, escalation, and termination of offending (e.g., Blumstein, Cohen, Roth, & Visher, 1986; Farrington & Wikström, 1993; LeBlanc & Fréchette, 1989). The likelihood of offending is significantly correlated to individual dispositions, for example, impulsiveness, and immediate social situations, for example, family conditions (e.g., Loeber & Farrington 1999; Wilson & Herrnstein, 1985). However, this research largely neglects the importance of the wider contexts in which criminal pathways are embedded. This includes meso- (e.g., communities) and macroenvironments (e.g., systems of welfare and public health provision, patterns of inequality, and residential segregation). The same holds for developmental research more generally, as pointed out by Brooks-Gunn, Duncan, Klebanov, and Sealand (1993): "The bulk of developmental research has focused on the most proximal environments, specifically the family and the peer group . . . and has largely ignored neighborhood contexts" (p. 354).

2. *Research on individual risk factors has largely failed to specify in any detail the causal mechanisms that link the risk factors to acts of crime and pathways in criminality.* Most research on individual development of offending uses the risk-and-protective-factors paradigm. Many individual and microenvironmental factors correlate with involvement in crime. These include, for example, impulsiveness, lack of guilt, broken family, poor parenting, parental criminality, child abuse, delinquent peers, and poor academic performance. However, "a major problem of the risk factor paradigm is to determine which risk factors are causes and which are merely markers or correlated with causes" (Farrington, 2000, p. 7).

3. *Research on environmental influences has largely failed to specify in any detail the causal mechanisms that link social context with crime and pathways in crime.* Offending rates vary by neighborhood context (e.g., Baldwin & Bottoms, 1976; Sampson & Groves, 1989; Shaw & McKay, 1969; Wikström, 1991; Wikström & Dolmén, 2001). Theories

have been developed to account for this relationship, most notably in the social disorganization/collective efficacy tradition, focusing on the effects of structural characteristics of neighborhoods (e.g., concentrated poverty, residential mobility, and population heterogeneity) on community social organization (e.g., levels of social capital, social integration/cohesion, and informal social control) and its association with offending and victimization (e.g., Kornhauser, 1978; Sampson, Raudenbush, & Earls, 1997). There seems to be a general agreement among researchers in this tradition that influences on offending behavior by community structural characteristics are largely mediated by dimensions of community social organization.

Research has also shown links between routine activities (e.g., the everyday organization of family life, work, and leisure) and crime (Cohen & Felson, 1979) and between lifestyles/individual routines and offending risks (Osgood, Wilson, O'Malley, Bachman, & Johnston, 1996; West & Farrington, 1977; Wikström, 2002). The community dimensions of routine activities and lifestyles research, however, have been seriously neglected (e.g., Bursik & Grasmick, 1993). The social disorganization/collective efficacy tradition implies the importance of routine activities and lifestyles (e.g., through the centrality of the concept of informal social control), but neither it nor routine activities/lifestyles research specify in any detail how social mechanisms link community organization and routines to criminal acts and pathways in crime (Wikström, 1998). Elliott et al. (1996) rightly observe that "the theoretical and empirical discussion of neighborhood effects is still at a rudimentary level" (pp. 389–390).

4. *Interactions between individual characteristics and community contexts in producing criminal acts and shaping pathways in crime are poorly understood.* Few studies have sought to disentangle the simultaneous effects of contextual and individual factors (e.g., Gottfredson, McNeill, & Gottfredson, 1991; Kupersmidt et al., 1995; Reiss & Rhodes, 1961). Wider contextual influences on pathways in crime, and interactions between contextual and individual influences, have scarcely been studied (cf. Loeber & Wikström, 1993; Wikström & Loeber, 2000). Much more is to be gained from integrating individual and environmental approaches than from their continued separate development (e.g., Farrington, Sampson, & Wikström, 1993; LeBlanc, 1997; Tonry, Ohlin, & Farrington, 1991). Sampson has noted that, "few studies have successfully demonstrated a unified approach to the individual and community level dimensions of crime" (Sampson, 1997, p. 32). Farrington observed that "researchers interested in neighbourhood influences have generally not adequately measured individual and family influences, just as researchers interested in individual and family influences have generally not adequately measured neighbourhood influences" (Farrington, 1993, p. 30).

5. *Existing approaches to crime prevention and policy are poorly integrated.* Existing community, developmental, situational, and criminal

justice approaches to crime control and prevention are poorly integrated, and based on an inadequate understanding of the interactions between individual and contextual factors. Crime prevention initiatives tend to target individuals, their development, or criminogenic situations (Wikström, Clarke, & McCord, 1995). Few integrated strategies have been formulated (cf. Wikström & Torstensson, 1999), and fewer have been implemented. And yet, "preventive strategies that are based on knowledge of 'kinds of individuals' in 'kinds of contexts' may have higher potential to be effective than strategies that pinpoint either the individual or the context" (Wikström & Loeber, 2000, p. 1203).

## CAUSAL MECHANISMS

It can be argued that the key objective of social science is to discover patterns in social life and offer explanations for them. To do so, we need to map out the correlates of social action and try to understand the underlying causal mechanisms at work. A causal mechanism may be viewed as a plausible (unobservable) process that links the cause and the effect (for discussions of social mechanisms, see Hedström & Swedberg, 1998). Some correlates of crime may be spurious associations, whereas others may help to identify what social mechanisms cause a particular social action. An important task is therefore to evaluate the correlates for their potential as representing causal mechanisms in relation to what constitutes social action.

The basic position taken here is that social actions, including criminal offending, ultimately are a result of individual choice and perception of alternatives, and that the key challenge for social science research is to understand the mechanisms by which individual characteristics and contextual factors, independently or in interaction, influence individual perceptions of alternatives and processes of choice. A key question for criminology then becomes, *What causal mechanisms make people consider and choose to act upon options that constitute acts of crime?* In this section we first briefly outline the causal mechanisms linking proximate factors and offending behavior. On this basis, we then go on to discuss the causal mechanisms linking the more distant (indirect) influence by the wider community context (structural and organizational characteristics) on offending behavior and pathways in crime.

### Proximate Causal Mechanisms

An act of crime may be seen as primarily caused by the individual's *reason* (motivation) to commit the particular act of crime, emerging from the interaction between the *individual's propensity* to engage in criminality and *the criminogenic features of the behavior setting* in which the individual

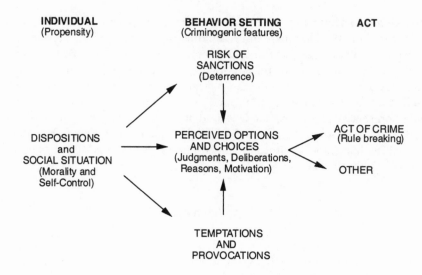

FIGURE 5.1. Unlawful acts: Proximate causal factors. Modified from Wikström (1998).

finds him- or herself (Figure 5.1). The motivational argument is basically that some types of behavior settings are more likely than other settings to make the individual see crime as an option and then to act upon such an option. The propensity argument is basically that different individuals in the same behavior setting will vary as regards their likelihood to see crime as an option and to act upon such an option.

The potential role in this of the community context is, at least, two-fold. First, it may influence (in the longer term) an individual's development of characteristics relevant to the (future) propensity to breach the rules of law and lifestyles that contribute to the shaping of pathways in criminality (e.g., by influencing processes of onset, duration, desistance, and escalation). Second, it may influence (in the short term) the prevalence of criminogenic behavior settings that confront individuals in their day-to-day living and therefore impact upon their motivation to offend.

## Acts of Crime

Acts of crime include a wide range of different types of behaviors (e.g., shoplifting, rape, tax evasion, assassinations). The only thing they have in common is that they are *the breaking of rules sanctioned by the state*. Explaining acts of crime is therefore ultimately about explaining why people choose to break a rule of law, not about why they chose to commit a specific act.[1] To explain acts of crime we do not necessarily need to be concerned with questions about why an act is considered a crime, and whether (morally) it is right or wrong that the particular act is criminalized.[2] This argument is easily extended to also include the explanation of violations of other socially defined rules and conventions.

## Reasons (Motivations)

The body and its biological makeup defines the individual. A human being has *agency* (powers to make things happen intentionally), which include committing acts of crime. Understanding *actions* (behavior under the person's guidance) is fundamentally about understanding individual *perception of options* and their *choices* (including the option to do nothing or just seeing one option).

It can be argued that the direct cause of social acts like crime is the *reason* (or motivation) a person has for committing the act (Davidson, 1980). An individual's reason for a particular act is traditionally viewed as made up of his or her *desires* (e.g., for gain, security, or respect[3]) and *beliefs* (e.g., about what actions would result in achieving gain, security, or respect), but should also, according to Schick (1991), include an *understanding* of the act and the situation (e.g., a person wants a CD player, he believes that he could obtain a CD player through shoplifting, but he doesn't see an act of theft as a way in which he would like to get a CD player). Schick (1997) refers to desires and beliefs as grounds for action and understandings as "the psychological context" (Schick, 1991, p. 84) or "our conceivings and labellings of the facts understood" (Schick, 1997, p. 23).[4]

Reasons for actions do not need to be wholly rational in the sense that they only result from evaluations of cost and benefits in relation to best possible future outcomes. They can (simultaneously) be more or less oriented toward the *past* (norms and habits), the *present* (judgments, problem solving), and the *future* (outcomes and consequences).[5] This is an important point since, although all actions involve some kind of choice, the choice may sometimes be more or less an expression of an individual norm or habit. For example, for many people the reason why they never or rarely see crime as an option may be that committing a crime is "something they just do not do," making fear of possible future negative consequences irrelevant to their choice whether or not to commit a crime.

It seems plausible to argue that reasons for action and their associated *emotions* (be they predominantly oriented toward the past, the present, or the future) emerge in situations and that they therefore primarily have to do with *within-individual variation* in motivation (although this is not the same as saying that different individuals are likely to react identically in the same setting). Philosophically oriented discussions of people's reasons for action do not pay much attention to the role of individual differences. However, it is conceivable that what reasons people have for their actions is largely a reflection of their set of individual characteristics (their *disposi-*

*tions* [e.g., skills, temperament, conscience], and their *immediate social situation* [e.g., financial and social resources, social bonds/attachments][6]) and the context in which they operate (the characteristics of the behavior settings they are confronted with). Individual characteristics and behavioral contexts may therefore be viewed as potential *causes of the motivation* for engaging in crime, that is, *indirectly causing offending behavior* through their impact on peoples desires, beliefs, and understandings.[7]

## Propensity

Although all individuals have the capability to commit acts of crime, there is a significant variation in individual involvement in criminality (e.g., Farrington, 2002; Moffitt, 1993; Wikström, 1987; Wolfgang & Figlio, 1972). It is plausible that part of this difference is due to more stable *between-individual variations* in the propensity to engage in acts of crime, that is, the readiness to react aggressively and to act upon desires in an unlawful way. From a holistic point of view, the individual propensity *to act unlawfully* may be thought of as primarily made up of specific cognitive and emotional characteristics that jointly determine morality and self-control. Individual *morality* may be defined in terms of an evaluative function of events in the world. It includes what the individual cares about, how strongly he or she cares about different things, how he or she thinks he or she should relate to other people, and what he or she considers as right and wrong (and associated feelings such as guilt and empathy[8]). For example, how important is it for him or her to follow the rules of the law regulating his or her relationship to others and their property? This is primarily a result of his or her internalized norms and social bonds.[9] Individuals' *self-control* may be defined as their capability to inhibit or interrupt a response as an effect of the executive functions of their brain (e.g., Barkley, 1997, pp. 51–58; Shonkoff & Phillips, 2000, pp. 93–123)—for example, their capability to resist acting upon a temptation or provocation that if carried through would constitute a breach of the law.[10]

An individual's morality has obvious implications for how he or she would see different *options* and what kind of options he or she might consider (his or her understandings of specific acts and situations), while the level of self-control has obvious implications for the individual's process of choice, that is, his or her degree of *reflection* and *deliberation* before making up his or her mind. Some individuals may never or only rarely consider breaking the law; others may have no or few problems with the thought of carrying out acts of crime. Some individuals may tend to act more on the spur of the moment; others may tend to more carefully consider the consequences of their actions. For example, it seems reasonable to assume that individuals who care strongly about following the law (and more broadly social conventions and rules) and who have high levels of self-control will less often feel motivated to act unlawfully than those for whom the reverse applies.[11]

If one accepts, at any given moment, that people vary in their propensity to engage in criminal activities, the key question then becomes *why* people vary in their morality and self-control (i.e., in their propensity to engage in crime) and what role, if any, community contexts play in generating individual differences in morality and self-control.

## Behavior Settings

The environment is all that is external to the person and that may influence (enable or constrain and guide) his or her actions, including offending behavior. Individuals' environments may be thought of as the configuration of *behavior settings*[12] (embedded in the wider cultural and structural behavioral context) that they are *exposed to* in the course of their day-to-day living. Individuals' encounters with behavior settings create *situations* (perception of options and prospects) in which the individuals may express their propensities by making judgments and choices resulting in actions.

It is plausible that some types of behavior settings are more likely than others to create situations in which individuals may act unlawfully. This assumption is consistent with the fact that crimes are far from randomly distributed in time and space, and that the occurrence of specific types of crimes tends to be linked to specific types of legal activities—for example, violence between strangers mostly occurs in the course of public entertainment activities (e.g., Block & Block, 1995; Wikström, 1991, pp. 229–231). The fact that even the most prolific offenders only spend a marginal proportion of their waking time offending underscores that behavior settings may play an important role in triggering unlawful actions (Wikström, 2002, p. 202). However, as pointed out by Farrington (2002, p. 690), "Existing research tells us more about criminal potential than about how that potential becomes the actuality of offending in any given situation."

What makes one behavior setting more *criminogenic* than another may largely be viewed as the extent to which it tends to produce *temptations* (perceived options to realize particular desires in an unlawful way), *provocations* (perceived attacks on the person's property, security, or respect that generates anger or similar emotional states that may promote unlawful aggressive responses), and *weak deterrence* (perceived low risks of detection, sanctions, etc., associated with acting unlawfully upon particular temptations or provocations present in the setting) (Wikström, 1998).

It is likely, in a given cultural and structural behavioral context (macroenvironment), that some types of behavior settings inherently produce higher levels than others of temptation, provocation, and deterrence.[13] However, it is as well plausible to assume that the extent to which individuals get tempted and provoked by a situation and the likelihood that they will act unlawfully upon such a temptation or provocation is dependent on their morality and self-control. It is further likely that the deterrent effect of a specific behavior setting is also dependent on the individual propensity to engage in crime. For example, for those with weak self-control the deterrent features of a behavior setting may not play such a great role for their choice of action since they may act more instantly with less concern for the future negative consequences of their current behavior (Wikström, 1995, 1996).

If one accepts the idea that behavior settings vary in their potential criminogenic characteristics, then the key question becomes *why* some behavior settings tend to be potentially more criminogenic than others (i.e., more often tend to create strong temptation or provocation and weak deterrence) and what role, if any, the wider community context has in producing behavior settings with more criminogenic characteristics (i.e., which tend to generate temptations or provocations and weak deterrence).

## Community-Level Causal Mechanisms

A *community* may be defined as the social and built environment of a common locality. There are no definite criteria for the geographical demarcation of a community. The community social environment consists of the patterns of social activities and social relationships in a locality. The community-built environment is the arrangement of buildings and spaces in a locality. The basic idea of most ecologically oriented approaches to the study of crime and pathways in criminality is that the community's structural characteristics affect the conditions for social life and control in the community and that this, in turn, has some bearing on (1) how people who grow up in the community will develop their individual characteristics relevant to their future propensity to offend and their lifestyles that shape pathways in criminality (*ecological context of development*), and (2) how people who live in the community will behave in daily life, including involvement in acts of crime (*ecological context of action*).

### Structural Characteristics

Communities vary widely in their structural characteristics. This includes variations in *residential population* characteristics and composition—for example, poverty, ethnic heterogeneity, family disruption, and residential stability. It also includes variation in the characteristics and layout of *buildings and spaces* and their related activities—for example, density and arrangement of space and presence of buildings and space for nonresidential use (Michelson, 1976). One might also add variations in the characteristics and composition of the *nonresidential population* of the area (e.g., those who work but do not live in the area, those who visit people who live in the area, or those who participate in activities taking place in the area). Variations in community structural characteristics are fundamentally a result of processes of *residential segregation* and *differential land use* which, in turn, are related to aspects of the wider political economy, such as means of production (technology), division of labor, and distribution of wealth (inequality) (e.g. Sampson, 1999, pp. 261–263; Wikström, 1998, p. 289).

We suggest here that the *social mechanisms* by which community structural characteristics, through their impact on the formation of the community social environment, influence individual development and actions may be summarized as *the three Rs*; resources, rules, and routines (Wikström, 1998, p. 284).[14] The basic argument is that *the community structure provides resources and rules that the residents can draw upon in their daily life, which in turn influence the patterning and content of their daily routines and the specific resources and rules associated with specific types of behavior settings generated by the community routines* (see Figure 5.2). The role of the community context for human action is thus that it constrains or facilitates and guides human action through the behavior settings created by the community routines and the specific resources and rules attached to particular behavior settings.

Although the importance of community resources and rules (and to a much lesser degree community routines) for the explanation of individual involvement in crime has long been recognized in community-oriented criminological research, *what has been missing is a concept that directly links the community context to individual development and actions* (Wikström, 1998). Behavior setting is a concept that may provide such a linkage.[15] As previously argued, it is in individuals' encounters with behavior settings that situations are created in which the individuals, depending on

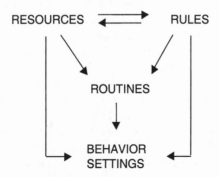

FIGURE 5.2. Behavior settings. Key social mechanisms of community structural-characteristic influences.

their characteristics, and the characteristics of the behavior setting, will perceive options, make choices, and take action.

## Resources

Community *resources* may be viewed as all the external social and economic support (by individuals and institutions) the residents in a community can draw upon in their day-to-day lives. They facilitate or constrain human development and action. The aggregate of individual and institutional resources in a community may be thought of as the *community capital* (Wikström, 1998). Communities vary in their level of resources (e.g., residents' social capital [i.e., their access to resourceful relationships they can draw upon] and their access to and quality of childcare, schools, and medical facilities). The concept of *disadvantage* is commonly used to describe communities with weak social and economic resources (e.g., Wilson, 1987). Community resources will have a general influence on the routine behavior of the residents of the community (e.g., their lifestyles).

Community resources are experienced and utilized by community residents in the behavior settings created by the community routines. It is plausible that the level of community resources (community capital) will have an impact on the residents' potential to develop their personal resources (human, financial, and social capital)[16] and to realize their desires. This, in turn, will have some influence on how individuals are likely to see their options and prospects in their day-to-day living, and therefore impact on the choices they make and their course of action.

## Rules

Community *rules* are all those norms and conventions (formal and informal) that the residents may be confronted with in their day-to-day life. They guide human development and action.[17] Communities may vary in their norms and conventions, their cohesiveness in values and expectations, and the degree to which norms and conventions are upheld by interventions and sanctions. The concept of *collective efficacy* has been suggested to describe the residents' willingness to intervene for the common good (i.e., their potential to exercise informal social control if needed) as the result of shared expectations and mutual trust in the community (Sampson, Morenoff, & Earls, 1999; Sampson et al., 1997).[18]

Community rules will have a general influence on the routine behavior of the residents of the community (e.g., their socialization practices). Community rules are communicated and upheld in behavior settings. It is plausible that community rules have an impact on the content and strength of the norms that are internalized and the social bonds that the residents in the community develop, and, in turn, what kind of desires and interests they have. This, in turn, will have some influence on how the individuals are likely to evaluate different options they perceive in their day-to-day living and the resulting course of action they may take.

It is generally assumed in the ecological literature that weak community resources (disadvantages) make it more difficult for residents to collectively create and uphold effective rules for behavior (collective efficacy).[19] However, it may also be argued that community rules (weak collective efficacy), in the longer run, may impact upon community resources (increased disadvantage), through the influence of high levels of disorder and crime on selective out-migration by more socially and economically resourceful residents and institutions (e.g., Sampson & Raudenbush, 1999: Skogan, 1990; Taub, Taylor, & Dunham, 1984).

## Routines

Community *routines* are the pattern of activities by time and place that occur in the community. Routine activities have been defined as "any recurrent and prevalent activities, which provide for basic population and individual needs" (Cohen & Felson, 1979, p. 593). They include activities related to family life, education, work, leisure, and transportation and are *manifested in the behavior settings they create* (e.g., family dinners, lectures, car manufacturing, tennis matches, and bus journeys). Routine activities are fundamentally generated by the necessity for individuals to cooperate to provide for their biological needs and social desires. They are broadly shaped by the community social environment through its provision of resources and rules. For example, one would expect some general differences between communities in socialization practices (routines) by their levels of disadvantage (resources) and their levels of collective efficacy (rules). The actual resources available to, and the rules guiding, activities in a particular behavior setting are also likely to vary between communities depending on their level of disadvantage and collective efficacy. For example, communities may vary by their level of disadvantage in the extent to which playgrounds are well equipped and kept up, and by their level of collective efficacy, to what extent playgrounds are well supervised.

It is plausible that the range and characteristics of behavior settings that individuals encounter in their day-to-day living as a result of the community routines will influence their development and actions because, as mentioned earlier, community rules are communicated and upheld, and community resources are experienced and utilized in the behavior settings.

## The Ecological Context of Development

Individual development occurs in an *ecological context* (a set of nested structures), and this context will impact on the course of development

(Bronfenbrenner, 1979; Moen, Elder, & Lúcher, 1995). In Bronfenbrenner's (1979) ecology of human development, it is the individual's day-to-day routines and activities, "the objects to which he responds and the people with whom he interacts on a face-to-face basis" (p. 7), that have a direct influence on his development. The community context has therefore only an *indirect* influence on individual development through its impact on shaping the form and content of the individual's day-to-day routines and activities.

*Place of residence* is an important determinant of ecological context. Modern societies, especially large urban areas, are highly segregated (e.g., Janson, 1980; Schwirian, 1974). *Segregation* means that the community structural characteristics, and thereby the community resources, rules, and routines, vary by areas of residence. This, in turn, means that the behavioral context (the configuration of behavior settings and their characteristics) that confronts the residents will vary by area of residence. Consider, for example, the difference in behavioral contexts between a homogeneous, residentially stable, and wealthy rural town and a heterogeneous, residentially unstable, and poor inner-city area.

The *neighborhood*, defined as the social and built environment surrounding the place of residence, is likely to have the greatest importance for the type and characteristics of the behavior settings the developing toddler and child is confronted with (e.g., Timms, 1971, pp. 31–32). Still, in adolescence, neighborhood-based behavior settings may for many youths be a significant part of their behavioral context,[20] while, for most people, it is less likely that the neighborhood will play an equally important role for their behavioral context in adulthood. In the widening world of the developing child and adolescent, their behavioral context will, as mentioned, generally expand outside their neighborhood, and therefore the need to take this fact into account when assessing community influences on development of individual characteristics and lifestyles increases with age.[21] This is something that has rarely been attempted in studies of neighborhood effects.

### Individual Development

As previously argued, individuals vary in their propensity to break the rules of the law and the key elements of this may be summarized as their morality and self-control. *Development* in the propensity to act unlawfully might therefore be defined as a lasting change in an individual's morality and self-control, making them more likely (in the future) to see acts of crime as an option and to act upon such options.[22] Individuals' variation in the propensity to engage in crime is likely to be a result of their *developmental history*, particularly their childhood and early adolescent development. The individual is not a passive recipient of environmental influences. Developmental outcomes will be a result of the *interaction* between the individuals and their environment (Magnusson, 1988, pp. 46–47). It is likely that the impact of the environment is strongest at the points in time when a particular developing characteristic has *its most rapid development* (e.g., Bloom, 1964; Earls & Carlson, 1995). It is further likely, as a result of an *increasing agency* through childhood (i.e., increasing physical and mental powers to intentionally make things happen), that individuals become generally more active and selective in relation to their environment, and therefore gradually enhance their potential to influence their own course of development.

## Community Socialization Practices and the Propensity to Act Unlawfully

Socialization has a key role when it comes to understanding individual development of morality and self-control (e.g., Aronfreed, 1968; Gottfredson & Hirschi, 1990; Kohlberg, 1984; Loeber & Stouthamer-Loeber, 1986; Martens, 1993). The role of the community context for community variation in socialization practices is a highly underresearched area. However, existing research suggests that it is likely that there is relevant variation in socialization practices by community context (e.g., Earls & Carlson, 1995; Furstenberg, Cook, Eccles, Elder, & Sameroff, 1999; Sampson, 1993, p. 165; Steinberg, Darling, Fletcher, Brown, & Dornbusch, 1995; Wikström & Loeber, 2000, p. 1130). In this section we discuss the potential role of the community context for community variation in socialization practices, and the resulting community variation in behavior settings that may promote the development of self-control and morality.

The main hypothesis here is that community capital and community collective efficacy influences (1) community socialization practices and (2) the specific resources available and rules guiding the particular types of behavior settings making up the socialization practice. This, in turn, determines the frequency with which children and adolescents in the community will encounter behavior settings having characteristics that may promote individual development of self-control and morality (Figure 5.3).

Community variation in *community capital* means that communities vary in the degree to which they can provide resources and services (e.g., time, money, and knowledge) to support families in their parenting role, over and above the resources of the individual family. Community variation in *collective efficacy* means that communities vary in the degree to which they can provide parental support by the monitoring and upholding of common rules in public and semipublic places, over and above the families' own capabilities to effectively monitor and react to rule violations outside the home.

*Socialization practices* include *family nurturing strategies* (e.g., the extent to which parents tend to prioritize activities that promote their children's health and their development of cognitive and emotional skills).

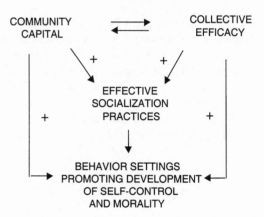

**FIGURE 5.3.** Behavior settings promoting development of self-control and morality: Community context influences.

They also include *family management techniques* (e.g., methods of discipline and extent of monitoring of children's activities) and *collective supervision* of children's behavior outside the home (e.g., neighbors' interventions and reactions to rule-breaking behavior).[23] While collective supervision clearly is a community factor, families nurturing their children, and particularly their management strategies, are also likely to be influenced by the community context in which families operate (e.g., Furstenberg, 1999, pp. 155–156; Sampson, 1997; Shonkoff & Phillips, 2000, pp. 225–296).

Strategies of family nurturing are likely to be most important for development outcomes in childhood (particularly for self-control), while family management techniques, and particularly the level of collective supervision, are likely to increase in their importance for development outcomes over late childhood and into adolescence. *Effective socialization practices* may be defined as those that create a high frequency of behavior settings that promote the development of self-control and morality. In communities where the socialization practices are effective, one would expect fewer children and adolescents to develop a strong propensity to act unlawfully.

Characteristics of behavior settings that may promote the development of *self-control* include settings with good nurturing, which, for example, may effect the child's development of executive functions; settings where rules for behavior and reactions to rule violations are consistent and foreseeable; and settings where long-term goals are encouraged over immediate gratification. Features of behavior settings that may promote the development of *morality* include those in which the developing child experiences that significant others show respect for him or her and for others and their property. It also includes behavior settings where the developing child or adolescent faces interventions and reactions when he or she shows no respect for others or their property.

The nature and strength of the impact of community socialization practices on individual development may be dependent on the *developmental phase* (since some characteristics tend to develop most strongly in certain, often early, phases, and the individual's agency increases by age), and the individual's previous *developmental history* (since development outcome is a result of the interaction between the individual and the environment, and therefore, at any given time, is dependent on the characteristics the individual has already developed). In general, this would suggest that *the impact of community context on individual development of self-control and morality (propensity) is likely to fade with age.*

### Community Lifestyles and Exposure to Criminogenic Behavior Settings

A *lifestyle* may be defined as the individual's preference for and active seeking out of particular sets of activities and related attributes. Not very much is known about the relationship between the community context and the development of particular lifestyles, although it is clear that lifestyles do tend to vary between communities (e.g., Michelson, 1976, pp. 61–94). Lifestyles are important because they represent individuals' *activity field*, thereby influencing exposure to different types of behavior settings. The link between community context and development of lifestyles is particularly interesting since persistent and serious offending may be strongly linked to particular types of lifestyles. In this section we discuss some tentative ideas about how the development of lifestyles may be influenced by the community context.

The main hypothesis here is that community capital and collective efficacy influence (1) the lifestyles of children and adolescents and (2) the specific resources available and rules guiding the particular types of behavior settings that make up their lifestyles. This will influence the frequency with which they are exposed to criminogenic behavior settings (i.e., settings entailing temptation or provocation and having weak deterrent qualities), and in turn, their involvement in crime and the shaping of pathways in criminality—for example, age of onset and escalation of seriousness of offending (Figure 5.4).

The types of lifestyles that appear to generate the most risk for involvement in offending are those in which children frequently socialize informally outside the home (Osgood et al., 1996; Sampson & Groves, 1989; West & Farrington, 1977, pp. 68–70; Wikström, 2002). It is plausible that children and adolescents living in more disadvantaged communities generally tend to socialize informally in semipublic and public settings more frequently than those living in more advantaged communities. This may depend on family and institutional resources and facilities in the community

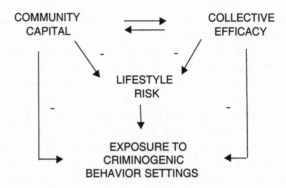

FIGURE 5.4. Exposure to criminogenic behavior settings: Community contextual influences.

to provide structured leisure time activities, but also the degree to which parents and others in the community generally tend to encourage children's and adolescent's involvement in structured leisure time activities (e.g., violin lessons, basketball practice, and theater visits). The latter may be seen partly as a function of the human and social capital among parents and other relevant actors (residents and functionaries) in the community.

However, there may also be reasons to believe that the risk generated by children's and youths' informal socialization outside the home may be dependent on other qualities of the community context. The community context may not only influence the degree to which children and adolescents socialize informally, but also the characteristics of the settings in which this happens. It seems reasonable to assume that informal socializing in communities with high levels of collective efficacy will generate less criminogenic behavior settings than in those communities with weak collective efficacy. For example, community levels of parental and collective monitoring of children's behavior in semipublic and public settings, and the likelihood that anyone will interfere against violations of norms and conventions in such settings, is likely to vary by community context.

Lifestyles in which children and youths spend significant time in *public and semipublic behavior settings* in which they *informally socialize* and are *unsupervised by adults*, in a behavioral context in which they *may express violations of norms and conventions without much risk of interference from others* (e.g., they can freely experiment with alcohol and drug use), may be considered *high-risk lifestyles*. Settings in which children and youths (at times) may socialize unsupervised are typically "street corners," "playgrounds," "parks," "fair grounds," and "shopping malls." For adolescents it may also include entertainment settings like "pubs and bars" and "discos." Behavior settings that are unsupervised by significant others and in which rule violations can take place without much risk of intervention and reaction from others may be particularly criminogenic (i.e., likely to create temptations and provocations and to have weak deterrent qualities). In communities where risky lifestyles are less prevalent, one would expect fewer children and adolescents to get involved in crime, particularly in frequent and serious criminality.

## Pathways in Criminality

Lifestyle formation and development is of particular interest in relation to pathways in criminality. A *pathway* may be defined as "a common pattern of development shared by a group of individuals, which is distinct from the behavioral development experienced by other groups of individuals" (Loeber, 1991, p. 98). A pathway in criminality may be seen as a stepping-stone process where the outcome of previous development influences the outcome of later development (Farrington, 1986). For example, initial criminality may influence the likelihood of later criminality, and the factors that influenced initial involvement in crime may be partly others than those influencing continuation in offending (Loeber & LeBlanc, 1990).

Individuals differ in the degree to which they *penetrate* pathways in crime, from those committing no crime to those who advance to the most serious forms of crime (Loeber & Farrington, 2001, pp. 7–8). Although there is not much research on community contextual influences on pathways in criminality, one study has shown that the degree of penetration varies by community context (with more penetration in disadvantaged communities), and therefore that it is possible that community contexts influence the level of penetration of a given pathway (Loeber & Wikström, 1993). One conceivable reason for this is that the type and characteristics of the behavior settings that children and adolescents encounter in areas that are disadvantaged and low in collective efficacy may more strongly facilitate and promote continued offending after the initial involvement. This may occur, for example, because of a higher exposure to settings of informal socialization unsupervised by adults and a behavioral context in which bystander intervention and reactions to offending may be less likely. It is also plausible that the more an individual penetrates a pathway in criminality, the more actively he or she will *seek out* behavior settings that will have criminogenic features. All in all, continuation and escalation in offending may be strongly influenced by lack of community capital and collective efficacy through its impact on lifestyles.

## ECOMETRICS

Typically, research into community influences on crime and offending behavior has used predefined administrative areas as units of analysis combined with official census data to measure community structural characteristics (e.g., Baldwin & Bottoms, 1976; Shaw & McKay, 1969; Wikström, 1991). More recent developments in *ecometrics*, the measurement and assessment of ecological settings, have included the use of contextual surveys (e.g., Sampson et al., 1997; Wikström & Dolmen, 2001) and systematic social observation, along with multilevel statistical methods evaluating and accounting for measurement error (Raudenbush & Sampson, 1999; Sampson & Raudenbush, 1999). In this section we discuss the analytical and methodological implications of this perspective for research designs in the study of community context influences on offending behavior.

It is commonly believed that the effects of community contexts on individual development and actions are weak in terms of proportion-explained variance. For example, Shonkoff and Phillips (2000, p. 332) report that "one striking result in broad-based studies of neighborhood effects on young children is that there are more differences in families and children *within* neighborhoods than *between* them" (italics in original). The findings are largely the same in studies specifically focusing on offending behavior (e.g., Gottfredson et al., 1991; Lizotte, Thornberry, Krohn, Chard-Wierschem, & McDowan, 1994; Simcha-Fagan & Schwartz, 1986). Against this background, it would be easy to draw the conclusion that the community context does not contribute much to individual variation in offending. However, there are several reasons why this reasoning is incorrect.

For one thing, variance components are descriptive statistics that reflect observed distributions rather than causal effects. For example, because of economic segregation, very few poor people, especially minorities, live in high-income areas. But experimental conditions that induce exogenous change such that poor people are assigned to better neighborhoods can still produce large causal effects even in the face of previously observed variance components that show little variation across contexts. Put simply, substantial causal effects of context are not incompatible with small intraclass neighborhood correlations (Duncan & Raudenbush, 2001; Sampson et al., 2002).

Second, what appear as individual characteristics at one point in time may, at least partly, have been a result of earlier community-context influences on the development of the particular characteristic. In fact, one can argue that the environment in which the individual grows up is more or less likely to have influenced the development of all individual characteristics relevant to offending behavior (e.g., Dishion, French, & Patterson, 1995, pp. 437–438; Shonkoff & Phillips, 2000, pp. 6–7). It follows that controlling for nonexogenous individual characteristics as a general strategy to determine community-context influences on individual criminality is a fundamentally flawed strategy. It is only when studying the role of the context of action that such an approach is warranted.[24]

Third, and relatedly, it may be argued that there is a need for a clearer analytical separation of the study of the role of the community context for development of propensity and its role in motivation for offending (i.e., context of action). In the former case (i.e., developmental context), it is predominantly the early development of individual characteristics relevant to future offending risks that is in focus. In the latter case (i.e., the action context), the focus is on how types of behavior settings, predominantly in late childhood and adolescence, influence the degree and nature of involvement in crime by individuals with different characteristics. From a developmental perspective, the two are obviously linked.

Fourth, in comparison with measures of individual characteristics, community-context measures are generally crude and less well developed. Raudenbush and Sampson (1999) argue that "without comparable standards to evaluate ecological assessments, the search for individual and ecological effects may overemphasise the individual component simply because the well-studied psychometric properties are likely to be superior to the unstudied ecometric ones" (p. 3). New standards are thus needed to bring community contextual measures up to the level that psychometric research has long operated under.[25]

Fifth, the use of predefined areas as a measure of residential community context does not take into account the fact that individuals living in a given community may vary in the exposure to their community characteristics and in their exposure to environments outside their residential community. For example, many behaviors of interest in criminology (e.g., stealing, smoking, taking drugs) unfold in places (e.g., schools, parks, center-city areas) outside of the residential neighborhoods in which the individuals involved in these behaviors live. This is a problematic scenario for neighborhood research seeking to explain contextual effects on individual differences in behavior since it excludes variations in the individuals' activity fields within their neighborhoods, but also the environmental effect by the individuals' activity field outside their neighborhoods, which, as previously argued, expand by age and may be particularly important in adolescence. A technique that may be useful to help overcome this problem is what has been called space–time budgets.

## Space–Time Budgets

A technique to study the individuals' participation in behavior settings is to use what is called time budgets or time diaries (see Pentland, Harvey, Lawton, & McColl, 1999 for an overview of time–budget studies). Typically, such studies involve interviewing the subjects about their activities over a time period (e.g., a day or a week) divided into time segments (e.g., by the hour). The subjects are basically questioned about *what they were doing* (e.g., eating), *with whom* (e.g., with parents), and *at what place* (e.g., at home). This information makes it possible to study the range and characteristics of behavior settings in which the individual participates. As claimed by Robinson (1999, p. 48), time budgets "represent complete accounts of daily activity" and they "allow one to generate estimates of how much societal time is spent on the complete range of human behaviour."

As suggested by Wikström (2002), time budget techniques can be complemented by questions regarding the *geographical location* of subject's activity (e.g., by predefined areas such as census tracts). This enables the researcher to directly link community context features to individual behavior settings. This may be useful in two ways. First, by taking random samples of the population in predefined areas, the data from a space–time budget study gives information on what kind of behavior settings a particular community context is likely to generate. Second, on the individual level, it tells us to what degree an individual is exposed to the various types of behavior settings generated by the community context, and also the individual exposure to behavior settings outside his or her residential community. The latter, for example, makes it possible to control for individual exposure to the neighborhood environment and environments outside the neighborhood when trying to assess contextual influences.[26]

## CROSS-LEVEL INTERACTIONS

We conclude this chapter by stressing the importance of studying cross-level interaction effects and offering a set of tentative hypotheses concerning the general nature and direction of community-context influences on individual development and action relevant to offending behavior. The relationship between individual characteristics and community-context characteristics in influencing offending behavior and its development is a highly neglected area of research. And yet, the community-level theory we have advanced here suggests that *the study of cross-level interactions may be the most promising avenue advancing knowledge about the role of the community context in crime causation.*

### Context of Development: From Development of Propensity to Realization of Propensity

Our theory suggests that the nature and strength of community-context influences (levels of community capital and collective efficacy) on the individual development of propensity and motivation to offend *varies by developmental phase.* We hypothesize *that the community influences on development of propensity decrease from infancy to adolescence, while its influence on motivation increases from infancy to adolescence.*

The main suggested reason for the decrease by age in the influence of community socialization practices on the development of propensity to offend is that many cognitive and emotional characteristics that determine morality, and particularly self-control, have their strongest development early in life and that they thereafter tend to stabilize (e.g., Shonkoff & Phillips, 2000; Tangey & Fischer, 1995). It seems reasonable, as we have previously argued, that the environmental impact on development of individual characteristics is at is strongest during the periods when the particular characteristics have their most rapid development.[27] We would expect to find a community effect, particularly on the early development of self-control and morality; *we specifically expect to find higher rates of children developing low self-control and weak morality among those living in areas with weak community capital and low collective efficacy.*

The community-context influence on individual motivation to offend (through its supply of criminogenic behavior settings) is dependent on the extent to which the individual participates in settings with criminogenic features. As children grow older, their activity fields expand outside the home, and therefore their risk to be exposed to criminogenic behavior settings in their neighborhood and also in the wider community outside their neighborhood increase. It is against this background, we argue, that the role of the community context as an influence on individual's motivation to offend increases, particularly over the childhood period. In this process the community-context influence on lifestyle formation is particularly relevant. It should be stressed that lifestyle formation is not independent of community socialization practices but is partly a consequence of them. We would expect to find a community effect on late childhood and adolescent lifestyle formation; *we expect to find higher rates of adolescents developing risky lifestyles among those living in areas with weak community capital and low collective efficacy.*

### Context of Action: Community-Context Influences on Motivation to Offend Vary Inversely by Individual Propensity to Offend

We argue that the nature and strength of community-context influences on motivation to offend *is dependent on the individual's previous developmental history* (determining his or her current propensity). We specifically hypothesize that *the community strength of impact on motivation to offend varies inversely by the individual propensity to offend.* That is, the community context has the strongest influence on individual motivation to offend for those with the weakest propensity to offend. They will be the individuals for whom exposure to strong situational inducements occasionally may make them act unlawfully. On the other hand, individuals who have developed a strong propensity to offend will be less affected by the community-context supply of criminogenic behavior settings. That is so because they are more likely to be active in seeking out good opportunities to offend. In other words, their offending is more about high propensities than about strong situational inducement.

Although very little research exists on the interaction between individual characteristics and community context in determining offending, two recent studies lend some support to the assumption that the community context of action may have its strongest impact on individuals with weaker propensity to offend. In these two studies it was shown that community levels of disadvantage had the strongest effect, respectively, (1) on *adolescent onset in serious offending* (Wikström & Loeber, 2000) and (2) on *prevalence of adolescent offending* (Wikström, 2002) for the most well-adjusted youths, while there were no significant difference by community disadvantage for the most poorly adjusted youths.[28]

## CONCLUSION

In this chapter we have argued that advancement in the understanding of the role of community context in crime causation requires better theorizing of social mechanisms that link community context to individual development and acts, improved "ecometrics," and a focus of study on cross-level interactions. A key premise of our discussion has been that the types and characteristics of the behavior settings in which the individual actually participates influence individual action and development most directly. We have also argued that the supply of types and characteristics of behavior settings vary by community contextual features such as the level of community capital and collective efficacy (see Figure 5.2). We have particularly highlighted the importance of behavior settings relating to socialization practices and lifestyle formation (see Figures 5.3 and 5.4). We have stressed the importance of perceptions of alternatives and processes of choice for individual acts of crime (see Figure 5.1). Finally, we believe that advancing the study of community-level influences on individual development and social action requires the use of more adequate methods to study both individual routines (e.g., space–time budgets) and community-level mechanisms (ecometrics), coupled with a rigorous focus on the analyses of cross-level interactions.

Several implications for research design flow from the logic of our position. To test ecological or community effects on the development of propensity, multilevel longitudinal designs are obviously essential. Studying development *in context* is the operative strategy; much lip service is given to this as desirable in criminology, but very little empirical research actually exists that is at all relevant. To test hypotheses of the context of social action, both longitudinal and cross-sectional designs are appropriate, as long as the context is directly measured. Experiments where behavior settings and ecological contexts are randomly manipulated are especially intriguing as a way to test causal hypotheses of the sort proposed in this chapter.

## ACKNOWLEDGMENTS

This article was completed while the authors were fellows at the Center for Advanced Study in the Behavioral Sciences, Stanford. We gratefully acknowledge the financial support provided by the William and Flora Hewlett Foundation, Grant No. 2000-5633.

## NOTES

1. However, the reasons for committing a certain act may also be the reason, or a part thereof, for breaking a law.
2. But, of course, this is in its own right a very important topic. However, it is highly plausible that societies at a given state of development, by and large, will be similar in what core types of behavior they tend to criminalize (e.g., Newman, 1976).
3. See Wrong (1994, pp. 70–109).
4. Schick (1997) gives the following criminological-relevant example of what he means by understandings: "The man who rapes and the man who doesn't are the same in their beliefs and desires. They both believe that a show of force might frighten some women into having sex with them, and they both want sex. They differ in their understandings. The rapist sees rape as raw, rough sex, as tough-guy sex, the way he likes it. The other sees rape as a violation. He wants sex, but not violation. and so the way he understands rape doesn't connect with what he wants, which means that he isn't moved to rape" (p. 19).
5. For an in-depth discussion of dimensions of human agency, see Emirbayer and Mische (1998).
6. For the importance of social bonds/attachments, see, for example, Durkheim (1961) and Hirschi (1969).
7. Individual and contextual characteristics, independently or interacting, may be viewed as causes of individuals' reasons to engage in crime if, when manipulated, they through some plausible mechanism will produce some change in people (in the short or longer term) relevant to how they perceive options and make choices in particular settings regarding whether or not to breach a rule of law.
8. Zahn-Waxler and Robinson (1995) talk about guilt, shame, and empathy as moral emotions.
9. Morality covers many more actions than those that are considered unlawful. In this context, however, we are concerned with moral aspects of unlawful acts, that is, the extent to which the individual finds different regulations of the law as right or wrong (depending on internalized norms), and whether the individual cares about, and how strongly he or she cares about, following the rules of law (depending on social bonds). It should be stressed that morality is used here in a nonjudgmental sense, that is, it refers to the correspondence between individual and collective norms and conventions. For example, weak individual morality refers to a low correspondence to what people in general care about

and find to be right or wrong. Similarly, as regarding morality and the law, weak morality refers to a low correspondence between what is regulated in the law and what the individual cares about and finds to be right or wrong. The importance of taking morality seriously when trying to understand "compliance with legal rules" has recently been well argued by Bottoms (2002).

10. Shonkoff and Phillips (2000, p. 116) state that "there is a growing consensus among researchers as to what executive functions entail: self-regulation, sequencing of behavior, flexibility, response inhibition, planning, and organization of behaviour." The roles of psychotic disorders like schizophrenia for offending may be highly relevant in this context but will not be specifically discussed in this chapter.

11. The idea that individuals' involvement in crime is dependent on the extent to which they are "vulnerable to temptations of the moment" (i.e., vary in their degree of self-control) is prominent in contemporary criminology and has most strongly been advocated by Gottfredson and Hirschi (1990, p. 87). The use of the term *self-control* by Gottfredson and Hirschi has a wider connotation than the one applied here, and involves aspects of what here has been defined as belonging to morality.

12. Barker (1968) originally suggested the concept of behavior setting. *Behavior settings* have been defined as naturally occurring units with standing patterns of behavior and a physical milieu that surrounds or encloses the behavior (Moss, 1976, pp. 214–216). They are located in time and space. Examples may be pub drinking sessions, classes/lectures, youths socializing on street corners, and family dinners. It is important to stress, as Schoggen (1989, p. 31) does, that "a standing pattern of behavior is not a characteristic of the particular individuals involved; it is an extra-individual behavior phenomenon; it has unique and stable characteristics that persist even when current inhabitants of the setting are replaced with others."

13. The degree to which given types of behavior settings create temptation, provocation, and weak deterrence may be related to the characteristics of the wider cultural and structural context in which it is embedded. This implies that this may vary between nations and in the same nation over time.

14. Giddens's (1979, 1984) theory of structuration stresses the importance of rules, resources, and routines for understanding social life. However, his discussion of these concepts differs in many respects from ours.

15. Dishion, French, and Patterson (1995, pp. 428–429, 450–455) are among the few that have stressed the importance of behavior settings for antisocial behavior. However, in their discussion the use of the concept is very broad, including as behavior settings all from neighborhoods to classrooms.

16. Human capital (e.g., skills), financial capital (e.g., money), and social capital (e.g., resourceful relationships the actor can draw upon) all refer to resources, albeit of different character (see, e.g., Coleman, 1990).

17. It can be argued that rules may sometimes act as resources.

18. Kohlberg attaches a strong role to the environment in its influence on individual actions of a moral character. He talks about "sense of community, solidarity and cohesion attained in a group" (1984, p. 265) as the moral atmosphere, and argues that "moral action usually takes place in a social group context, and that context usually has a profound influence on the moral decision making of

individuals. Individual moral decision-makings in real life are almost always made in the context of group norms or group decision-making processes. Moreover, individual moral action is often a function of these norms and processes" (p. 263).

19. For example, Kornhauser (1978) argues that social disorganization, defined as lack of "a structure through which common values can be realized and common problems solved " (p. 63), emerges in poor, residentially unstable, and heterogeneous communities because it is difficult to realize common values among the residents, due to such factors as poor communication resulting from residents' diverse and changing cultural backgrounds and experiences, but also because the social institutions, due to factors such as lack of money, skills, and personal investments by residents, tend to be inadequate, isolated from each other, and unstable. Poorly functioning social institutions and a lack of common values among community residents result in poor informal social controls and defective socialization, which, in turn, causes high rates of offending by community residents. See also Sampson, Morenoff, and Earls (1999).

20. A recent time–budget study of 14- to 15-year-olds in the city of Peterborough, UK, showed that the youths, on average, spent 38% of their waking time in the home, 20% in other places in their neighborhood, 28% in their school and, not including time spent in their school, 14% outside their neighborhood (Wikström, 2002).

21. This also has some implications for what structures are relevant as indirectly influencing their day-to-day life. Aber, Gephart, Brooks-Gunn, and Connell (1995, p. 54) suggest "that in early childhood, the neighborhood influences children's development primarily by its effects on parents. A secondary effect could be formed through the quality of care provided by other major caregivers (who are typically members of the community). In middle childhood and adolescence, the effects of neighborhoods on development may be mediated by a new set of factors, primarily school and peers. Finally, in early and late adolescence, still other factors are hypothesized to mediate neighborhoods' effects on development. Possibilities include direct contact with certain 'neighborhood processes' like adult monitoring of youth, as well as broader institutional and cultural processes like the operation of the labor market, the justice system, and the beliefs and values that guide family formation."

22. Bronfenbrenner (1979, p. 3) has in general terms defined *development* as "a lasting change in the way in which a person perceives and deals with his environment."

23. Farrington (2002, p. 681) stresses that "the belief that offending is wrong, or a strong conscience, tends to be built up if parents are in favour of legal norms, if they exercise close supervision over their children, and if they punish socially disapproved behaviour using love-oriented discipline. Antisocial tendencies can also be inhibited by empathy, which may develop as a result of parental warmth and loving relationships. The belief that offending is legitimate, and anti-establishment attitudes generally, tend to be built up if children have been exposed to attitudes and behaviour favouring offending (e.g., in a modelling process), especially by members of their family, friends and in their communities."

24. A common strategy in multilevel research is to estimate a model whereby a host

of individual, familial, peer, and school variables are entered as controls along-side current neighborhood characteristics of residence. But this strategy con-founds the potential importance of both long-term community influences and mediating developmental pathways regarding children's personal traits and dis-positions, learning patterns from peers, family socialization, school climate, and more. Put differently, static models that estimate the direct effect of current neighborhood context on a particular outcome (e.g., delinquency, level of aca-demic achievement) may be partitioning-out relevant variance in a host of me-diating and developmental pathways of influence.

25. A full discussion of this methodological paradigm is found in Raudenbush and Sampson (1999).

26. A related issue concerns approaches to assessing how individuals perceive alter-natives and make choices in particular behavior settings. One way to tap this may be the use of scenarios in which the subjects are asked to report the alter-native they see and the choices they are likely to make in different kinds of hy-pothetical behavior settings presented to them. This would, for example, enable the researcher to study variation between communities in individual perception of options and choices relating to acts of crime in similar types of behavior set-tings. The aim of scenario-based research is to try and create as much as possi-ble real-life situations. In criminological research, scenarios have predomi-nantly been used in deterrence research (see, e.g., Nagin, 1998).

27. Although we do not claim that there are no further developments later in life of individual characteristics relevant to individual propensity to offend. In partic-ular, it is plausible that changes in the individual's immediate social situation (e.g., his or her attachments) may influence his or her morality (particularly what he or she cares about).

28. In these studies propensity to offend was measured by a composite risk-protec-tive construct including key individual disposition and immediate social situa-tion variables.

## REFERENCES

Aber, J. L., Gephart, M. A., Brooks-Gunn, J., & Connell, J. P. (1997). Development in context: Implications for studying neighborhood effects. In J. Brooks-Gunn, G. J. Duncan, & J. L. Aber (Eds.), *Neighborhood poverty: Context and consequences for children* (Vol. 1, pp. 41–64). New York: Russell Sage Foundation.

Aronfreed, J. M. (1968). *Conduct and conscience: The socialization of internalized control over behavior.* New York: Academic Press.

Baldwin, J., & Bottoms, A. E. (1976). *The urban criminal.* London: Tavistock.

Barker, R. G. (1968). *Ecological psychology: Concepts and methods for studying the environ-ment of human behavior.* Stanford, CA: Stanford University Press.

Barkley, R. A. (1997). *ADHD and the nature of self-control.* New York: Guilford Press.

Block, R., & Block, C. (1995). Space, place and crime: Hot spot areas and hot spot places of liquor-related crime. In J. E. Eck & D. Weisburd (Eds.), *Crime and place* (pp. 145–183). Washington, DC: National Academy Press.

Bloom, B. S. (1964). *Stability and change in human characteristics.* New York: Wiley.

Blumstein, A., Cohen, J., Roth, J. A., & Visher, C. A. (1986). *Criminal careers and career crimi-nals* (Vol. 1). Washington, DC: National Academy Press.

Bottoms, A. E. (2002). Morality, crime, compliance and public policy. In A. E. Bottoms & M. Tonry (Eds.), *Ideology, crime and criminal justice: A symposium in honour of Sir Leon Radzinowicz* (pp. 20–51). Cullompton: Willian.

Bronfenbrenner, U. (1979). *The ecology of human development*. Cambridge, MA: Harvard University Press.

Brooks-Gunn, J., Duncan, G. J., Klebanov, P. K., & Sealand, N. (1993). Do neighborhoods influence child and adolescent development? *American Journal of Sociology, 99*(2), 353–395.

Bursik, R. J., & Grasmick, H. G. (1993). *Neighborhoods and crime*. New York: Lexington Books.

Cohen, L. E., & Felson, M. (1979). Social-change and crime rate trends: Routine activity approach. *American Sociological Review, 44*(4), 588–608.

Coleman, J. S. (1990). *Foundations of social theory*. Cambridge, MA: Belknap Press of Harvard University Press.

Davidson, D. (1980). *Essays on actions and events*. Oxford, UK: Clarendon Press.

Dishion, T. J., French, D. C., & Patterson, G. R. (1995). The development and ecology of antisocial behavior. In D. Cicchetti & D. J. Cohen (Eds.), *Developmental psychopathology: Vol. 2: Risk, disorder, and adaptation* (pp. 421–471). New York: Wiley.

Duncan, G. J., & Raudenbush, S. W. (1999). Assessing the effects of context in studies of child and youth development. *Educational Psychologist, 34*(1), 29–41.

Durkheim, E. (1961). *Moral education*. New York: Free Press.

Earls, F., & Carlson, M. (1995). Promoting human capability as an alternative to early crime prevention. In P.-O. Wikström, R. V. Clarke, & J. McCord (Eds.), *Integrating crime prevention strategies: Propensity and opportunity* (pp. 141–168). Stockholm: Fritzes.

Elliott, D. S., Wilson, W. J., Huizinga, D., Sampson, R. J., Elliott, A., & Rankin, B. (1996). The effects of neighborhood disadvantage on adolescent development. *Journal of Research in Crime and Delinquency, 33*(4), 389–426.

Emirbayer, M., & Mische, A. (1998). What is agency? *American Journal of Sociology, 103*(4), 962–1023.

Farrington, D. P. (1986). Stepping stones to adult criminal careers. In D. Olweus, J. Block, & M. R. Yarrow (Eds.), *Development of antisocial and prosocial behaviour: Research, theories and issues* (pp. 359–384). New York: Academic Press.

Farrington, D. P. (1993). Have any individual, family, or neighbourhood influences on offending been demonstrated conclusively? In D. P. Farrington, R. J. Sampson, & P.-O. Wikström (Eds.), *Integrating individual and ecological aspects of crime* (pp. 7–37). Stockholm: Allmänna Förlaget.

Farrington, D. P. (2000). Explaining and preventing crime: The globalization of knowledge. The American Society of Criminology 1999 presidential address. *Criminology, 38*(1), 1–24.

Farrington, D. P. (2002). Human development and criminal careers. In M. McGuire, R. Morgan, & R. Rainer (Eds.), *The Oxford handbook of criminology* (pp. 657–701). Oxford, UK: Clarendon Press.

Farrington, D. P., Sampson, R. J., & Wikström, P.-O. (Eds.). (1993). *Integrating individual and ecological aspects of crime*. Stockholm: Allmänna Förlaget.

Farrington, D. P., & Wikström, P.-O. (1993). Criminal careers in London and Stockholm: A cross-national comparative study. In E. Weitekamp & H. J. Kerner (Eds.), *Cross-national and longitudinal research on human development* (pp. 65–89). Dordrecht, The Netherlands: Kluwer.

Furstenberg, F. F. Jr., Cook, T. D., Eccles, J. S., Elder, G. H. Jr., & Sameroff, A. (1999). *Managing to make it*. Chicago: University of Chicago Press.

Giddens, A. (1979). *Central problems in social theory*. London: Macmillan.

Giddens, A. (1984). *The constitution of society*. Cambridge, UK: Polity Press.

Gottfredson, D. C., & Hirschi, T. (1990). *A general theory of crime*. Stanford, CA: Stanford University Press.

Gottfredson, D. C., McNeil, R. J., & Gottfredson, G. D. (1991). Social area influences on delinquency: A multilevel analysis. *Journal of Research in Crime and Delinquency, 28*(2), 197–226.

Hedstrom, P., & Swedberg, R. (1998). *Social mechanisms: An analytical approach to social theory.* Cambridge, UK: Cambridge University Press.

Hirschi, T. (1969). *Causes of delinquency.* Berkeley and Los Angeles: University of California Press.

Janson, C. G. (1980). Factorial social ecology: An attempt at summary and evaluation. *Annual Review of Sociology, 6,* 433–456.

Kohlberg, L. (1984). *Essays on moral development: Vol. 2. The psychology of moral development.* San Francisco: Harper & Row.

Kornhauser, R. R. (1978). *Social sources of delinquency.* Chicago: University of Chicago Press.

Kupersmidt, J. B., Griesler, P. C., Derosier, M. E., Patterson, C. J., & Davis, P. W. (1995). Childhood aggression and peer relations in the context of family and neighborhood factors. *Child Development, 66*(2), 360–375.

LeBlanc, M. (1993). Prevention of delinquency: An integrative multilayered control based perspective. In D. P. Farrington, R. J. Sampson, & P.-O. Wikström (Eds.), *Integrating individual and ecological aspects of crime* (pp. 279–314). Stockholm: Allmänna Förlaget.

LeBlanc, M. (1997). A generic control theory of the criminal phenomena: The structural and dynamic statements of an integrative multilayered control theory. In T. P. Thornberry (Ed.), *Developmental theories of crime and delinquency* (pp. 215–286). New Brunswick, NJ: Transaction Press.

LeBlanc, M., & Fréchette, M. (1989). *Male criminal activity from childhood through youth.* New York: Springer-Verlag.

Lizotte, A. J., Thornberry, T. P., Krohn, M. D., Chard-Wierschem, D. C., & McDowan, D. (1994). Neighborhood context and delinquency: A longitudinal analysis. In E. M. G. Weitekamp & H. J. Kerner (Eds.), *Cross-national longitudinal research on human development and criminal behavior* (pp. 217–227). Dordrecht, The Netherlands: Kluwer.

Loeber, R. (1991). Questions and advances in the study of developmental pathways. In D. Cicchetti & S. Toth (Eds.), *Rochester symposium on developmental psychopathology III* (pp. 97–115). Rochester, NY: Rochester University Press.

Loeber, R. (1996). Development continuity, change, and pathways in male juvenile problem behaviors and delinquency. In J. D. Hawkins (Ed.), *Delinquency and crime: Current theories* (pp. 1–27). Cambridge, UK: Cambridge University Press.

Loeber, R., & Farrington, D. P. (1999). *Serious and violent juvenile offenders: Risk factors and successful interventions.* Thousand Oaks, CA: Sage.

Loeber, R., & Farrington, D. P. (2001). *Child delinquents: Risk factors, interventions, and service needs.* Beverly Hills, CA: Sage.

Loeber, R., & Leblanc, M. (1990). Toward a developmental criminology. *Crime and Justice: A Review of Research, 12,* 375–473.

Loeber, R., & Stouthamer-Loeber, M. (1986). Family factors as correlates and predictors of juvenile conduct problems and delinquency. *Crime and Justice: A Review of Research, 7,* 29–149.

Loeber, R., & Wikström, P.-O. (1993). Individual pathways to crime in different types of neighborhoods. In D. P. Farrington, R. J. Sampson, & P.-O. Wikström (Eds.), *Integrating individual and ecological aspects of crime* (pp. 169–204). Stockholm: Allmänna Förlaget.

Magnusson, D. (1988). *Individual development from an interactional perspective.* Hillsdale, NJ: Erlbaum.

Martens, P. L. (1993). An ecological model of socialization in explaining offending. In D. P. Farrington, R. J. Sampson, & P.-O. Wikström (Eds.), *Integrating individual and ecological aspects of crime* (pp. 109–151). Stockholm: Allmänna Förlaget.

Michelson, W. (1976). *Man and his urban environment.* Reading, MA: Addison-Wesley.

Moen, P., Elder, G. H. Jr., & Lúcher, K. (1995). *Examining lives in context.* Washington, DC: American Psychological Association.

Moffitt, T. E. (1993). Adolescence-limited and life-course-persistent antisocial behavior: A developmental taxonomy. *Psychological Review, 100*(4), 674–701.

Moss, R. H. (1976). *The human context: Environmental determinants of behavior.* New York: Wiley.

Nagin, D. S. (1998). Criminal deterrence research at the outset of the twenty-first century. In *Crime and justice: A review of research* (Vol. 23, pp. 1–42). Chicago: University of Chicago Press.

Newman, G. (1976). *Comparative deviance.* New York: Elsevier.

Osgood, D. W., Wilson, J. K., O'Malley, P. M., Bachman, J. G., & Johnston, L. D. (1996). Routine activities and individual deviant behavior. *American Sociological Review, 61*(4), 635–655.

Pentland, W. E., Harvey, A. S., Lawton, M. P., & McColl, M. A. (1999). *Time use research in the social sciences.* New York: Kluwer Academic/Plenum.

Raudenbush, S. W., & Sampson, R. J. (1999). Ecometrics: Toward a science of assessing ecological settings, with application to the systematic social observation of neighborhoods. *Sociological Methodology, 29,* 1–41.

Reiss, A. J. (1986). Why are communities important in understanding crime? In A. J. Reiss & M. Tonry (Eds.), *Crime and justice: A review of research* (Vol. 8, pp. 1–34). Chicago: University of Chicago Press.

Reiss, A. J., & Rhodes, A. L. (1961). The distribution of juvenile-delinquency in the social-class structure. *American Sociological Review, 26*(5), 720–732.

Robinson, J. P. (1999). The time-diary method. In W. E. Pentland, A. S. Harvey, M. P. Lawton, & M. A. McColl (Eds.), *Time use research in the social sciences* (pp. 47–90). New York: Kluwer Academic/Plenum.

Sampson, R. J. (1993). Family and community-level influences on crime. In D. P. Farrington, R. J. Sampson, & P.-O. Wikström (Eds.), *Integrating individual and ecological aspects of crime* (pp. 153–168). Stockholm: Allmänna Förlaget.

Sampson, R. J. (1997). The embeddedness of child and adolescent development: A community-perspective on urban violence. In J. McCord (Ed.), *Violence and childhood in the inner city* (pp. 31–77). Cambridge, UK: Cambridge University Press.

Sampson, R. J. (1999). What "community" supplies. In R. F. Ferguson & W. T. Dickens (Eds.), *Urban problems and community development* (pp. 241–292). Washington, DC: Brookings Institution Press.

Sampson, R. J., & Groves, W. B. (1989). Community structure and crime: Testing social-disorganization theory. *American Journal of Sociology, 94*(4), 774–802.

Sampson, R. J., Morenoff, J. D., & Earls, F. (1999). Beyond social capital: Spatial dynamics of collective efficacy for children. *American Sociological Review, 64*(5), 633–660.

Sampson R. J., Morenoff, J. D., & Gannon-Rowley, T. (2002). Assessing "neighborhood effects": Social processes and new directions in research. *Annual Review of Sociology, 28,* 443–478.

Sampson, R. J., & Raudenbush, S. W. (1999). Systematic social observation of public spaces: A new look at disorder in urban neighborhoods. *American Journal of Sociology, 105*(3), 603–651.

Sampson, R. J., Raudenbush, S. W., & Earls, F. (1997). Neighborhoods and violent crime: A multilevel study of collective efficacy. *Science, 277*(5328), 918–924.

Schick, F. (1991). *Understanding action.* Cambridge, UK: Cambridge University Press.

Schick, F. (1997). *Making choices: A recasting of decision theory.* Cambridge, UK: Cambridge University Press.

Schoggen, P. (1989). *Behavior settings.* Stanford, CA: Stanford University Press.

Schwirian, K. P. (1974). *Comparative urban structure.* Lexington, MA: D.C. Heath.

Shaw, C., & McKay, H. (1969). *Juvenile delinquency and urban areas.* Chicago: University of Chicago Press.

Shonkoff, J. P., & Phillips, D. A. E. (2000). *From neurons to neighborhoods: The science of early childhood development.* Washington, DC: National Academy Press.

Simcha-Fagan, O., & Schwartz, J. E. (1986). Neighborhood and delinquency: An assessment of contextual effects. *Criminology, 24*(4), 667–703.

Skogan, W. G. (1990). *Disorder and decline.* New York: Free Press.

Steinberg, L., Darling, N. E., Fletcher, A. C., Brown, B. B., & Dornbusch, S. M. (1995). *Authoritative parenting and adolescent adjustment: An ecological journey.* In P. Moen, G. H. Elder, Jr., & K. Lúcher (Eds.), *Examining lives in context* (pp. 423–466). Washington, DC: American Psychological Association.

Tangney, J. P., & Fischer, K. W. (1995). *Self-conscious emotions: The psychology of shame, guilt, embarrassment, and pride.* New York: Guilford Press.

Taub, R. P., Taylor, D. G., & Dunham, J. D. (1984). *Paths of neighborhood change: Race and crime in urban America.* Chicago: University of Chicago Press.

Timms, D. W. G. (1971). *The urban mosaic.* Cambridge, UK: Cambridge University Press.

Tonry, M., Ohlin, L. E., & Farrington, D. P. (1991). *Human development and criminal behavior.* New York: Springer-Verlag.

West, D., & Farrington, D. P. (1977). *The delinquent way of life.* London: Heineman.

Wikström, P.-O. (1987). *Patterns of crime in a birth cohort* (Report No. 24). Stockholm: University of Stockholm, Department of Sociology.

Wikström, P.-O. (1991). *Urban crime, criminals and victims.* New York: Springer-Verlag.

Wikström, P.-O. (1995). Self-control, temptations, frictions and punishment: An integrated approach to crime prevention. In P.-O. Wikström, J. McCord, & R. V. Clarke (Eds.), *Integrating crime prevention strategies: Propensity and opportunity* (pp. 7–38). Stockholm: Fritzes.

Wikström, P.-O. (1996). Causes of crime and crime prevention. In T. Bennett (Ed.), *Preventing crime and disorder* (pp. 115–158). Cambridge, UK: University of Cambridge, Institute of Criminology.

Wikström, P.-O. (1998). Communities and crime. In M. Tonry (Ed.), *The handbook of crime and punishment* (pp. 269–301). New York: Oxford University Press.

Wikström, P.-O. (2002). *Adolescent crime in context.* Cambridge, UK: University of Cambridge, Institute of Criminology.

Wikström, P.-O., Clarke, R. V., & McCord, J. (1995). *Integrating crime prevention strategies: Propensity and opportunity.* Stockholm: Fritzes.

Wikström, P.-O., & Dolmén, L. (2001). Urbanisation, neighbourhood social integration, informal social control, minor social disorder, victimisation and fear of crime. *International Review of Victimology, 8,* 121–140.

Wikström, P.-O., & Loeber, R. (2000). Do disadvantaged neighborhoods cause well-adjusted children to become adolescent delinquents? *Criminology, 38,* 1109–1142.

Wikström, P.-O., & Torstensson, M. (1999). Local crime prevention and its national support: Organisation and direction. *European Journal on Criminal Policy and Research, 7,* 459–481.

Wilson, J. Q., & Herrnstein, R. J. (1985). *Crime and human nature.* New York: Touchstone Books.

Wilson, W. J. (1987). *The truly disadvantaged: The inner city, the underclass, and public policy.* Chicago: University of Chicago Press.

Wolfgang, M., & Figlio, R. M. (1972). *Delinquency in a birth cohort.* Chicago: University of Chicago Press.

Wrong, D. H. (1994). *The problem of order: What unites and divides society?* New York: Free Press.

Zahn-Waxler, C., & Robinson, J. (1995). Empathy and guilt: Early origins of feelings and responsibility. In J. P. Tangney & K. W. Fischer (Eds.), *Self-conscious emotions: The psychology of shame, guilt, embarrassment, and pride.* New York: Guilford Press.

# PART III

# TARGETED CAUSAL MODELS

# *Development of Conduct Problems during the Preschool Period*

# 6

# Starting at the Beginning

*Exploring the Etiology of Antisocial*
*Behavior in the First Years of Life*

KATE KEENAN
DANIEL S. SHAW

The activation and regulation of emotions and behavior are critical to healthy physical and psychological development. We operationalize the regulation of emotions and behaviors as the ability to control the intensity of a response to the environment and the ease of recovery from the response. We hypothesize that deficits in regulation are part of all forms of psychopathology, including antisocial behavior. Atypical patterns of emotional activation may also play a key role in psychopathology, but in this chapter we focus on the regulation of emotions. Learning to regulate emotions and behaviors is a process that begins early in life. Thus, stimuli and experiences that elicit negative emotions and behaviors, such as frustration, anger, defiance, and aggression, are necessary components to the learning process since they provide the young child and his or her caregivers with the opportunity to develop more adaptive behaviors that increase emotional and behavioral regulation. When there are significant impediments to the development of such strategies, an accumulation of suboptimal emotional and behavioral functioning results. In this chapter we posit that, for many children, antisocial behavior is the result of individual differences in regulatory capacities and impediments in the appropriate early socialization of emotional and behavioral regulation.

Developmental psychologists have long studied the caregiver's role in early childhood socialization. Such investigations have focused on constructs such as the internalization of moral standards (e.g., Kochanska,

1995), the management of frustration (e.g., Calkins & Johnson, 1998), and the development of empathy (Zahn-Waxler, Radke-Yarrow, Wagner, & Chapman, 1992). In this chapter we review literature demonstrating conceptual and empirical links between these developmental processes and factors associated with antisocial behavior in children and adolescents. There is, however, little interdisciplinary effort in generating useful paradigms for studying the link between these early socialization experiences and the development of antisocial behavior (see Landy & Peters, 1992, and Shaw & Bell, 1993, for exceptions). We believe that the risk for the development of antisocial behavior is the result of both individual deficits in the capacity to regulate emotions and behaviors and a caregiving environment that exacerbates these individual deficits by not providing the appropriate level of developmental guidance in important socialization processes. A comprehensive approach to articulating and testing etiological theories of antisocial behavior will draw on developmental, clinical, and biological approaches to measuring and conceptualizing individual differences.

In this chapter we begin by outlining typical and atypical development in emotional and behavioral regulation and the socialization of these competencies during two developmental periods: infancy and toddlerhood. We then propose two common pathways to early-onset antisocial behavior, both of which should be considered highly exploratory, as data to support such pathways are quite minimal. The first begins with an irritable infant in a caregiving environment that errs on the side of overstimulation, whereas the second begins with an underaroused infant in a caregiving environment that tends toward understimulation. Mechanisms by which these early infant characteristics progress to problematic toddler and preschool behavior are proposed. It is a primary goal of this chapter to argue for the salience of the first years of life for preventing chronic antisocial behavior for many children, and to shift the perception of an "early-intervention" time frame from elementary school to infancy and toddlerhood. Whereas most current theories of the etiology of conduct and antisocial behavior focus on the preschool period and later, we believe that the origins of such behaviors actually begin in infancy.

## DEFINING THE TERM "REGULATION" OF EMOTIONS AND BEHAVIORS

The terms "emotion regulation" and "emotional dysregulation" are used frequently in developmental and developmental psychopathology literature. There is no consensus on how to operationally define this construct, although competing hypotheses are currently being tested (e.g., Keenan, Gunthorpe, & Young, 2002). We propose using the term "emotion regulation" (and "emotion dysregulation") as opposed to the terms "difficult temperament" or "negative emotionality" because the former promotes distinguishing among multiple components of emotionality, including the frequency with which a response is activated (i.e., threshold), the intensity of the response, efforts at decreasing the response, and the latency to recovery. Although there are likely to be significant associations among these components, assessing individual differences in *each* of these areas of emotional functioning may reveal meaningful subgroups of children with regard to risk for antisocial behavior.

There is evidence to support differentiating components of emotional functioning. First, different brain mechanisms are involved in the activation of stress responses versus the homeostatic feedback control of such a response. For example, research on the role of the hypothalamic–pituitary–adrenal (HPA) axis on the stress response has demonstrated that the hypothalamic paraventricular nucleus (PVN) is critical for HPA activation, whereas structures outside the hypothalamus, such as the hippocampus and the prefrontal cortex, provide controlling homeostatic feedback (Sapolsky, Krey, & McEwan, 1984; Sullivan & Gratton, 2002). Further, there is evidence that caregiving behaviors during the early part of development influence the efficacy of the feedback loop but do not influence the activation of the HPA system (Liu et al., 1997).

Second, there appear to be relatively robust individual differences from very early in life in the *intensity* of and the *latency to recover* from responses to stressful stimuli, including duration and intensity of crying, attempts at self-soothing, and cortisol response (Keenan, Gunthorpe, & Young, 2002; Stifter, Spinrad, & Braungart-Rieker, 1999). Even in contexts where there is very little variation in the elicitation of a response (e.g., blood draw), there are significant individual differences in the intensity and ease of recovery from the response as early as the first 2 days of life (Keenan, Gunthorpe, & Young, 2002). Moreover, we will review evidence from both human and animal literature that environmental factors are associated with indices of emotion regulation throughout infancy and toddlerhood, and perhaps even prenatally. Thus, we provide a mechanism by which deficits in emotion regulation emerge and are later exacerbated, leading to the development of psychopathology.

The third reason is that the regulation of emotions and behaviors is a primary method by which individuals with mental health problems are treated. Cognitive, behavioral, and psychopharmacological interventions typically target changes that are operationalized as increases in the regulation of attention or activity in the case of attention-deficit/hyperactivity disorder, physiological arousal in the case of anxiety disorders, and depressogenic cognitions in the case of mood disorders. One could argue, therefore, that a goal of mental health services is to develop and implement methods for constructively managing individual differences along dimensions such as attention, activity, arousal, and negative emotions.

For these reasons, we use the terms "emotion regulation" and "emotion dysregulation" and operationally define them in terms of latency to, intensity of, and the ability to self-soothe and recover from a response that involves negative emotions. In this chapter we review studies that use these operational definitions, but also supplement the literature review with studies in which broader constructs of negative emotionality or difficult temperament are used, given that relatively few studies have tested hypotheses that involve specific dimensions of emotion regulation. The studies are divided into two developmental periods: infancy and toddlerhood, with each section containing data on typical and atypical development of regulatory skills, factors in the caregiving environment that affect such skills, the socialization of these skills, and sex differences in the development and socialization of emotional and behavioral regulation. The emergence of sex differences in developmental vulnerabilities, such as emotion dysregulation, has implications for understanding the etiology of psychopathology, including antisocial behavior. If the reported sex differences in the prevalence of antisocial behavior are valid, then understanding how and when boys' and girls' behavioral and emotional functioning diverge may facilitate the development of testable hypotheses about etiology.

## REGULATION OF EMOTIONS AND BEHAVIORS DURING INFANCY

Individual differences in the capacity to regulate arousal in response to stimuli are present at birth. In many studies, these individual differences have been operationalized as the *intensity* of behavioral and biological responses to stimuli and the *latency* to return to baseline behavioral and biological functioning after the stressor (Gunnar, Connors, Isensee, & Wall, 1988; Keenan, Gunthorpe, & Young, 2002; Spangler & Scheubeck, 1993; Thompson, 1994). Two important areas of research relevant to the regulation of arousal in infancy are research on temperamental differences and studies of biological (e.g., cortisol) and behavioral responses to known stressors (e.g., inoculation).

Indices of emotion regulation via measures of temperament are present in many studies of typical and atypical development of children. Most developmental psychopathology research has focused on a "proneness to distress" or a "difficultness" factor that reflects both negative affect and difficulty with self-regulation of that affect (Rothbart & Ahadi, 1994). Although the methods of assessment of these dimensions vary across studies, the construct appears to be relatively robust and stable over the first few months and even into later infancy. For example, Bates (1992) defined temperamental difficultness via factor analysis, the result of which included items representing frequency and intensity of negative emotion and difficulty being soothed. This factor remained distinct from other temperamental dimensions from 6 to 24 months.

In typically developing infants, regulation of behavior, as demonstrated by more stable periods of sleep and wakefulness and less frequent crying and irritability, proceeds at a fairly rapid rate in the first year of life (St. James-Roberts & Plewis, 1996). The increase in regulatory skills is concurrent with other developmental gains, including increases in social communication and motor skills, which provide the infant with opportunities to signal to the caregiver that she wants to be held, or to crawl toward a desired object, thereby engaging in regulatory strategies (Kopp, 1989). Similar results have been generated through research on the role of neuroendocrine functioning. In normal development, habituation to a negative stimulus such as separation from a caregiver or inoculation is associated with a lessened cortisol response over time (Gunnar, Connors, & Isensee, 1989; Gunnar, Hertsgaard, & Larson, 1992; Lewis & Ramsay, 1995a; Ramsay & Lewis, 1994).

The results from studies on the stability of very early individual differences in emotion and behavioral regulation are mixed. For example, individual differences in cortisol reactivity, which is usually defined as the change in cortisol levels from prestressor to poststressor, are often reported to be only modestly stable and limited in their predictive utility across developmental periods (Gunnar, Brodersen, & Krueger, 1996; Lewis & Ramsay, 1995b). On the other hand, some behavioral constructs, such as the ease with which distress is elicited and the intensity of negative affect in neonates, have been associated with later measures of the same construct (Larson, DiPietro, & Porges, 1987, as cited in Rothbart, Derryberry, & Posner, 1994; Matheny, Riese, & Wilson, 1985). Crockenberg and Smith (1982) reported that neonatal irritability measured in the first 2 weeks of life was significantly associated with observations of latency to calm at 1 and 3 months of age.

Part of the inconsistency in the stability of individual differences in regulation of arousal in infancy is due to the challenge of developing reliable and valid definitions of infant emotion regulation and/or dysregulation given the number of systems involved, the variability in how quickly various systems react to stressors, the impact of the pre- and postnatal environments, and the absence of a consensus on what constitutes "maladaptive" infant behavior. *Emotion dysregulation* has been defined as an inability to respond to stimuli with well-maintained control (Keenan, 2000). In a well-regulated infant, modulated changes in emotions, behavior, and neuroendocrine functioning allow optimal responding to stimuli. In an emotionally dysregulated infant, transitions to states or responses to stimuli are accompanied by unmodulated changes in behavior, emotions, or neuroendocrine functioning. A lack of modulation could be manifest in many ways, including a response that is too weak, a response that is too intense, or one that is too long in duration.

Thus, although there appear to be reliable and meaningful differences in regulatory abilities in infancy, how well those individual differences map onto later problems with emotional and behavioral functioning has not been adequately explored.

## FACTORS AFFECTING EMOTIONAL AND BEHAVIORAL REGULATION IN INFANCY

Since the increasing capacity for self-regulation is part of a normal maturation process, it is expected that factors affecting the normal development of the fetus or neonate may also interrupt or impede other maturational processes. With regard to regulation of emotion and behavior, there is evidence that medically high-risk neonates have deficits in their self-regulatory capacities. For example, Mayes, Bornstein, Chowarska, Haynes, and Granger (1996) compared arousal levels in 36 cocaine-exposed and 27 non-cocaine-exposed, predominately African American, 3-month-old infants. Arousal was measured by behavioral state (alert or crying), affect (negative, positive, or neutral), and attention. There were no significant differences between the two groups on baseline measures of these three indices of arousal. In response to a novel stimulus, however, cocaine-exposed infants displayed more negative affect and cried more often and longer than non-cocaine-exposed infants.

Mode of delivery has been associated with later dysregulation of the stress response, with deliveries requiring forceps resulting in a greater increase in cortisol and longer duration of crying in response to inoculation at 4 months (Taylor, Fisk, & Glover, 2000). Maternal psychological experiences during pregnancy have also been associated with poor regulation of the stress response. Keenan, Grace, and Gunthorpe (2002) found that mothers who reported experiencing a greater number of life stressors during pregnancy had neonates who were observed to have greater difficulty with self-soothing than mothers with fewer life stressors.

It is possible, however, that what appears to be an association between prenatal factors and infant emotion and behavioral regulation is actually better understood as a genetic predisposition for deficits in regulation that are expressed in the mother as high levels of life stress, and in the infants as poor modulation of neuroendocrine functioning or difficulty being soothed. Some evidence for the direct association between altered stress reactivity in neonates and the prenatal environment has been generated from animal studies. Weinstock (1997) has documented less optimal responses to *stress*, defined as heightened behavioral reactivity, in rat pups whose mothers were exposed to stress during the first trimester of pregnancy. Schneider and Moore (2000) reported similar findings in primates: infants who were exposed to stress prenatally showed poorer neurobehavioral functioning at birth and poorer behavioral response to novelty later in life. Prenatal cocaine exposure in the rodent has been associated with delays in attaining developmental milestones (Tonkiss, Shumsky, Shultz, Almeida, & Galler, 1995) and longer duration of aggression responses in males (Johns & Noonan, 1995).

In summary, teratological and maternal psychological factors appear to be associated with differences in infant emotional regulation. In the human, there is still debate as to what this association reflects: the importance of insults during fetal development or the inherited predisposition for deficits in emotion and behavior regulation. Moreover, there is evidence to suggest that early parenting behavior during infancy and the early toddler period explains more variance in later emotional and behavioral functioning than pre- and perinatal factors, including prenatal drug exposure (Beeghly & Tronick, 1994; Shaw, Bell, & Gilliom, 2000; Wakschlag & Hans, 1999). This research is reviewed in the following section.

## SOCIALIZATION OF EMOTIONAL AND BEHAVIORAL REGULATION IN INFANCY

There is a substantial amount of data supporting an association between the early caregiving environment and the development of emotion regulation during infancy (Field, Healy, Goldstein, & Guthertz, 1990; Gable & Isabella, 1992; Spangler, Schieche, Ilg, Maier, & Ackerman, 1994). During this developmental period, caregiver responsiveness to the infant appears to have significant implications for social development. "Responsiveness" generally refers to a caregiver's ability to engage at a behavioral and emotional level that is consistent with the infant's needs and refers to the quality, pacing, developmental level, and consistency of responding. Thus, a child who appropriately communicates distress requires a different type of responsiveness than a child who is contentedly exploring toys. As postulated and demonstrated by researchers of attachment styles (Ainsworth, 1979; Erickson, Sroufe, & Egeland, 1985), contingent and sensitive responding to an infant's needs is believed to be an important step in the development of self-regulatory skills. For example, responsively soothing a distressed infant may be a first step in helping an infant learn to manage negative emotion.

A few studies have demonstrated the effect of caregiving on biological and behavioral regulation of emotional arousal. Gable and Isabella (1992) reported that maternal behavior during the first month of life explained unique variance in the regulation of arousal, including use of head orientation, gaze aversion, and facial expression, in 4-month-olds, even after controlling for the infant's ability to regulate arousal at 1 month. Spangler and colleagues (1994) demonstrated that healthy infants with average skills in self-regulation developed signs of behavioral and biological dysregulation when exposed to insensitive caregiving. For example, infants of highly insensitive mothers at 3 and 6 months had significantly higher increases in cortisol level from baseline to post-mother–child interaction, but no significant differences in baseline cortisol values than infants of sensitive caregivers. By 9 months, however, infants whose mothers were rated as insensitive had *both* higher baseline levels of cortisol and greater cortisol reactivity.

During the second half of the first year, as cognitive changes in the infant increasingly allow him or her to form more stable images of caregiver behavior and predictability, several research teams have uncovered an association between maternal unresponsiveness and later externalizing problems (Shaw & Winslow, 1997). Direct observations of maternal responsiveness have also shown cross-sectional and longitudinal associations with externalizing problems, particularly for boys (Gardner, 1987). Using a model of mother–infant interaction based on the mother's ability to match the intensity of the infant's attention-seeking behavior, Martin, Maccoby, and Jacklin (1981) found that, for boys only, low maternal responsiveness at 10 months was associated with lower rates of compliance at 22 months and higher rates of coercive child behavior at 42 months, results that have been replicated by Shaw and colleagues (Shaw, Keenan, & Vondra, 1994; Shaw et al., 1998) on two occasions using two independent samples of high-risk children. Thus, throughout the first year of life, caregiver behavior is associated with concurrent and later behavioral and emotional regulation.

## SEX DIFFERENCES IN EMOTIONAL AND BEHAVIORAL REGULATION

Most research on sex differences in behavioral indices of infant emotion regulation has revealed few differences (Gunnar, Porter, Wolf, Rigatuso, & Larson, 1995; Keenan & Shaw, 1997; Prior, Smart, Sanson, & Oberklaid, 1993). For example, in a sample of 100 healthy infants, no sex differences were observed in level of distress or the strategies the infants used to regulate distress (e.g., distraction, escape attempts) during frustration tasks at 5, 10, and 18 months (Stifter & Jain, 1996). Nor were there sex differences in the effectiveness of different strategies on reduction of negative emotions (Stifter & Braungart, 1995). Martin, Wisenbaker, Baker, and Huttunen (1997) reported no significant sex differences on maternal reports of frequency and intensity of negative emotion at 6 months of age. In the Australian Temperament Project (Prior et al., 1993), girls and boys were rated equally on dimensions of infant irritability, intensity, reactivity, and overactivity. In a sample of neonates from low-income environments, no sex differences were found with regard to irritability assessed at 10 days of life (van den Boom & Gravenhorst, 1995). Similarly, Keenan, Gunthorpe, and

Young (2002) reported no sex differences in cortisol reactivity to a stressor in healthy newborns.

There are some reports in which early sex differences are reported, however. Gunnar and colleagues (1995) reported that 6-month-old boys scored higher on the "distress to limitations" factor than did girls. Davis and Emory (1995) found significant sex differences in neonates' cortisol reactivity. The majority of findings, however, appear to support greater similarity between girls and boys than differences.

Surprisingly, relations between parenting behaviors in the first year of life and child sex are often not examined. Of the few studies that exist, the effects are not particularly strong. Rosen, Adamson, and Bakeman (1992) observed mother–infant dyads during exposure to novel stimuli in a social-referencing paradigm. There were no differences in how mothers of boys and mothers of girls affectively communicated happiness, but there were differences in how they communicated fear. Mothers of girls showed less intense affect when communicating fear than mothers of boys. This sex difference in maternal behavior was followed by a sex difference in infant behavior during the fear task, in which girls evidenced more avoidance of the novel stimuli than boys.

Weinberg, Tronick, Cohn, and Olson (1999) examined sex differences in infant expression and maternal response during the still-face paradigm, in which the caregiver is instructed to alternate between episodes of typical face-to-face interaction and a flat, expressionless face. Although boys showed more distress during the still face than girls, there were no observed sex differences in maternal behavior. Similarly, Braungart-Reiker, Garwood, Powers, and Notaro (1998) found little effect of infant gender on the quality of the parent–infant behavior or parental sensitivity to infant emotion during the still-face paradigm.

Sex effects of parental socialization of infant emotion may be revealed in other contexts, however. McHale (1995) reported that sex of infant was associated with the emotional tone of parental interactions. Parents were observed during play with their infant sons or daughters. Among maritally distressed families, parents of boys were more likely to manifest hostile and competitive coparenting. Maritally distressed parents of girls were more like to evidence discrepant parenting with regard to expressions of warmth and level of involvement, such that one parent's involvement was coupled with the other parent's detachment. Thus, in the context of marital dissatisfaction, the quality of the parenting behaviors with infants appeared to vary between parents of girls and parents of boys.

In summary, sex differences in the capacity to regulate emotions and behaviors, and in the socialization of emotional and behavioral regulation, appear to be minimal. There may, however, be subtle differences in the types of emotion regulation strategies used by parents of infant girls and boys.

## EMOTIONAL AND BEHAVIORAL REGULATION DURING TODDLERHOOD

From the end of infancy to the beginning of the preschool period there are major developmental changes in self-concept, beginning with self-recognition, proceeding to self-evaluation (including making self-evaluative and referential statements), and then to the development of conscience (Stipek, Gralinski, & Kopp, 1990). These developmental gains in self-concept are associated with increases in the awareness of social demands on the self, including compliance requests by caregivers (Kochanska, Coy, & Murray, 2001). As comprehension regarding "dos' and "don'ts" increases, so does noncompliance (Kaler & Kopp, 1990). In one cross-sectional study (Klimes-Dougan & Kopp, 1999), rates of noncompliance in response to a clean-up task rose from 68% of 18-month-olds to 97% of 30-month-olds.

There is also evidence of increasing rates of aggression during this developmental period. Tremblay and colleagues (1999) reported that many aggressive behaviors began to emerge toward the end of the first year of life. By 17 months, close to half of children are reported to push others, a quarter reportedly kick others, and approximately 15% of children have bitten others (Tremblay et al., 1999). In general, physical aggression increases in frequency until about the age of 2 years, at which point there is a slow but steady decline into the school-age period (Tremblay et al., 1996).

Efforts at regulating negative emotions develop during toddlerhood, and individual differences in this capacity are present (Grolnick, Bridges, & Connell, 1996). Kagan, Snidman, and Arcus (1998) have focused on the ability to regulate behavioral and emotional reactivity to stimuli designed to elicit fear. Clear individual differences in emotion regulation are present in the toddler period, with some evidence of the stability of such individual differences to later ages (Kagan et al., 1998). There is also evidence that, over time, most toddlers increase the use of strategies that are associated with decreases in negative emotion such as self-comforting and requesting help from caregivers earlier than younger toddlers (Kopp, 1989).

Despite the fact that behaviors reflecting poor emotional and behavioral regulation are relatively common during this developmental period, one can differentiate subsets of toddlers who show extremely high rates of aggression, noncompliance, and deficits in emotion regulation. For example, Keenan and colleagues (Keenan, Shaw, Walsh, Delliquadri, & Giovannelli, 1997; Keenan, Shaw, Delliquadri, Giovannelli, & Walsh, 1998) used observational methods for identifying toddlers who were highly aggressive and noncompliant. Those toddlers continued to show deficits in these areas at later periods in toddlerhood and preschool, and were more likely to be diagnosed with a disruptive behavior disorder at age 5.

In Shaw, Owens, Giovannelli, and Winslow's (2001) cohort of low-income boys, 63% of boys identified at or above the 90th percentile on the Child Behavior Checklist (CBCL; Achenbach, 1992) Externalizing factor at age 2 remained above the 90th percentile at age 5. At age 6, 62% remained in the clinical range. Importantly, false negative rates were relatively low. Only 13% of boys below the 50th percentile on externalizing problems at age 2 moved into the clinical range at age 5.

In addition, individual differences in intensity of distress is associated with other developmental vulnerabilities such as poor problem-solving behaviors. For example, 2-year-olds who demonstrated distress in response to frustration were more likely to display aggression, and were less likely to use instrumental behaviors to overcome their distress, than toddlers who did not display high levels of distress (Calkins & Johnson, 1998).

Thus, extreme deficits in emotional and behavioral regulation during the toddler period are associated with less optimal concurrent functioning and future behavioral and emotional problems.

## FACTORS AFFECTING EMOTIONAL AND BEHAVIOR REGULATION DURING TODDLERHOOD

It is somewhat artificial to identify only a few factors that are relevant to emotional and behavioral regulation in toddlerhood given that all developmental processes are better conceptualized as interrelated. However, in an effort to be parsimonious, we focus on two that we propose have particular relevance for toddler regulation of negative affect, aggression, and noncompliance and for later antisocial behavior: language and empathic responding.

Language is a primary means by which parents and other socializing agents affect children's behavior. For most children, there is a tremendous growth in language development during the second year of life. This increase in the ability to communicate occurs during a time of evolving autonomy and is an important component for both the child and the parent in navigating this challenging period of development. For the child, frustration is likely to be reduced when needs are more easily met, while the parent may feel more efficacious in her or his ability to understand and communicate expectations to this child. We hypothesize that language is a primary means by which children learn to solve problems nonaggressively and effectively decrease negative emotions such as anger, fear, and sadness. Thus, typical language development may be advantageous to both child and parent in reducing stress and facilitating the socialization process. Delayed language, on the other hand, may increase stress at the individual and dyadic level and impede normal socialization.

A few studies have demonstrated an association between poor language skills in early childhood and early disruptive behavior problems. Coy, Speltz, DeKlyen, and Jones (2001) reported that low Verbal IQ and language skills were associated with poor social problem solving and encoding of social situations in preschool boys. Stansbury and Zimmermann (1999) demonstrated that delayed language in preschoolers was associated with suboptimal emotion socialization behaviors by parents, which in turn was associated with externalizing and internalizing problems. Stowe, Arnold, and Ortiz (2000) found that language functioning was associated with observed disruptive behavior in a preschool classroom and teacher-reported social problems, but only for boys. Finally, in one prospective study, language development in the first 2 years of life was associated with registered criminality in adulthood (Stattin & Klackenberg-Larsson, 1993).

The ability to take another's perspective is a cognitive-emotional skill that evolves during the toddler period. A large part of this learning occurs in the context of aggression and rule violation. Caregivers tend to focus on the impact of such behaviors on others as a means of disciplining. Thus, normative aggression and noncompliance serve as important catalysts for the development of aspects of perspective taking, including empathy. By the end of the preschool period children have internalized rules that are associated with being able to inhibit behavior, follow rules, and manage negative emotions (Kochanska, Murray, & Coy, 1997). Most typically, developing preschool children have a basic understanding of the impact of their behavior on others and can control their behavior based on internalized social norms (Kochanska et al., 1997).

Empathic responses to others' distress also emerge during the toddler period. Zahn-Waxler and colleagues (1992) have observed increases in the frequency of behaviors directed toward reducing another's distress during the second year of life. In addition, toddlers begin to evidence attempts at understanding another person's distress. Interestingly, as they got older, toddlers were less likely to show empathic concern when distress occurred as a result of their own behavior (Zahn-Waxler et al., 1992).

There are clearly individual differences in empathic capacities during this developmental period. These differences appear to be associated with deficits in emotional and behavioral regulation. For example, in a longitudinal study from preschool to late elementary school, Hastings, Zahn-Waxler, Robinson, Usher, and Bridges (2000) reported a significant interaction effect of individual differences in empathy and disruptive behavior at preschool age on the stability and severity of disruptive behavior at school age.

Such individual differences in empathy can be explained in part by other developmental and cognitive competencies. Cognitively, the ability to generate hypothetical alternatives is just emerging during this period (Reznick, Corley, & Robinson, 1997). Language skills also affect the development of empathy, given that much of the socialization of empathic responding occurs via language. Thus, by toddlerhood there is likely to be interrelations among these developmental competencies, although this has yet to be tested.

## SOCIALIZATION OF EMOTIONAL AND BEHAVIORAL REGULATION DURING TODDLERHOOD

Researchers studying the relations between caregiving and children's behaviors and emotions in the preschool period have identified several characteristics of parenting related to children's behavior such as parental involvement, hostility, consistency, and harsh discipline (Gardner, 1987; Zahn-Waxler, Iannotti, Cummings, & Denham, 1990). For example, Pettit and Bates (1989) demonstrated that low rates of maternal positive involvement during infancy and toddlerhood strongly predicted children's disruptive behavior at age 4. Renken, Egeland, Marvinney, Mangelsdorf, and Sroufe (1989) showed that maternal hostility and abuse when children were 42 months old predicted children's aggression during elementary school.

Some research on parenting during the toddler period has attempted to assess how patterns of parental response to toddler behaviors and emotions affect later development of aggressive and disruptive behavior. For example, Shaw and colleagues (1998) found that toddlers of parents who were observed as rejecting during a clean-up task demonstrate an increased risk for conduct problems at age 3.5. Furthermore, a composite score of observed rejecting parenting at ages 1.5 and 2 differentiated clinically significant levels of boys' conduct problems at ages 5 and 8 according to *both* parent and teacher reports (Shaw et al., 2001).

Bates, Pettit, Dodge, and Ridge (1998) assessed the outcome in late childhood of difficult and nondifficult preschoolers in the context of authoritative and passive parents. Toddlers who scored high on resistance to control (e.g., those who were socially unresponsive, dominating, impulsive) with passive parents had the worst outcome in terms of subsequent parent- and teacher-rated externalizing problems at school age. Campbell, Pierce, Moore, Marakovitz, and Newby (1996) reported that observations of negative maternal control and maternal self-report of negative discipline at age 4 predicted externalizing problems at age 9, even after controlling for earlier behavior problems. In a cross-sectional study of 2- to 4-year-old children, Kochansaka and Aksan (1995) demonstrated that the level of mutual positive affect is associated with higher rates of compliance and greater internalization of rules.

Thus, how parents respond to negative emotions and behaviors during the toddler period significantly appears to affect the continuity of such problems even after controlling for variation in toddler behavior.

## SEX DIFFERENCES IN BEHAVIORAL AND EMOTIONAL
## REGULATION DURING TODDLERHOOD

There are several studies documenting few sex differences in behavioral and emotional regulation during the toddler period (e.g., Prior et al., 1993; Stifter & Jain, 1996). However, there do appear to be sex differences in developmental competencies and the strategies used to regulate behaviors and emotions. In a community-based study by Briggs-Gowan, Carter, Moye Skuban, and McCue Horwitz (2001), mothers reported that girls showed higher levels of compliance, empathy, and mastery motivation than boys. This finding of greater competencies among girls than boys has also been reported in studies of language development and functioning (Morisset, Barnard, & Booth, 1995) and emotional perspective taking (Zahn-Waxler, Radlke-Yarrow, Wagner, & Chapman, 1992). Such competencies may affect aspects of behavioral and emotional regulation. For example, Raver (1996) reported no sex differences in the frequency of displays of negative emotion among 2-year-olds in response to different types of stressors. There were sex differences, however, in the types of strategies that girls and boys used during the stress tasks. Girls tended to seek comfort from their mothers when distressed more often than boys. Boys, on the other hand, used distraction (i.e., diverting their attention away from the stressor), more than girls.

The study of discipline practices in early childhood also has revealed interesting sex differences that appear to directly influence behavioral and emotional regulation. For example, Smetana (1989) observed "moral" and "conventional" transgressions between 36 toddlers and their mothers and between the toddlers and their peers. *Moral transgressions* were defined as acts that violated the rights or welfare of others, including object conflicts and aggression. *Conventional transgressions* were defined as breaking familial or cultural rules or conventions. Mothers of girls responded to their daughters' moral transgressions by pointing out the consequences that the transgression would have on the peer, whereas mothers of boys responded with punishment. Similarly, Ross, Tesla, Kenyon, and Lollis (1990) observed maternal interventions in object-related conflicts between toddler peers. Although mothers generally intervened in favor of the peer over their own child, mothers of boys favored their own children three times as often as mothers of girls.

In summary, there appear to be reciprocal effects between sex of child and parenting behaviors. The data thus far indicate that differences in parenting as a result of the child's sex are more pronounced in toddlerhood than in infancy. This may be because sex differences in certain competencies, such as language fluency, empathy, and compliance, appear to emerge in toddlerhood, thus affecting parenting behaviors. On the other hand, sex differences in these competencies may in part be the result of subtle differences in parenting behaviors during infancy. Continued exploration of how such sex differences emerge may lead to a better understanding of how to facilitate positive development in these areas for both girls and boys.

## TWO PATHWAYS TO ANTISOCIAL BEHAVIOR FROM INFANCY TO PRESCHOOL

We have thus far provided theoretical and, when available, empirical evidence for the importance of individual differences in and the socialization of emotional and behavioral regulation to the development of antisocial behavior. In this section we hypothesize that there are two primary pathways that lead to different types of antisocial behavior. Following the work of Dodge and Coie (1987), the first type of behavior is characterized as *reactive*, which we define as antisocial behavior that is predominately a response to an event (e.g., aggression in response to limit setting, noncompliance in response to perceived unfairness). The second type is *proactive*, which we define as antisocial behavior that occurs as a result of achieving a specific antisocial goal (e.g., lying to deceive). Whereas Dodge and Coie focused specifically on aggression, we propose expanding the distinction to encompass other manifestations of disruptive behavior such as stealing, noncompliance, and rule violations. Essentially we view disruptive behavior problems as stemming from either emotional and behavioral overarousal or emotional and behavioral underarousal, which can be observed as early as the first year of life. These two pathways are conceptualized as addressing some of the heterogeneity in antisocial behavior originating in early childhood, although they are by no means comprehensive and do not include factors more relevant for later starter periods such as peer deviance, parental monitoring, and neighborhood climate.

The hypothesized pathway to reactive antisocial behavior (Figure 6.1) begins with an irritable infant who is unable to respond to typically occurring external and internal stimuli such as diaper changes and hunger cues with well-modulated arousal. These infants have more intense responses to stress as measured by crying, heart rate, and cortisol changes, and have a longer latency to recover than the average infant. The high levels of negative emotion are often accompanied by poorly coordinated motor activity that may further increase the level of arousal. Because these infants cry more frequently and intensely than most infants, and appear motorically hyperactive, we believe that caregivers have a hard time reading their cues. For example, they may misinterpret arm extensions as an attempt to push the caregiver away. Crying that is not rhythmic may interfere with feeding, leading the caregiver to postpone feeding despite the infant's significant hunger. This pattern of poor communication on the part of the infant and unsuccessful caregiver attempts at managing the distressed infant has three primary negative sequelae. First, caregivers try to avoid situations that may

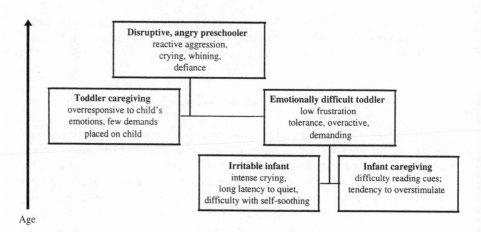

**FIGURE 6.1.** Pathway to reactive antisocial behavior.

result in distress on the part of the infant because they feel ineffective in managing intense negative affect. Second, caregivers tend to respond quickly to the first signs of distress in a way that dampens the affect, with the goal of preventing escalation of negative affect. These two consequences reduce the number of opportunities the parent has for developing appropriate skills for helping her or his infant manage negative emotions.

The third negative sequela is a limitation in the opportunity for the infant to experience negative emotion, thus preventing the infant from developing strategies to constructively express and manage emotional distress. Some of these strategies are self-generated, including self-soothing mechanisms such as sucking and attention shifting. However, the potentially more important strategies are interpersonal, that is, using a caregiver to help identify the source of distress and to develop a strategy to manage the distress. This process begins at birth and continues throughout development. The capacity to identify and analyze the source of distress and generate strategies changes substantially with the accumulation of developmental competencies such as cognitive, language, and social competencies. But the skills developed in infancy serve as building blocks upon which these later developing skills are placed, leading to even greater maturity in emotion regulation.

When a child enters the toddler period without basic skills in self-soothing or without patterns of interaction with the caregiver that effectively manage distress, emotional functioning can become increasingly dysregulated. As stated earlier, typical challenges of the toddler period include increases in autonomous behavior as well as greater awareness and understanding of limit setting by adults. Thus, toddlers encounter a greater number of intra- and interpersonal experiences that are likely to elicit frustration, anger, and sadness than infants. A toddler who was unable to develop appropriate regulatory skills in infancy meets these increasingly challenging experiences with poorly modulated emotional and behavioral responses, such that a caregiver is confronted with both intense emotions and aggressive and destructive behaviors. As a result, constructive socialization of aggression and noncompliance is impeded; many caregivers continue to avoid setting limits and providing structure in an effort to reduce the frequency of intense emotional outbursts and negative interactions. Without such supports and structure, prosocial development is also delayed. The child thus enters the preschool period with an accumulation of deficits and a lack of development of prosocial behaviors. In this pathway, preschool antisocial behavior is characterized primarily by oppositionality and aggression that mainly occurs in response to an event, whereas covert behaviors, such as stealing and lying to deceive, are much less common.

The second hypothesized pathway begins with an infant who is underaroused by stimuli. This type of infant may be conceptualized as a "quiet" infant who rarely cries and who seems to be relatively unaffected by external stimuli. Such infants may also show minimal behavioral and biological reactions to low levels of stimulation, so that they may appear unresponsive to the caregiver. The caregiver may respond by reducing her or his level of interaction with this child either because the efforts feel unreciprocated or because the infant is seen as self-sufficient. Thus, the level of interaction decreases. This pattern, however, reflects another form of miscommunication between the infant and the caregiver. The infant may actually require greater levels of stimulation to achieve a state that allows him or her to be engaged and interact with the caregiver. Activation of that aroused and alert state by the caregiving environment may help the infant access an optimal level of arousal more quickly and easily, whereas less frequent activation of alert states may lead to greater deviation from normative levels of arousal. In addition, the infrequent interaction between the infant and the caregiver deprives the dyad of opportunities for developing patterns of communication upon which to build.

As this infant moves into toddlerhood, she or he lacks a foundation for constructively using the caregiver to help manage problems and achieve goals. As the toddler engages in greater exploration of the environment, the caregiver will begin to impose limits and rules. However, the dyad's earlier lack of experience in regulating behaviors and emotions puts them at a disadvantage for negotiating this new developmental challenge. The toddler may appear to be unresponsive to parental behavior and be described as persistent in a way that indicates a disregard of others. A caregiver who experiences her child as unresponsive may be at risk for exerting less effort at socializing both positive and negative behaviors, making it even more difficult to exert control when necessary. Without the successful application of appropriate disciplinary strategies, the caregiver may at times use more severe or harsh strategies. In addition, the toddler may not experience levels of fear arousal that help to reduce some negative behaviors. For example, fear of getting hurt or of eliciting a negative response from one's caregiver often serves to reduce the probability of a toddler engaging in a dangerous or prohibited behavior. A child whose level of fear arousal is chronically low may not experience a level of arousal high enough and uncomfortable enough to inhibit such behaviors.

By the end of the toddler period, the dyad is now in a difficult position for preparing the child for preschool. The child does not have experience in using adults to guide his or her behavior and his or her pattern of response to stimuli is not one that normally deters children from engaging in risky behavior. The toddler–caregiver relationship may have been characterized by underinvolvement and lack of warmth. Thus positive affect may also be less likely to be expressed by the child. Such a child enters the preschool period with negative behaviors that are fairly resistant to normative socialization efforts by peers and teachers and a lack of socially engaging behaviors. The child's lack of emotional engagement may further distance socializing agents (e.g., teachers), resulting in decreasing opportunities for developing prosocial skills. Although children on this second pathway may be described as having both oppositional and conduct problems, the oppositional behaviors consist primarily of overt forms of defiance and disregard for authority, and the conduct problems include covert behaviors and cruelty to others that is carried out in a deliberate, proactive way.

The two models would be incomplete without acknowledging factors that compromise the quality of early caregiving. The effects of many caregiving environment factors such as parental depressive symptoms, parental conflict, and low social support on child emotional and behavioral regulation are believed to be at least partially accounted for by parenting practices (Keenan, 2000; Shaw & Bell, 1993; Shaw et al., 2000). If childrearing methods place children at greater risk for conduct problems, factors that compromise the quality of very early caregiving need to be examined. Research on parental adjustment and intrafamily factors, such as parental depression (Zahn-Waxler, Iannotti, Cummings, & Denham, 1990), parental conflict (Jouriles et al., 1991), parenting hassles (Crnic & Greenberg, 1990), and social support (Crnic, Greenberg, Ragozin, Robinson, & Basham, 1983) all indicate significant associations with child conduct problems. Some of these correlates (e.g., maternal depression and life stressors) have also demonstrated associations with very early deficits in emotion regulation. It is likely that progression along the above pathways is moderated by a lack of resources in the caregiving environment, which reduce the caregiver's ability to actively engage in behaviors that support emotional and behavior regulation.

## EVIDENCE FOR THE PROPOSED PATHWAYS

There are a number of studies that provide support for the contribution of deficits in emotion regulation in infancy and later disruptive behavior. These studies are highly useful in piecing together evidence for the salience of early child characteristics, caregiving behaviors, and the interaction of the two. In terms of the contribution of infant emotional and behavioral regulation to later antisocial behavior, a few studies exist in which components of the proposed model have been tested. Stifter and colleagues (1999) reported that the intensity of distress and the capacity to regulate distress at 5 months were both associated with different forms of noncompliance at 30 months. A sample of 100, full-term, healthy infants was recruited through a local community hospital. At 5, 10, and 18 months, infants were observed during laboratory assessments during which behavioral reactivity and regulation was observed. Regulatory behaviors during frustration tasks were coded from videotapes and included orientation toward mother or other objects, trying to escape, and self-comforting. At 30 months, compliance during developmental testing, cleanup, and electrode placement was observed. Noncompliance behaviors included active defiance (e.g., whining, reacting with anger) and passive noncompliance (e.g., ignoring requests). Infants who were considered low reactors to stress and high regulators were more likely to ignore maternal requests as toddlers. In contrast, infants who were high reactors and poor regulators were more likely as toddlers to respond to maternal requests with anger and irritability. Thus, these results support our hypothesis that different patterns of reactivity (high and low) in infancy are associated with different patterns of later antisocial behavior.

A number of longitudinal studies provide some support for the second pathway. For example, two studies have demonstrated relations between early measures of fearlessness and later antisocial behavior. These studies are relevant given the potential association between underarousal in infancy and fearlessness or sensation seeking in toddlerhood. Colder, Mott, and Berman (2002) used data from the children of the National Longitudinal Study of Youth (NLSY) participants to test the predictive utility of two dimensions of infant temperament, activity level and fearfulness, to later externalizing and internalizing problems at school age. High activity level and low fearfulness measured within the first year of life was associated with increases in behaviors such as cheating and lying, purposeful destruction of property, and arguing from 4 to 8 years for boys, whereas all other combinations of those two temperamental dimensions were not associated with changes in those types of antisocial behaviors.

Similar to the findings of Colder and colleagues, Shaw, Gilliom, Ingoldsby, and Nagin (2003) found evidence for the influence of early child fearlessness on the course of early conduct problems. A semiparametric mixture model was applied to a sample of 284 low-income boys to model developmental trajectories of overt conduct problems from ages 2 to 8. Follow-up analyses indicated that persistent problem behaviors were associated with high child fearlessness and high maternal rejecting parenting.

In a third study, conducted by Olson, Bates, Sandy, and Lanthier (2000), 168 infants were followed from age 6 months to age 17 years. Maternal report of frequency and intensity of negative emotionality, sootheability, resistance to control, and parenting behaviors were hypothesized as the primary precursors to later antisocial behavior. Mothers and teachers completed behavior checklists from entry to school through adolescence. Overall, main effects of maternal perceptions of toddlers' resistance to control and lack of emotional responsiveness and lack of observed warmth in the mother–infant interaction were found for child and adolescent externalizing problems.

## POTENTIAL SEX DIFFERENCES IN THE PROPOSED PATHWAYS

We (Keenan & Shaw, 1997) proposed earlier that although there appear to be few sex differences in rate or type of behavioral and emotional problems in infancy and toddlerhood, sex differences emerge during the latter part of the preschool period, with girls showing somewhat of a decrease in the overall rate of problem behaviors. Furthermore, we proposed that there are two primary explanations for the lower rates of problems with behavioral and emotional regulation in the preschool period among girls than among boys. First, there are significant sex differences in language development and empathic responding, with girls showing more developed skills in these areas than boys in early childhood. These developmental competencies, we argued, positively affected parents' socialization of behavioral and emotional regulation. Second, we posited that the socialization of sex differences resulted in a greater effort on the part of parents to extinguish manifestations of aggression, overt noncompliance, and irritability in girls, but not in boys. Although we believe that the potentially greater focus of encouraging empathic responding and compliance in girls may carry with it risk for other types of deficits in emotion regulation, such as depression (Keenan & Hipwell, 2002), girls' transitions to the preschool period appear to be facilitated by these developmental and social processes. In summary, the socialization of emotional and behavioral regulation during the toddler period appears to be less challenging for girls than for boys.

With regard to the proposed model, we expect similar findings with regard to less persistence across development among girls than among boys. This hypothesis follows from the data supporting the emergence and solidification of social competencies during the preschool period. Thus, we expect less predictive utility from infant over- or underarousal to later reactive and proactive antisocial behavior in girls than in boys.

When we do find predictive utility of infant behavior and emotion to preschool functioning in girls, we propose that the overaroused model (Figure 6.1) will be the more common pathway for girls for several reasons. First, when girls do manifest antisocial behavior, they tend to have higher rates of comorbid negative emotion (e.g., depression and anxiety symptoms) than do boys (Loeber & Keenan, 1994). Thus, it is possible that the most common pathway to antisocial behavior for girls includes difficulty with managing negative emotion early in life.

Second, the greater press for parents to socialize girls to internalize rules and consider how their behavior effects others is sufficiently strong to interrupt the early signs of disruptive behavior that are common to the underaroused pathway (Figure 6.2), including persistence, disregard for rules and punishment, and sensation-seeking behaviors. For example, Maccoby, Snow, and Jacklin (1984) reported that mothers of infant girls increased their effort at completing a problem-solving task when their daughters were not complying, whereas mothers of boys did not increase their effort. Kerig, Cowan, and Cowan (1993) observed that parents of daughters were more likely to respond positively to compliance behaviors than parents of sons. In contrast, the press to socialize girls not to display negative emotionality appears to be less strong than for boys, although the data is mixed depending on whether the negative emotion is fear or irritability. For example, parents appear more accepting of shyness in girls than

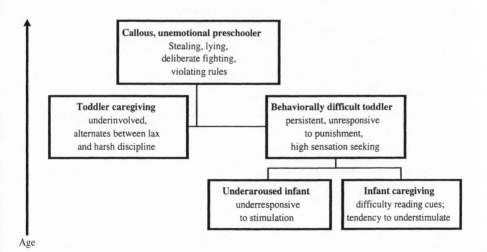

FIGURE 6.2. Pathway to proactive antisocial behavior.

in boys (Simpson & Stevenson-Hinde, 1985). This rather indirect data leads us to argue that the majority of girls with early-onset antisocial behavior will be better conceptualized as having followed the reactive pathway.

## FUTURE TESTS OF THE PROPOSED MODEL

Broadly speaking, there is evidence for the contribution of both early child characteristics and factors in the caregiving environment to the development of antisocial behavior. What has yet to be tested is the predictive utility of more objective measures of individual differences in emotion regulation in infancy, and the specificity of parenting behaviors that exacerbate the deficits inherent in problematic emotion regulation. In addition, there have been no models that posit that an early bifurcation in the quality of dysregulation (i.e., under- vs. overarousal) accounts for heterogeneity in later disruptive and antisocial behavior. A complete test of the proposed model would begin with an assessment of the prenatal environment, with specific attention paid to the factors that have already been demonstrated to be associated with the neonate's capacity for regulating arousal, including prenatal exposure to teratogens and maternal stress in both animals and humans (see Figure 6.3). Assessment of these experiences throughout

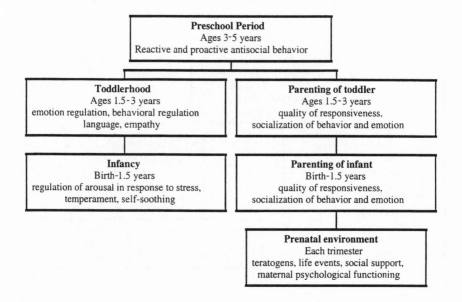

FIGURE 6.3. Complete developmental model from the prenatal environment to the preschool period.

the pregnancy may help identify whether specific periods of fetal development may be more sensitive to such factors than others, as has been found in the animal literature (e.g., Weinstock, 1997). During the period of infancy (birth–age 1.5 years) regular systematic assessment of patterns of arousal to known stressors and maternal perceptions of the infant's average ability to regulate arousal (i.e., temperament) should be assessed. Parenting behaviors in response to the infant's arousal to a stressor and in the context of a nonstressful interaction will generate data on both the response to intense emotion and the more typical emotional tone that characterizes the parent–infant dyad. In toddlerhood, continued assessment of emotionality and behavioral response to high and low stress should be conducted, as should assessment of parenting behaviors in both contexts. Finally, at the level of preschool development, a range of reactive and proactive antisocial behaviors should be measured across home, school, and peer contexts.

We note, however, that one necessary component to the model is the reliable and valid differentiation between under- and overarousal to stress, and reactive and proactive antisocial behavior. Some work has been done on the latter construct. Dodge and Coie (1987) have developed a teacher report measure of reactive and proactive aggression. Their work, however, has focused almost exclusively on aggression in school-age children, and is limited in the number of items used to measure each construct (three for each). The utility of their reactive and proactive constructs over and above the current DSM categories of oppositional defiant disorder and conduct disorder has been questioned (Waschbusch, Willoughby, & Pelham, 1998). Although oppositional defiant disorder and conduct disorder symptoms include behaviors that could be conceptualized as reactive or proactive, the current diagnostic system for disruptive behavior disorders does not allow for a systematic assessment of the salience of emotional and behavioral over- or underarousal in the manifestation of oppositional defiant disorder and conduct disorder symptoms.

Keenan and Wakschlag (2002) have described a research agenda aimed at exploring the validity of symptoms of disruptive behavior disorders in preschool children. As part of this research, a more systematic assessment of reactive and proactive antisocial behaviors according to parent and teacher report will be conducted, as well as observations of emotional and behavioral regulation in the context of tasks designed to elicit negative emotion. Thus, the reliability and validity of reactive and proactive antisocial behavior constructs will be tested.

Similarly, the literature on emotional regulation in infancy is not sufficiently developed for testing the proposed hypotheses. There has been a bias toward operationalizing overarousal despite the fact that there is a substantial group of infants who demonstrate an imperceptible change in their level of arousal in response to stimuli that elicit emotional response in most infants (e.g., Keenan, Gunthorpe, & Young, 2002). Thus, more effort needs to be directed at testing alternatives to defining different forms of under- and overarousal in infancy. Keenan, Gunthorpe, and Young (2002) have collected data on 100 neonates whose mothers live in low-income environments. Within 48 hours of birth, objective measures of regulation of arousal were collected as well as information on the mothers' experiences with stressors during pregnancy. These babies have been seen every 6 months up until the age of 2. Information on maternal perception of temperament, regulation of arousal both biologically and behaviorally, stressors in the caregiving environment, observed parenting behavior, and early emerging behavioral and emotional problems were gathered. In this study, we have begun exploring operational definitions of over- and underarousal by examining patterns of cortisol reactivity at birth. We plan to continue examining individual patterns of arousal both behaviorally and biologically and to test their association with later deficits in emotional and behavioral regulation.

In conclusion, we propose a theory of the etiology of antisocial behavior that focuses on early deficits in emotion regulation as a causal factor. The caregiving environment further modifies individual differences in early emotion regulation. Although our model can be categorized as a "child effects" model, we do acknowledge that extremely negative caregiving environments can negatively affect infants and toddlers whose initial capacity for emotion regulation was quite strong. Alternatively, highly supportive caregiving environments can result in the development of optimal emotional and behavioral regulation skills, even in the context of earlier dysregulation. We therefore believe that our proposed model that includes assessing individual differences in infant regulation and factors in the caregiving environment that directly affect regulatory skills will account for more variance in later antisocial behavior than models that are focused on either caregiving environments (e.g., social learning theory models) or individual differences (e.g., population variation in genotypes).

## ACKNOWLEDGMENTS

This chapter was prepared with support from Grant Nos. K01 MH-01484 and R01 MH62437 to Dr. Keenan and Grant No. K02 MH-01666 to Dr. Shaw from the National Institute of Mental Health. We would like to thank Drs. Benjamin Lahey and Terrie Moffit for their constructive feedback on an earlier draft.

## REFERENCES

Achenbach, T. M. (1992). *Manual for Child Behavior Checklist: 2–3 and 1992 profile.* Burlington, VT: University of Vermont.
Ainsworth, M. S. (1979). Infant–mother attachment. *American Psychologist, 34*, 932–937.
Bates, J. E. (1992). *Infant Characteristics Questionnaire.* Bloomington: Indiana University.

Bates, J. E., Pettit, G. S., Dodge, K. A., & Ridge, B. (1998). Interaction of temperamental resistance to control and restrictive parenting in the development of externalizing behavior. *Developmental Psychology, 34*, 1–14.

Beeghly, M., & Tronick, E. Z. (1994). Effects of prenatal exposure to cocaine in early infancy: Toxic effects on the process of mutual regulation. *Infant Mental Health Journal, 15*, 158–175.

Braungart-Reiker, J., Garwood, M. M., Powers, B. P., & Notaro, P. C. (1998). Infant affect and affect regulation during the still-face paradigm with mothers and fathers: The role of infant characteristics and parental sensitivity. *Developmental Psychology, 34*, 1428–1437.

Briggs-Gowan, M. J., Carter, A. S., Moye Skuban, E., & McCue Horwitz, S. (2001). Prevalence of social–emotional and behavioral problems in a community sample of 1- and 2-year-old children. *Journal of the American Academy of Child and Adolescent Psychiatry, 40*, 811–819.

Calkins, S. D., & Johnson, M. C. (1998). Toddler regulation and distress to frustrating events: Temperamental and maternal correlates. *Infant Behavior and Development, 21*, 379–395.

Campbell, S. B., Pierce, E. W., Moore, G., Marakovitz, S., & Newby, K. (1996). Boys' externalizing problems at elementary school age: Pathways from early behavior problems, maternal control, and family stress. *Development and Psychopathology, 8*, 701–719.

Colder, C. R., Mott, J. A., & Berman, A. S. (2002). The interactive effects of infant activity level and fear on growth trajectories of early childhood behavior problems. *Development and Psychopathology, 14*, 1–24.

Coy, K., Speltz, M. L., DeKlyen, M., & Jones, K. (2001). Social-cognitive processes in preschool boys with and without oppositional defiant disorder. *Journal of Abnormal Child Psychology, 29*, 107–119.

Crnic, K. A., & Greenberg, M. T. (1990). Minor parenting stresses with young children. *Child Development, 61*, 1628–1637.

Crnic, K. A., Greenberg, M. T., Ragozin, A. S., Robinson, N. M., & Basham, R. B. (1983). Effects of stress and social support on mothers and premature and full-term infants. *Child Development, 57*, 209–217.

Crockenberg, S. B., & Smith, P. (1982). Antecedents of mother–infant interaction and infant irritability in the first three months of life. *Infant Behavior and Development, 5*, 105–119.

Davis, M., & Emory, E. (1995). Sex differences in neonatal stress reactivity. *Child Development, 66*, 14–27.

Dodge, K. A., & Coie, J. D. (1987). Social-information processing factors in reactive and proactive aggression in children's peer groups. *Journal of Personality and Social Psychology, 53*, 1146–1158.

Erickson, M. F., Sroufe, L. A., & Egeland, B. (1985). The relationship between quality of attachment and behavior problems in preschool in a high-risk sample. *Monographs of the Society for Research in Child Development, 50*(1–2), 147–166.

Field, T., Healy, B., Goldstein, S., & Guthertz, M. (1990). Behavior–state matching and synchrony in mother–infant interactions of nondepressed versus depressed dyads. *Developmental Psychology, 26*, 7–14.

Gable, S., & Isabella, R. A. (1992). Maternal contributions to infant regulation of arousal. *Infant Behavior and Development, 15*, 95–107.

Gardner, F. E. (1987). Positive interaction between mothers and conduct-problem children: Is there training for harmony as well as fighting? *Journal of Abnormal Child Psychology, 15*, 283–293.

Grolnick, W. S., Bridges, L. J., & Connell, J. P. (1996). Emotion regulation in two-year-olds: Strategies and emotional expression in four contexts. *Child Development, 67*, 928–941.

Gunnar, M. R., Brodersen, L., & Krueger, K. (1996). Dampening of adrenocortical responses during infancy: Normative changes and individual differences. *Child Development, 67*, 877–889.

Gunnar, M. R., Connors, J., & Isensee, J. (1989). Lack of stability in neonatal adrenocortical reactivity because of rapid habituation of the adrenocortical response. *Developmental Psychobiology, 22*, 221–233.

Gunnar, M. R., Connors, J., Isensee, J., & Wall, L. (1988). Adrenocortical activity and behavioral distress in human newborns. *Developmental Psychobiology, 21*, 297–310.

Gunnar, M. R., Hertsgaard, L., & Larson, M. (1992). Cortisol and behavioral responses to repeated stressors in the human newborn. *Developmental Psychobiology, 24*, 487–505.

Gunnar, M. R., Porter, F. L., Wolf, C. M., Rigatuso, J., & Larson, M. C. (1995). Neonatal stress reactivity: Predictions to later emotional temperament. *Child Development, 66*, 1–13.

Hastings, P. D., Zahn-Waxler, C., Robinson, J., Usher, B., & Bridges, D. (2000). The development of concern for others in children with behavior problems. *Developmental Psychology, 36*, 531–546.

Johns, J. M., & Noonan, L. R. (1995). Prenatal cocaine exposure affects social behaviour in Sprague–Dawley rats. *Neurotoxicology and Teratology, 17*, 569–576.

Jouriles, E. N., Murphy, C. M., Farris, A. M., Smith, D. A., Richters, J. E., & Waters, E. (1991). Marital adjustment, parental disagreements about child rearing, and behavior problems in boys: Increasing the specificity of the marital assessment. *Child Development, 62*, 1424–1433.

Kagan, J., Snidman, N., & Arcus, D. (1998). Childhood derivatives of high and low reactivity in infancy. *Child Development, 69*, 1483–1493.

Kaler, S. R., & Kopp, C. B. (1990). Compliance and comprehension in very young toddlers. *Child Development, 61*, 1997–2003.

Keenan, K. (2000). Emotion dysregulation as a risk factor for psychopathology. *Clinical Psychology: Science and Practice, 7*, 418–434.

Keenan, K., Grace, D., & Gunthorpe, D. (2002). *Examining stress reactivity in neonates: Relations among cortisol activity, behavior, and prenatal factors.* Unpublished manuscript, Department of Psychiatry, University of Chicago.

Keenan, K., Gunthorpe, D., & Young, D. (2002). Patterns of cortisol reactivity in African-American neonates from low-income environments. *Developmental Psychobiology, 41*, 1–13.

Keenan, K., & Hipwell, A. (2002). *Preadolescent clues to understanding depression in girls.* Unpublished manuscript, Department of Psychiatry, University of Chicago.

Keenan, K., & Shaw, D. S. (1994). The development of aggression in toddlers: A study of low-income families. *Journal of Abnormal Child Psychology, 22*, 53–78.

Keenan, K., & Shaw, D. S. (1997). Developmental and social influences on young girls' behavioral and emotional problems. *Psychological Bulletin, 121*, 97–113.

Keenan, K., Shaw, D. S., Delliquadri, E., Giovannelli, J., & Walsh, B. (1998). Evidence for the continuity of early problem behaviors: Application of a developmental model. *Journal of Abnormal Child Psychology, 26*, 443–454.

Keenan, K., Shaw, D. S., Walsh, B., Delliquadri, E., & Giovannelli, J. (1997). DSM-III-R disorders in preschoolers from low-income families. *Journal of the American Academy of Child and Adolescent Psychiatry, 36*, 620–627.

Keenan, K., & Wakschlag, L. (2002). Can a valid diagnosis of disruptive behavior disorder be made in preschool children? *American Journal of Psychiatry, 159*, 351–358.

Kerig, P. K., Cowan, P. A., & Cowan, C. P. (1993). Marital quality and gender differences in parent–child interaction. *Developmental Psychology, 29*, 931–939.

Klimes-Dougan, B., & Kopp, C. B. (1999). Children's conflict tactics with mothers: A longitudinal investigation of the toddler and preschool years. *Merrill-Palmer Quarterly, 45*, 226–241.

Kochanska, G. (1995). Children's temperament, mothers' discipline, and security of attachment: Multiple pathways to emerging internalization. *Child Development, 66*, 597–615.

Kochanska, G., & Askan, N. (1995). Mother–child mutually positive affect, the quality of child compliance to requests and prohibitions, and maternal control as correlates of early internalization. *Child Development, 66*, 1–13.

Kochanska, G., Coy, K. C., & Murray, K. T. (2001). The development of self-regulation in the first four years of life. *Child Development, 72*, 1091–1111.

Kochanska, G., Murray, K., & Coy, K. (1997). Inhibitory control as a contributor to conscience in childhood: From toddler to early school age. *Child Development, 68,* 263–277.

Kopp, C. B. (1989). Regulation of distress and negative emotion. *Developmental Psychology, 25,* 343–354.

Landy, S., & Peters, R. D. (1992). Toward an understanding of a developmental paradigm for aggressive conduct problems during the preschool years. In R. D. Peters, R. J. McMahon, & V. L. Quinsey (Eds.), *Aggression throughout the life span* (pp. 1–30). Newbury Park, CA: Sage.

Lee, C. L., & Bates, J. E. (1985). Mother–child interaction at age two and perceived difficult temperament. *Child Development, 56,* 1314–1325.

Lewis, M., & Ramsay, D. S. (1995a). Developmental changes in infants' responses to stress. *Child Development, 66,* 657–670.

Lewis, M., & Ramsay, D. S. (1995b). Stability and change in cortisol and behavioral response to stress during the first 18 months of life. *Developmental Psychobiology, 28,* 419–428.

Liu, D., Diorio, J., Tannenbaum, B., Caldji, C., Francis, D., Freedman, A., Sharma, S., Pearson, D., Plotsky, P. M., & Meaney, M. J. (1997). Maternal care, hippocampal glucocorticoid receptors, and hypothalamic–pituitary–adrenal responses to stress. *Science, 277,* 1659–1662.

Loeber, R., & Keenan, K. (1994). The interaction of conduct disorder and its comorbid conditions: Effects of age and gender. *Clinical Psychology Review, 14,* 497–523.

Maccoby, E. E., Snow, M. E., & Jacklin, C. N. (1984). Children's dispositions and mother–child interaction at 12 and 18 months: A short-term longitudinal study. *Developmental Psychology, 20,* 459–472.

Martin, J. A., Maccoby, E. E., & Jacklin, C. N. (1981). Mothers' responsiveness to interactive bidding and nonbidding in boys and girls. *Child Development, 52,* 1064–1067.

Martin, R., Wisenbaker, J., Baker, J., & Huttunen, M. (1997). Gender differences in temperament at six months and five years. *Infant Behavior and Development, 20,* 339–347.

Matheny, A. P., Riese, M. L., & Wilson, R. S. (1985). Rudiments of infant temperament: Newborn to 9 months. *Developmental Psychology, 21,* 486–494.

Mayes, L. C., Bornstein, M. H., Chawarska, K., Haynes, O. M., & Granger, R. H. (1996). Impaired regulation of arousal in 3-month-old infants exposed prenatally to cocaine and other drugs. *Development and Psychopathology, 8,* 29–42.

McHale, J. P. (1995). Coparenting and triadic interactions during infancy: The roles of marital distress and child gender. *Developmental Psychology, 31,* 985–996.

Morisset, C. E., Barnard, K. E., & Booth, C. L. (1995). Toddlers' language development: Sex differences within social risk. *Developmental Psychology, 31,* 851–865.

Olson, S. L., Bates, J. E., Sandy, J. M., & Lanthier, R. (2000). Early developmental precursors of externalizing behavior in middle childhood and adolescence. *Journal of Abnormal Child Psychology, 28,* 119–133.

Pettit, G., & Bates, J. (1989). Family interaction patterns and children's behavior problems from infancy to 4 years. *Developmental Psychology, 25,* 413–420.

Prior, M., Smart, M. A., Sanson, A., & Oberklaid, F. (1993). Sex differences in psychological adjustment from infancy to 8 years. *Journal of the American Academy of Child and Adolescent Psychiatry, 32,* 291–304.

Ramsay, D. S., & Lewis, M. (1994). Developmental change in infant cortisol and behavioral response to inoculation. *Child Development, 65,* 1491–1502.

Raver, C. C. (1996). Relations between social contingency in mother–child interaction and 2-year-old's social competence. *Developmental Psychology, 32,* 850–859.

Renken, B., Egeland, B., Marvinney, D., Mangelsdorf, S., & Sroufe, L. A. (1989). Early childhood antecedents of aggression and passive-withdrawal in early elementary school. *Journal of Personality, 57,* 257–281.

Reznick, J. S., Corley, R., & Robinson, J. (1997). A longitudinal twin study of intelligence in the second year. *Monographs for the Society for Research in Child Development 62*(1, Serial No. 249).

Rosen, W. D., Adamson, L., & Bakeman, R. (1992). An experimental investigation of infant social referencing mothers' messages and gender differences. *Developmental Psychology, 28,*
1172–1178.

Ross, H., Tesla, C., Kenyon, B., & Lollis, S. (1990). Maternal intervention in toddler peer conflict: The socialization of principles of justice. *Developmental Psychology, 26,* 994–1003.

Rothbart, M. K., & Ahadi, S. A. (1994). Temperament and the development of personality. *Journal of Abnormal Psychology, 103,* 55–66.

Rothbart, M. K., Derryberry, D., & Posner, M. I. (1994). A psychobiological approach to the development of temperament. In J. E. Bates & T. D. Wachs (Eds.), *Temperament: Individual
differences at the interface of biology and behavior* (pp. 83–116). Washington, DC: American Psychological Association.

Sapolsky, R. M., Krey, L. C., & McEwan, B. S. (1984). Glucocorticoid-sensitive hippocampal
neurons are involved in terminating the adrenocrotical stress response. *Proceedings of the
National Academy of Sciences, 81,* 6174–6177.

Schneider, M. L., & Moore, C. F. (2000). Effect of prenatal stress on development: A nonhuman
primate model. In C. A. Nelson (Ed.), *The effects of early adversity on neurobehavioral
development* (pp. 201–244). Mahwah, NJ: Erlbaum.

Shaw, D. S., & Bell, R. Q. (1993). Developmental theories of parental contributors to antisocial
behavior. *Journal of Abnormal Child Psychology, 21,* 493–518.

Shaw, D. S., Bell, R. Q., & Gilliom, M. (2000). A truly early starter model of antisocial behavior
revisited. *Clinical Child and Family Psychology Review, 3,* 155–172.

Shaw, D. S., Gilliom, M., Ingoldsby, E. M., & Nagin, D. (2003). Trajectories leading to school-
age conduct problems. *Developmental Psychology, 39,* 189–200.

Shaw, D. S., Keenan, K., & Vondra, J. I. (1994). Developmental precursors of externalizing
behavior: Ages 1 to 3. *Developmental Psychology, 30,* 355–364.

Shaw, D. S., Owens, E. B., Giovannelli, J., & Winslow, E. B. (2001). Infant and toddler pathways
leading to early externalizing disorders. *Journal of the American Academy of Child and
Adolescent Psychiatry, 40,* 36–43.

Shaw, D. S., Owens, E. B., Vondra, J. I., Keenan, K., & Winslow, E. B. (1996). Early risk factors
and pathways in the development of early disruptive behavior problems. *Development and
Psychopathology, 8,* 679–700.

Shaw, D. S., & Winslow, E. B. (1997). Precursors and correlates of antisocial behavior from infancy to preschool. In D. M Stoff & J. Breiling (Eds.), *Handbook of antisocial behavior*
(pp. 148–158). New York: Wiley.

Shaw, D. S., Winslow, E. B., Owens, E. B., Vondra, J. I., Cohn, J. F., & Bell, R. Q. (1998). The development of early externalizing problems among children from low-income families: A
transformational perspective. *Journal of Abnormal Child Psychology, 26,* 95–107.

Simpson, A. E., & Stevenson-Hinde, J. (1985). Temperamental characteristics of three- to four-
year-old boys and girls and child–family interactions. *Journal of Child Psychology and
Psychiatry, 26,* 43–53.

Smetana, J. G. (1989). Toddlers' social interactions in the context of moral and conventional
transgressions in the home. *Developmental Psychology, 25,* 499–508.

Spangler, G., & Scheubeck, R. (1993). Behavioral organization in newborns and its relation to
adrenocortical and cardiac activity. *Child Development, 64,* 622–633.

Spangler, G., Schieche, M., Ilg, U., Maier, U., & Ackerman, C. (1994). Maternal sensitivity as an
external organizer for biobehavioral regulation in infancy. *Developmental Psychobiology,
27,* 425–437.

Stansbury, K., & Zimmerman, L. K. (1999). Relations among child language skills, maternal
socializations of emotion regulation, and child behavior problems. *Child Psychiatry and
Human Development, 30,* 121–142.

Stattin, H., & Klackenberg-Larsson, I. (1993). Early language and intelligence development and
their relationship to future criminal behavior. *Journal of Abnormal Psychology, 102,* 369–
378.

Stifter, C. A., & Braungart, J. M. (1995). The regulation of negative reactivity in infancy: Function and development. *Developmental Psychology, 31,* 448–455.

Stifter, C. A., & Jain, A. (1996). Psychophysicological correlates of infant temperament: Stability of behavior and autonomic patterning from 5 to 18 months. *Developmental Psychobiology, 29,* 379–391.

Stifter, C. A., Spinrad, T. L., & Braungart-Rieker, J. M. (1999). Toward a developmental model of child compliance: The role of emotion regulation in infancy. *Child Development, 70,* 21–32.

Stipek, D. J., Gralinski, J. H., & Kopp, C. B. (1990). Self-concept development in the toddler years. *Developmental Psychology, 26,* 972–977.

St. James-Roberts, I., & Plewis, I. (1996). Individual differences, daily fluctuations, and developmental changes in amounts of infant waking, fussing, crying, feeding, and sleeping. *Child Development, 67,* 2527–2540.

Stowe, R. M., Arnold, D. H., & Ortiz, C. (2000). Gender differences in the relationship of language development to disruptive behavior and peer relationships in preschoolers. *Journal of Applied Developmental Psychology, 20,* 521–536.

Sullivan, R. M., & Gratton, A. (2002). Prefontal cortical regulation of hypothalamic–pituitary–adrenal function in the rat and implications for psychopathology. *Psychoneuroendocrinology, 27,* 99–114.

Taylor A., Fisk, M. N., & Glover, V. (2000). Mode of delivery and subsequent stress response. *Lancet, 355,* 120.

Thompson, R. A. (1994). Emotion regulation: A theme in search of definition. In N. Fox (Ed.), The development of emotion regulation, *Monographs of the Society for Research in Child Development, 59*(Serial No. 2–3, 25–52).

Tonkiss, J., Shumsky, J. S., Shultz, P. L., Almeida, S. S., & Galler, J. A. (1995). Prenatal cocaine but not prenatal malnutrition affects foster mother–pup interactions in rats. *Neurotoxicology and Teratology, 17,* 601–608.

Tremblay, R. E., Boulerice, B., Harden, P. W., McDuff, P., Perusse, D., Pihl, R. O., & Zoccolillo, M. (1996). Do children in Canada become more aggressive as they approach adolescence? In Human Resources Development Canada & Statistics Canada (Eds.), *Growing up in Canada: National Longitudinal Survey of Children and Youth* (pp. 127–137). Ottawa, Ontario, Canada: Statistics Canada.

Tremblay, R. E., Japel, C., Perusse, D., Boivin, M., Zoccolillo, M., Montplaisir, J., & McDuff, P. (1999). The search for the age of "onset" of physical aggression: Rousseau and Bandura revisited. *Criminal Behavior and Mental Health, 9,* 8–23.

van den Boom, D., & Gravenhorst, J. (1995). Prenatal and perinatal correlates of neonatal irritability. *Infant Behavior and Development, 18,* 117–121.

Wakschlag, L. S., & Hans, S. L. (1999). Relation of maternal responsiveness during infancy to the development of behavior problems in high-risk youths. *Developmental Psychology, 35,* 569–579.

Waschbusch, D. A., Willoughby, M. T., & Pelham, W. E. (1998). Criterion validity and the utility of reactive and proactive aggression: Comparisons to attention deficit hyperactivity disorder, oppositional defiant disorder, conduct disorder, and other measures of functioning. *Journal of Clinical Child Psychology, 27,* 396–405.

Weinberg, M. K., Tronick, E., Cohn, J. F., & Olson, K. L. (1999). Gender differences in emotional expressivity and self-regulation during early infancy. *Developmental Psychology, 35,* 175–188.

Weinstock, M. (1997). Does prenatal stress impair coping and regulation of the hypothalamic–pituitary–adrenal axis? *Neuroscience and Biobehavioral Reviews, 21,* 1–10.

Zahn-Waxler, C., Iannotti, R. J., Cummings, E. M., & Denham, S. (1990). Antecedents of problem behaviors in children of depressed mothers. *Development and Psychopathology, 2,* 271–292.

Zahn-Waxler, C., Radke-Yarrow, M., Wagner, E., & Chapman, M. (1992). Development of concern for others. *Developmental Psychology, 28,* 126–136.

# 7

# Why Socialization Fails
## The Case of Chronic Physical Aggression

### RICHARD E. TREMBLAY

This chapter is divided into four main sections. The first section addresses *the taxonomic issue*. I explain why my focus is on the causes of chronic physical aggression rather than on the causes of conduct disorder, serious juvenile delinquency, or antisocial behavior. The second part deals with *the descriptive issue*. Present knowledge on the development of physical aggression from early childhood to adulthood is summarized. The third part deals with *the causal issue*. I describe variables that may have a causal role in the development of chronic physical aggression. The fourth and final part deals with *the test of causal hypotheses*. I formulate hypotheses and suggest research designs to test these hypotheses. For readers who are in a hurry or who have no patience for long-winded discussions of terms and definitions, the first two sections are summarized in the following two paragraphs.

Section I explains that the taxonomies we are presently using to find causes of antisocial behavior, and eventually prevent these behaviors, were created before *a thorough developmental description* of the behaviors we define as antisocial, delinquent, or disordered. I suggest that we need to understand both the development and causes of subtypes of antisocial behavior to decide if they can be aggregated or not. Following this logic, I focus in the rest of the chapter on the development and causes of one subtype, physical aggression.

In section II, I argue that the development of physical aggression occurs in a way that is the opposite of what most recent sociological and psychological theories propose. The evidence we now have on the lifespan development of physical aggression suggests that this behavior is unlearned rather than learned. Physical aggression appears during infancy as a natural way of expressing anger and as a natural instrument to achieve goals—for example, taking an object from someone else. During their development most children learn to use alternative strategies to express anger and achieve their goals. Those who do not will become increasingly dangerous for others as they grow older, because they become physically stronger and more cognitively skilled. Thus, to find the causes of chronic physical aggression, we need to ask "why an individual has not learned to inhibit physical aggression," rather than ask "why he has learned to physically aggress." It follows that to prevent the development of chronic physical aggression we need to ask "how an individual can learn to inhibit physical aggression" rather than "how we can prevent him from learning to aggress." This view of the development of the most feared antisocial behavior, physical violence, obviously challenges a number of well-received ideas in criminology and developmental psychopathology. Physical aggression is not an illness that one "catches," it is a natural behavior that one learns to "control."

## PROBLEMS WITH OUR TAXONOMIES

*As is well known, the development of a taxonomy of the phenomenon to be studied is a necessary first step in scientific enquiry.*
                                        —QUAY (1999, p. 3)

In the invitation to write this chapter authors were asked to "advance specific *hypotheses* about the *causes* of conduct disorder and serious juvenile delinquency." The editors stated that "a great deal has been learned about the correlates of conduct disorder and serious delinquency, but we have made much less progress towards understanding its *causes*. Because understanding causation should lead to important breakthroughs in prevention, it is essential that the field focus more on causal factors and causal mechanisms."

There are many reasons why we have not made much progress towards understanding "causes" of conduct disorder and serious juvenile delinquency. I believe that the two most important ones are related, first to the operational definition of the outcome for which we want to find the causes, second to the lack of true experiments. All undergraduate students learn that testing hypotheses concerning causes implies the use of properly designed experiments, and part of a well-designed experiment involves adequate operational definition of the manipulated variables and the outcome.

Bearing this in mind, it will certainly come as a surprise to undergraduate students to read that 21st century developmental psychopathology is still confronted with serious problems of definition. The preparation of this book serves as a good example. Consider that, of the 14 researchers in developmental psychopathology who accepted the invitation to write a chapter on "*causes* of *conduct disorder* and *serious juvenile delinquency*," only two used in their tentative titles the term "conduct disorder," and none included the term "serious juvenile delinquency," in their title, although two titles included the term "serious delinquency," one included the term "delinquency," and another included the term "juvenile delinquency." Of the nine titles that did not include the terms "conduct disorder" or "delinquency," eight used the term "antisocial" and two used the term "aggression." The ninth title simply did not include any outcome!

Considering this variety of terms, most undergraduates who understand the request made by the editors will likely come to the conclusion that conduct disorder, delinquency, and antisocial behavior are synonyms, and that the terms "serious" and "juvenile" are possibly meaningless. However, I may be underestimating the young people who enter the field today. They may be wiser than I was when I entered the field in 1967 as a graduate student working on the treatment of juvenile delinquents. At that time the following books were among the classics: Powers and Witmer's (1951) *An Experiment in the Prevention of Delinquency*, Redl and Wineman's (1951) *The Aggressive Child*, and Robins's (1966) *Deviant Children Grown Up*. The words "aggressive," "deviant," and "delinquent" entered my mind as synonyms, and it took me many years to realize that this confusion was a serious handicap to understanding the development and causes of the phenotypes I was paid to study. I have since come to believe that we cannot find the causes of "delinquency," "antisocial behavior," and "conduct disorder" because each aggregates heterogeneous types of behaviors that possibly have different causes.

The term "delinquency" presents a further problem for those who take a developmental approach. A delinquent is by definition someone who breaks the law. Laws concerning juveniles are made by taking into account age, that is, development. Thus an 11-year-old who physically attacks someone will be considered delinquent in some jurisdictions and not delinquent in others. Many investigators of delinquent behavior have simply decided not to use the legal age to define who is and who is not delinquent. Thus an 11-year-old who physically attacks someone in a state where age 12 is the official delinquency age will still be labeled delinquent for the purpose of the study. But ask these investigators if they are willing to label "delinquent" a 2- or 3-year-old who physically attacks someone and most will refuse to use that term for a young child. The question then is, at what age will they accept use of the dangerous label? At 3, 4, 5, 6, 7, 8, or 9 years of age? In 1998, the U.S. Office of Juvenile Justice and Delinquency Prevention created a study group on "very young offenders." As a member of that group I am proud to say that we found the answer. We decided that children between the ages of 7 and 12 would be labeled "child delinquents"

(Loeber & Farrington, 2001). Why age 7? Well, why not? Doesn't the Bible have age 7 as the "age of reason"?

The "age" problem also exists in determining when juvenile delinquency ends and adult criminality begins. Should it be 21, 18, 16, or less? Should it depend on the behavior, on its consequence, on emotional maturity, or on cognitive development? In his discussion of this topic, which he titles "That Malice Which Is to Supply Age," Zimring (1998) cites a story from Sir William Blackstone (1857) which led to the title: "[A] boy of ten years old was convicted on his own confession of murdering his bedfellow, there appearing in his whole behavior plain tokens of a mischievous discretion; and, as sparing this boy merely on account of his tender years might be of dangerous consequence to the public, by propagating a notion that children might commit such atrocious crimes with impunity, it was unanimously agreed by all the judges that he was a proper subject of capital punishment. But, in all such cases, the evidence of that malice which is to supply age, ought to be strong and clear beyond all doubt and contradiction."

I suggest that we should stop using legal terms to define behaviors for developmental studies, especially if we are looking for causes. The term "delinquent" should be used for studies that specifically aim to address legal issues. Consider the further difficulty of operationalizing the terms of reference that we were given concerning delinquency: "serious juvenile delinquency." Not only do we have to use jurisdictions that have the same definition of delinquency with reference to age and type of behavior, but also we need jurisdictions that have the same age definition of "juvenile" and the same definition of "serious." Does the word "serious" apply to the actual behavior or to its consequences? Is a physical attack "serious" only when it draws blood? Do we need a dead body? Can we label a 6-year-old who kills a classmate with a gun a "serious juvenile delinquent"? Does it depend on the legal consequences? Discussing predictions of a new generation of youth violence in the United States, Zimring (1998) explicitly shows how what he calls "compounded distortions" of numbers and adjectives led from studies of youth with police contact in Philadelphia in the1950s to predictions of an army of young superpredators in the whole of the United States in 2010.

The behaviors that are generally included in "delinquency" scales include three large a priori categories: (1) the property offenses that can be classified into a vandalism category and a theft category, each of which can also be subclassified into an overt and a covert category, that is, acts of vandalism and theft can be done openly or by taking every precaution to hide the behavior; (2) the person offenses that can be subdivided into physical, verbal, and indirect aggression, and then subclassified into proactive and reactive, that is, to initiate the attack or to attack as a response to an attack; and (3) the status offenses that involve subcategories such as running away from home; not going to school; consumption of alcohol, drugs, and tobacco; driving under age; and having sex under age.

The term "conduct disorder" (CD) is generally used with reference to the American Psychiatric Association (APA) classification of mental disorders. It has been widely used since the 1980s, and sophisticated interview protocols were created to facilitate its assessment in epidemiological and clinical studies (e.g., Angold et al., 1995; Shaffer, Fisher, Dulcan, & Davies, 1996). The DSM-IV manual (American Psychiatric Association, 1994) states that CD "is one of the most frequently diagnosed conditions in outpatient and inpatient mental health facilities for children" (p. 88). Considering its prevalence, the methodological sophistication of the assessment tools, and its social relevance, one would expect a well-established taxonomy. Unfortunately, this is not the case. Over a period of 14 years (1980–1994) the guidelines of the APA went from five categories of CD (undersocialized aggressive, undersocialized nonaggressive, socialized aggressive, socialized nonaggressive, atypical; DSM-III, American Psychiatric Association, 1980), to three categories (solitary aggressive, group, undifferentiated; DSM-III-R, American Psychiatric Association, 1987), and finally to two categories (childhood-onset, adolescent-onset; DSM-IV, American Psychiatric Association, 1994). CD covers essentially the same symptoms as "delinquency." The DSM-IV specifies four categories that can be mapped onto the categories listed above: (1) aggression to people and animals; (2) destruction of property; (3) deceitfulness or theft; and (4) serious violations of rules. To be classified CD, an individual has to meet at least three of 15 criteria. This procedure can lead to extremely different types of CD cases. For example, compare the following four cases, where each case is a 15-year-old male: case A has run away from home at least twice, and from age 12 has been truant from school and often stays out at night despite parental prohibitions; case B often initiates physical fights with peers, uses a knife to intimidate peers, and forces girls into sexual activity; case C deliberately sets fires, vandalizes schools, and is cruel to animals; case D breaks into homes, shoplifts, and uses stolen credit cards. The four cases do not share any CD symptoms, but will receive the same diagnoses and investigators will be looking for common "causes." However, a 15-year-old male who regularly steals while confronting his victims, but does not manifest any of the other 14 DSM-IV criteria, will be picked up by the police, placed in a detention center for juvenile delinquents, but will not be considered a CD case.

The term "antisocial" is less associated with a professional group than the terms "conduct disorder" (psychiatrists) and "delinquent" (lawyers and criminologists). This may be the reason why eight of the original 14 authors of this book used the term in their original title. The *American Heritage Dictionary* (1985) defines "antisocial" in the following way: "1. Shunning the society of others, not sociable; 2. Opposed or hostile to the established social order; marked by or engaging in behavior that violates accepted mores: drug abuse and other antisocial activity" (p. 116). Coie and Dodge (1998) in their review of research titled "Aggression and Antisocial Behavior" in the most recent edition of the *Handbook of Child Psychology* included in their definition of antisocial behavior the following categories of behavior: aggressive behaviors, noncompliance with adults, delinquency, substance abuse, cheating, early and risky sexual activity, and vandalism (p. 781).

There was much work in the 1970s and 1980s showing moderate levels of correlation among all these forms of deviant behaviors during adolescence (e.g., Elliott, Huizinga, & Ménard, 1989; Jessor & Jessor, 1977). However, such correlations may reflect the fact that there are a small number of individuals who use many forms of antisocial behaviors at a given point in time, with most other individuals using only subsets. If correlations were to be used as the ultimate criteria for identifying a behavior disorder, we would probably use the terms "externalizing," or "disruptive," or "overt" to include at least "oppositional behavior," "hyperactivity," "conduct disorder," "physical aggression," and "delinquency." Other "antisocial" behaviors, such as cheating, stealing, substance abuse, early and risky sexual behavior, and vandalism would also be correlated, but they would not fit the title of the dimension well (externalizing or disruptive or overt) since they tend to be "covert" behaviors. More than a decade ago Magnusson and Bergman (1990) and others (e.g., Cairns, Cairns, & Neckerman, 1988; Pulkkinen & Tremblay, 1992) argued that we needed to take a "person" rather than a "variable" approach to categorize individuals at a given point in time. Recent methods of data analysis coupled with data sets including frequent measurements from early childhood to adulthood now provide sophisticated means of examining taxonomies of antisocial behavior from a developmental perspective (e.g., Baillargeon et al., 2001; Broidy et al., 2003; Nagin & Tremblay, 2001a). I suggest that we reexamine our taxonomies, first by analyzing the development of different forms of antisocial behavior from early childhood to adulthood, and secondly by using experiments to test to what extent these different forms of antisocial behavior have the same causes. When this work is completed, we will have solid grounds upon which to build our taxonomies.

## PHYSICAL AGGRESSION

The editors of the present book specifically asked us (1) to advance explicit, disconfirmable causal hypotheses, and (2) to provide specific descriptions of the crucial studies needed to confirm or disconfirm the hypotheses. To comply with this request, and follow the logic described in the preceding section, I decided to focus on the causes of chronic physical aggression (see Coie & Dodge, 1998; Tremblay, 2000a).

## What Is Physical Aggression?

Physical aggression is often used as the flagship of the antisocial–delinquent–conduct disorder domain. The public worries about juvenile delinquents because they are perceived to be a physical threat. Funding for research on juvenile delinquency and CD increases when juveniles commit homicide, not when they run away from home, shoplift, or are truant from school. The editors of the present book probably had this issue in mind when they asked us to address "conduct disorder and *serious* juvenile delinquency." I will address three key issues concerning the operationalization of physical aggression before summarizing research on its development: specificity, seriousness, and intentionality.

### The Specificity Issue

There is a huge scientific literature on aggressive behavior. Unfortunately, the problem of operationalizing aggressive behavior has significantly limited progress in understanding its development and its causal factors (Tremblay, 2000a). The best illustration of this problem is the content of the "aggression" scales that have been used over the past decades. The most popular scales contain a mix of behaviors that range from physical aggression to attention seeking and disobedience. For example, the "aggressive" scale of the Child Behavior Checklist (CBCL; Achenbach & Edelbrock, 1983) includes the following: "argues, brags, demands attention, disobeys, poor peer relations, jealous, lies, shows off, stubborn, moody, sulks, loud." This "aggressive" scale has 23 items with only two that refer clearly to physical aggression and two others that could be interpreted as physical aggression. Peer rating "aggression" scales have the same problem. The "aggression" scale for the Columbia County Study, one of the few large longitudinal studies specifically aimed at understanding the development of aggressive behavior (Huesmann, Eron, Lefkowitz, & Walder, 1984; Lefkowitz, Eron, Walder, & Huesmann, 1977), includes the following items: disobeys teacher, gives dirty looks, makes up stories and lies, does things that bother others, gets in trouble. Again, only two of the 10 items could be interpreted as physical aggression: starts fights, pushes and shoves.

The DSM-IV assessment for CD has the advantage of including six out of the 15 criteria that describe physical aggressions toward humans. A seventh item describes physical cruelty toward animals. Note that both criteria dealing with cruelty specify "physical" cruelty. Some studies of aggression confound physical and mental cruelty, the later being much more difficult to measure. Unfortunately, there is no provision for a CD diagnosis specifically for individuals who use physical aggression. Such diagnoses existed in the DSM-III versions. Interestingly, Lahey et al. (1998) reported that those classified as "childhood-onset" CD, according to the DSM-IV criteria, scored positive on some of the physical aggression criteria significantly more often than the "adolescent-onset" cases did.

## The Seriousness Issue

Studies of aggressive behavior in species other than humans have tended to use definitions based on topographical qualities of the behavior, that is, the actual behavior characteristics of the "aggressor" (Hartup & deWit, 1974; Tremblay, 2000a). However, definitions of aggressive behavior for research on humans tend to focus either on the impact of the behavior on the victim (seriousness) or on the intention of the aggressor. Those who focus on the impact will ask whether the behavior has or could have hurt the victim. For example, in their review of research on aggression, Loeber and Stouthamer-Loeber (1998) chose the following definition: "aggression is defined as those acts that inflict bodily or mental harm on others" (p. 242). The word "serious" is often used to qualify the negative impact of the behavior on the victim. This approach to defining aggression can be compared to the way children make moral judgments before the age of reason: it is not the behavior that is wrong, but its consequence (see Turiel, 1998). This approach will of course lead to the conclusion that a punch from a 6-foot, 250-pound, 16-year-old is more serious than a punch from a 5-foot, 100-pound, 16-year-old, and that a punch from a 24-month-old weakling is not really an act of aggression.

## The Intentionality Issue

In their review of research on aggression, Coie and Dodge (1998) followed the definition used by Parke and Slaby (1983), which refers to the possible negative consequence of the act, but stresses the intent: "behavior that is aimed at harming or injuring another person or persons" (p. 550). The "intent" criterion has significantly limited the study of the early development of aggressive behavior. If "intent" is required for an action to be considered "aggressive," then young children who do not understand that their behavior can hurt another cannot be considered "aggressive" (see, e.g., Kagan, 1974). This argument is similar to the "age of reason" argument for declaring someone "delinquent." In the recent case of a 6-year-old boy who gunned down a 6-year-old girl in his classroom, one of the frequently asked questions was, "Did the boy really understand what he had done?" (Did Kayla Have to Die?, 2000). One could add, "Did he really understand what dying means?" and "At what age do humans really understand what dying means?" Goethe's (1774/1993) Werther asks before committing suicide, "To die! What does that mean?" (p. 155).

Thus, most studies of the origins of aggression have kept away from preschool children, who are too weak to hurt others and not cognitively able to understand right from wrong. For example, Lefkowitz et al. (1977, p. 36) reported that "the initial goal of the [Columbia County longitudinal] study was to select a representative sample of American children, seven to nine years old, and to investigate the factors that might influence the development of aggression." In his presidential speech to the International Society for Research on Aggression, 30 years after the start of the study, one of the principal investigators concluded that aggression appeared to "crystallize" around 8 years of age (Eron, 1990). Nine years later, referring to a longitudinal study of youth from ages 6 to 15 years of age, Nagin and Tremblay (1999) reported that the peak level of physical aggression was at age 6.

We seem to be slowly learning that to investigate the developmental origins of human behavior, we need to start at the beginning. What would happen to research on aggressive behavior in nonhuman species if intent were required to declare an animal aggressive? Does a hen intend to hurt when she pecks another to get at her food? Does a 12-month-old girl intend to hurt when she pushes another to grab her toy? The intent criterion is a problem not only for infants and nonhuman species. Behavior, which is driven by anger and fear, is generally not under the control of one's will, even during adulthood. Many, if not most, of the aggressive behaviors following intense frustration are impulsive behaviors that were not intended. Gray (1971, 1982) proposed that a "fight–flight system" controlled the behavioral reactions to unconditioned punishment and nonreward. Lewis, Alessandri, and Sullivan (1990) showed that by 4 months of age infants clearly expressed facial anger reactions to frustrations. A few months later the infant will have better control over his limbs and will hit and kick when he becomes angry (Goodenough, 1931; Tremblay et al., 1999).

## The Development of Chronic Physical Aggression

For the purpose of this essay I have chosen to define *physical aggression* as the use of behaviors, similar to the following, in antagonistic interactions with other humans: hitting, slapping, kicking, biting, pushing, grabbing, pulling, shoving, throwing objects at another, beating, twisting, choking. Some scales use terms such as "fighting" and "bullying" to summarize these behaviors. Threatening to physically aggress and use of objects to aggress is also included in the definition (see Blurton-Jones, 1972; McGrew, 1972; Restoin et al., 1985; Straus, 1979). *Chronic physical aggression* (CPA) is defined as a tendency throughout childhood and adolescence to use physical aggression more frequently than the large majority of a birth cohort. Based on studies that will be described below, it can be expected that the group of CPA males and females in a birth cohort of industrialized countries would include approximately 5% of the cohort. The inclusion of a reference group to define "chronic" ensures that we are taking into account variations due to cohort effects and cultural context. Reference groups should also be divided into males and females to take into account important sex differences in developmental trajectories of physical aggression, as will be described later. I also included in the definition a relatively long developmental period (childhood and adolescence) to clearly indicate that the focus is not on individuals who show occasional problems with physical aggression. The "explicit, disconfirmable causal hypotheses" I propose exclude, for example, cases such as a highly physically aggressive adolescent who did not show high levels of physical aggression during childhood. According to the available data, such cases are probably rare and should not be confounded with chronic cases from childhood to adolescence (Brame, Nagin & Tremblay, 2001; Broidy et al., 2003; Nagin & Tremblay, 1999; Nagin & Tremblay, 2003). An important limit to the phenotype that I address is that it is not subdivided into subcategories of physical aggression, such as proactive and reactive (Dodge, Lochman, Harnish, Bates, & Pettit, 1997; Poulin & Boivin, 2000; Vitaro, Gendreau, Tremblay, & Oligny, 1998). I could not make such divisions because, to my knowledge, there is no published work on the developmental trajectories of subtypes of physical aggression from early childhood to preadolescence.

At the end of the 1980s the U.S. National Academy of Sciences assembled a group of world experts to form a "Panel on the Understanding and Control of Violent Behavior." The report (Reiss & Roth, 1993) summarized the state of knowledge and concluded that:

> Modern psychological perspectives emphasize that aggressive and violent behaviors are *learned* responses to frustration, that they can also be learned as instruments for achieving goals, and that the learning occurs by observing models of such behaviors. Such models may be observed in the family, among peers, elsewhere in the neighborhood, through the mass media, or in violent pornography, for example. (p. 7, emphasis in original)

This interpretation of the research literature appears to be an attempt to summarize what we know about the proximal and distal causes of "aggressive and violent behaviors." The *distal causes* refer to the development of aggressive behavior in humans. The *proximal causes* refer to the stimulus for an aggressive act. The distal cause is attributed to "learning." Humans would not use "aggressive and violent behaviors" if they had not learned to do so. The mechanism by which they learn, according to the Academy of Sciences report, is imitation. If they could not imitate or if they had no one to imitate, they would not have learned to use aggression, and thus could not use it. The proximal causes are frustration and goal achievement. Once they have learned to use aggression, they will use it when they are frustrated or when they want to achieve a goal.

To find the distal causes, that is, the causes for the development of aggressive behavior, one needs to have a good idea of that development. The "learning" hypothesis does indeed appear to fit the association that has been shown between age and crime. Labeled the "age–crime curve," it highlights the fact that delinquent behaviors increase substantially during adolescence. This age–crime curve was described as long ago as the early 19th century (see Figure 7.1, from Quetelet, 1869), and has been replicated regularly since in industrialized countries (see Elliott, 1994; Farrington, 1987). Note that Quetelet in 1869 was differentiating types of antisocial behavior. The usual psychological and sociological "causal" explanation for the age–crime curve is that, as children grow older, they are more and more negatively influenced by their environment. Learning to physically aggress through imitation from models found in the family, among peers, in the neighborhood, and the media is presumed to have reached its peak toward the middle or end of adolescence (e.g., Anderson & Bushman, 2002; Bushman & Anderson, 2001; Huesmann & Miller, 1994; Johnson, Cohen, Smailes, Kasen, & Brook, 2002).

The fact that the frequency of these behaviors starts decreasing during adulthood is generally explained by the positive impact of major life events such as military service, marriage, and employment (for a review, see Laub & Sampson, 2001), and by the impact of physical maturation

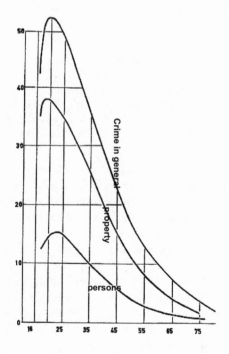

FIGURE 7.1. Crimes in France during the 19 years from 1826 to 1844 (Quetelet, 1869).

or "aging" (Laub & Sampson, 2001; Quetelet, 1833). However, the age–crime curve does not include most of the physical aggression that occurs among couples and toward their children, both of which start before cohabitation and continue well into adulthood (e.g., Brendgen, Vitaro, Tremblay, & Lavoie, 2001; Moffitt, Robins, & Caspi, 2001; Stets & Straus, 1989).

The social impact (seriousness) of antisocial behavior during adolescence captured the attention of investigators and theoreticians to the point that the developmental antecedents to these problems of adolescence where largely neglected. Over the past 40 years some studies attempted to identify childhood problems that could "explain" the adolescent problems (e.g., Huesmann et al., 1984; Loeber, Farrington, Stouthamer-Loeber, & Van Kammen, 1998; Raine, 2002; Robins, 1966; Tremblay, Pihl, Vitaro, & Dobkin, 1994; West & Farrington, 1973; White, Moffitt, Earls, Robins, & Silva, 1990). However, these studies were trying to identify the causes of a phenomenon that had yet to be fully described. Is it true that the frequency of physical aggression increases with age from birth to the end of adolescence? How many different developmental trajectories of physical aggression are there? To a large extent the description of the phenomenon had not been done before we jumped into the game of testing "causes" with correlations.

A few studies did monitor physical aggression with repeated measures over many years (for a review, see Tremblay, 2000a). Most of these longitudinal studies followed subjects from childhood to adolescence, but some monitored physical aggression during early childhood and from early childhood to school entry. Figure 7.2 describes hypothetical trajectories of physical aggression from birth to adulthood. The trajectories are hypotheses because, to my knowledge, no one to date has described the trajectories of physical aggression from early childhood to adulthood. The results from large prospective longitudinal studies in Canada, New Zealand, and the United States on samples of different ages were used for the Figure 7.2 trajectories. There seems to be four basic trajectories, indicating (1) that most children start using physical aggression in infancy (e.g., Hay, Castle, & Davies, 2000; Keenan & Wakschlag, 2000; Tremblay et al., 1999); (2) that there is an increase in frequency of physical aggression up to the third or fourth year after birth (Côté, Vaillancourt, et al., 2002; Tremblay, 2000b; Tremblay et al., 2002); (3) that the frequency from then on decreases steadily up to adolescence (Brame et al., 2001; Broidy et al., 2003; Cairns, Cairns, Neckerman, Ferguson, & Gariépy, 1989; Côté, Vaillancourt, et al., 2002; Lacourse et al., 2002; Nagin & Tremblay, 1999); (4) that those on the CPA trajectory may show a decline during childhood and an increase during preadolescence and adolescence, which would still be lower than the infancy peak (see Brame et al., 2001; Broidy et al., 2003; Côté, Vaillancourt, et al., 2002; Lacourse et al., 2002; White, Bates, & Buyske, 2001); (5) that by adulthood all humans probably have substantially desisted in

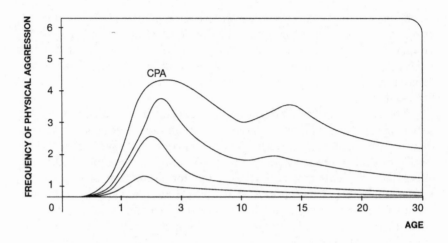

FIGURE 7.2. Age–physical aggression curves (hypothesized).

their frequency of physical aggression compared to their peak during early childhood; (6) that there is no indication of a significant group of children who have low levels of physical aggression in early childhood and later start using physical aggression with a frequency that is similar to the CPA group; (7) that males tend to use physical aggression more frequently than females, and that the differences between the sexes are smallest in early childhood, but increase rapidly during the preschool years (Broidy et al., 2003; Cairns et al., 1989, Côté, Vaillancourt, et al., 2002); and (8) that there is a group of girls with relatively high levels of physical aggression from early childhood to the start of adolescence that we could label "chronic," although their level of physical aggression tends to be lower than the level of the chronic males (Broidy et al., 2003; Côté, Vaillancourt, et al., 2002), and they may not maintain a high level in adolescence. In-deed, the Broidy et al. (2003) analyses suggests that physical aggression during adolescence may be substantially reduced in girls, even for the chronic cases, and White et al. (2001) report that they did not conduct tra-jectory analyses on their sample of girls ($N = 682$) followed from 12 to 31 years of age because the number of girls with serious delinquency was too small. The physically aggressive behaviors used in their study (assault, fighting with weapons or in a gang, armed robbery) may not capture the type of physical aggressions adolescent girls and young women engage in. These problems clearly show that we need much more data on different forms of physical aggression in girls during adolescence and adulthood to decide what we mean by "female CPA."

The latter descriptions of the development of physical aggression from early childhood to early adulthood lead me to the following conclusions:

1. If children learn to physically aggress, they do so during infancy. It is more likely that behaviors such as pushing, pulling, hitting, kicking, throwing, and beating are all spontaneous behaviors, like crying, sucking, sitting up, standing, walking, running, and putting objects to one's mouth. These behaviors appear with neuromotor maturation, and become instruments at the service of basic drives such as hunger, anger, and affiliation.

2. Rather than learning to physically aggress, children appear to be learning *not* to physically aggress. Some seem to learn rapidly, others appear to take more time, and some appear not to learn very well before the end of adolescence (compare curves in Figure 7.2). The latter group is the one we identify as the "chronic" cases. They are most probably at highest risk of chronic physical aggression during adulthood, but we have to leave this part of the story for the day when there will be more evidence to rely on.

3. Children who have learned to regulate physical aggression are not children who *never* use physical aggression, they are children who use it *less often* than those who have not learned. If humans do not need to learn to physically aggress, all humans are at risk of using physical aggression given the appropriate circumstances. Nicolson (1955) applied this idea to human evolution in his book *Good Behaviour*: "The stages by which mankind progresses towards reasonableness and a sense of values is not a stairway of continual ascent. There are frequent relapse" (1955, pp. 9–10).

4. To find the causes of chronic physical aggression we will have to find (a) mechanisms that explain how humans learn to regulate physical aggression during early childhood, during childhood, during adolescence, and during adulthood; (b) mechanisms that explain the failure to learn to regulate physical aggression during early childhood; (c) mechanisms that explain failure to learn to regulate physical aggression during childhood by those who did not learn during early childhood; and (d) mechanisms that explain failure to learn to regulate physical aggression during adolescence and early adulthood by those who did not learn during early childhood and childhood.

## THE CAUSES OF CHRONIC PHYSICAL AGGRESSION (HANDLE WITH CARE)

*Oh, why did you have to be born with this violent temper, this uncontrollable clinging passion for everything you touch!*
—GOETHE (1774–1993, p. 138)

Kraemer et al. (1997) suggested a terminology to differentiate *causes* (causal risk factors), from *markers* (fixed and variable risk factors) and *cor-*

*relates* (concomitants and consequences) in psychiatric research. The aim of this chapter is to formulate hypotheses that could lead to the identification of causal risk factors of CPA, which can only be done by experimental research. To my knowledge, no such factors have yet been identified with the experimental procedure recommended by Kraemer et al. (1997). Most research has been correlational, and thus has led to the identification of fixed (e.g., sex) and variable (e.g., parenting style) risk factors, as well as to concomitant correlates (e.g., hyperactivity) and consequences (e.g., gang membership).

I differentiate the types of risk factors and putative causes according to their source and level of understanding (see Figure 7.3). The dichotomy individual/environmental is used to classify the sources. *Individual sources* are within the individual at the time they are measured. However, they have generally been influenced by external causes in the period preceding the assessment. *Environmental sources* are external to the individual at the time of measurement, but they have often been influenced by the individual in the period preceding the assessment. Among the individual factors and environmental factors there are facilitators and inhibitors of aggression. From a developmental perspective the internal inhibitors of physical aggression are weak during early childhood and generally increase with age. This strengthening of internal control will be enhanced by external inhibitors, but also depends on the strength of the internal and external facilitators of aggression. Within the individual I use four levels of causal factors: genetic, physiological, psychological (cognitive, emotional, moral), and behavioral. Within the environmental factors I use three levels: physical, psychological, and social.

Before describing some factors that could be causal factors of CPA according to some research evidence, I must admit that, except in extremely rare cases, I do not believe that we will find *the* causal factors of CPA, be they a gene, a brain structure, a cognitive function, an emotional organization, a moral propensity, a behavioral configuration, a parental disposition, a family feature, a neighborhood's social capital, or an environmental toxin. In the large majority of cases, those who have been exposed to many of these factors will not have a trajectory of CPA. In fact, all the evidence since Quetelet's work in the early 19th century suggests that even the chronic cases tend to reduce the frequency of their physical aggressions with time.

My present conviction is that during the early childhood of the large majority of children there are many causes that cumulate to promote children's regulation of physical aggression. Similarly, in a minority of cases, many causes cumulate to handicap regulation of physical aggression. Those who succeed in inhibiting physical aggression early are less likely to use physical aggression later on. Consequently, the later an individual manages to regulate physical aggression, the more likely he or she is to relapse. This

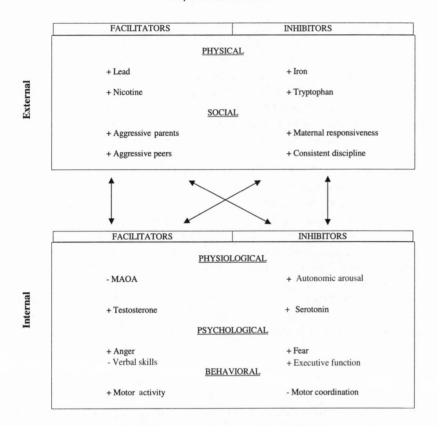

FIGURE 7.3. General model of factors and processes leading to increases or decreases in physical aggression. (Specific factors are only examples; see text.)

is probably due in part to the strength of the internal (physiological and psychological) facilitators and inhibitors, and in part to the environmental conditions (facilitators and inhibitors) in which individuals choose or are forced to live in. The multifactorial nature of causal factors that I postulate obviously presents a challenge to testing causal effects as outlined by Kraemer et al. (1997).

Because of space limitation it is impossible to describe all the factors for which there is evidence that they may contribute to a cumulative process of causal factors. I have instead selected factors that help to illustrate the process by which different levels of individual and environmental factors interact and possibly lead to an increased likelihood that regulation of physical aggression will or will not be learned. The choice of illustrative factors was based on my judgment that they may be among the most important causal factors during the early development of physical aggression.

## Individual factors

### Genetic Factors

Since all humans, like most other animals, appear to be using physical aggression early in life without having learned to do so, it seems likely that we are genetically programmed to hit, kick, and bite when needed, as we are apparently programmed to suck and to cuddle in the arms of the caregiver. This form of genetic effect must, however, be distinguished from genetic effects that could explain individual differences in the propensity to use physical aggression. There is indeed much variability in the early expression of physical aggression (Hay et al., 2000; Keenan & Wakschlag, 2000; Tremblay et al., 1999). This variability can be due to genetic and environmental factors. Few adequate studies have been done regarding genetic and environmental effects on frequency of physical aggression in humans. Many experimental and molecular genetic studies have been done with nonhumans (e.g., Maxson, 1996; Miczek, Maxson, Fish, & Faccidomo, 2001). Some molecular genetic studies have been done with humans (e.g., Bock & Goode, 1996; Caspi et al., 2002). A recent study of a twin sample at 19 months does suggest a relatively large genetic effect, and an effect of the environment that is unique to each twin in a pair (Dionne, Tremblay, Boivin, Laplante, & Pérusse, 2003). No common environmental effects were observed. Considering the association of physical aggression with many characteristics that have been shown to have some genetic basis (e.g., testosterone, temperament, personality, antisocial behavior), it would be extremely surprising to find that the variability in early physical aggression in humans is not associated with genetic variability. However, making a causal demonstration of genetic effects on chronic physical aggression in humans will be extremely difficult to do, except if genetic manipulation becomes relatively easy from a technical and an ethical point of view. Present twin and molecular genetic studies only provide correlational evidence of possible genetic effects.

### Physiological Factors

Physical aggression in animals and humans has been associated with a number of physiological characteristics that could facilitate or inhibit the use of physical aggression. Numerous studies have focused on hormones, neuromodulators, brain structures, and brain functioning.

Testosterone is a good example of the complexity involved in testing causal hypotheses concerning physiological factors with humans. Because males have much higher levels of testosterone than females, and because testosterone increases substantially during adolescence, reaches a peak during early adulthood, and then decreases with age, it has been suggested that testosterone could explain both the sex differences in antisocial behavior and the age–crime curve (e.g., Ellis & Coontz, 1990; Eysenck & Gudjonsson, 1989). However, as we have seen, the frequency of physical aggression does not follow the age–crime curve. Children have high levels of physical aggression long before their testosterone starts to rise during puberty. In fact, Schaal, Tremblay, Soussignan, and Susman (1996) showed that 13-year-old males with high levels of physical aggression since kindergarten had lower levels of testosterone than their peers. This phenomenon could be due to the fact that children with chronic physical aggression tend to be rejected by their peers. Indeed, much research has shown that levels of testosterone are highly influenced by the social status of an individual (Mazur & Booth, 1998). An alternative explanation for the association between testosterone and the age–crime curve would be that testosterone causes antisocial behavior that does not involve physical aggression. However, from a biological perspective, it would be surprising that increasing levels of testosterone during adolescence would cause increases in car thefts and running away from home, but not in frequency of physical aggression. Thus the association of testosterone and delinquent behavior during adolescence may be in large part an association between the fact that increases in testosterone during adolescence are associated with increase in physical size, and the latter is associated with less tolerance of deviant behavior by the environment.

There is, however, another mechanism by which testosterone could cause high levels of physical aggression. Testosterone levels during fetal life have been shown to play a role in programming brain circuits (Monaghan & Glickman, 1992; Rubinow & Schmidt, 1996). The differences in testosterone levels during fetal life can be due to both genetic factors and environmental factors (Archer, 1994; Harris, Vernon, & Boomsma, 1998; Meikle, Stringham, Bishop, & West, 1988). Animal studies of the organizing effect of testosterone on the brain during fetal life have reported associations with cognitive development, motor activity, aggression, and sexual orientation (e.g., Bachevalier & Hagger, 1991; Goy & McEwen, 1980). Studies with humans are evidently more difficult to do. The available evidence suggests that testosterone during the fetal life of humans also plays a role in creating cognitive and behavioral tendencies that may make it more difficult to learn to control physical aggression (Rubinow & Schmidt, 1996). For example, high testosterone levels have been linked to dominant behavior (Mazur & Booth, 1998) and cognitive functions, including verbal fluency (Christiansen & Knussmann, 1987; Dabbs, 1992; Finegan, Niccols, & Sitarenios, 1992; Jacklin, Wilcox, & Maccoby, 1988; Kimura & Hampson, 1994). It is easy to imagine that an infant who has a high need to dominate his or her environment (get his or her way), has poor cognitive abilities, and is less skilled at using language will be more likely to use physical aggression and less likely to learn to use his or her verbal skills to dominate. Sex differences in testosterone levels during fetal life would also explain sex differences in physical aggression. The increasing differences in physical aggression between males and females from early childhood to

adulthood would mirror other sex differences that increase during development, such as muscle mass, motor skills, and cognitive abilities (e.g.,
Hampson & Kimura, 1992).

Much research has also been done on aggression and the neurotransmitter serotonin (5-HT). There is good evidence from animal and human
studies that individuals with low levels of serotonin tend to be more impulsive and aggressive (e.g., Coccaro, 1996; Ferris, 1996; Hen, 1996; Higley et
al., 1996; LeMarquand, Benkelfat, Pihl, Palmour, & Young, 1999; Moffitt
et al., 1998; Raine, 2002). The work of Suomi and his colleagues (e.g.,
Higley, Linnoila, & Suomi, 1994; Suomi, 2002; Suomi, Chapter 13, this
volume) shows that rhesus monkeys with high levels of impulsivity and aggression (between 5% and 10% of a cohort) tend to have low levels of the
central serotonin metabolite (5-HIAA). During their early years these individuals tend to escalate play fighting into physically damaging aggression.
By adolescence they are at high risk of dying from wounds inflicted during
fights or from accidents. Young rhesus monkeys with low 5-HIAA appear
to be on a trajectory of chronic physical aggression that is similar to the
human children we have been studying. In fact, Constantino et al. (Constantino & Murphy, 1996; Constantino, Morris, & Murphy, 1997) have
shown that newborn humans from parents with a history of antisocial personality disorder have lower cerebrospinal fluid (CSF) 5-HIAA concentrations compared to newborns from families devoid of a history of antisocial
behavior. These infants were rated less sociable at 9 months and more disruptive at age 30 months. They would be expected to show high levels of
physical aggression and have more difficulty learning to regulate these behaviors. From the perspective of preventive interventions, it is important to
note that both medication and diet that increase serotonin level have been
shown to decrease agonistic behavior and increase affiliative behavior
(Chamberlain, Ervin, Pihl, & Young, 1987; Coccaro & Kavoussi, 1997;
Fava et al., 1997; Knutson et al., 1998; Moskowitz, Pinard, Zuroff,
Annable, & Young, 2001; Raleigh & McGuire, 1991).

*Psychological Factors*

There has been much research on the cognitive, emotional, and moral correlates of aggressive behavior (see Coie & Dodge, 1998; Tremblay &
LeMarquand, 2001). I will use research on anger control and executive
functioning as examples of the early role of psychological factors in learning to regulate physical aggression. Anger is one of a small group of physiological states labeled "primary emotions" that can be observed in infants
(Lewis, 1993). The other primary emotions are contentment, joy, interest,
surprise, distress, sadness, disgust, and fear. Anger is typically expressed
when a goal is not achieved or when the activity toward a goal is blocked
(Stein & Jewett, 1986; Lewis et al., 1990). Clear expressions of anger following frustration in a learning situation have been described as early as 8

weeks after birth (Lewis et al., 1990; Lewis, Sullivan, Ramsay, & Alessandri, 1992). The authors suggest that these experiments demonstrate that 8-week-old infants perceive links between means and ends, that anger or sadness tends to follow inability to achieve goals, and that there are early individual differences in goal-oriented behavior and expression of anger and sadness. With a longitudinal study of children from 9 to 33 months of age, Kochanska (2001) has shown that the majority of children show a decrease in angry reactions from 14 to 33 months, while a minority show an increase. One would expect that infants who invest more energy in pursuing goals and have more intense anger reactions are more at risk of using physical aggression to achieve their goals and in reaction to frustration.

The term "executive function" has been used to refer to deliberate problem solving, that is, the regulation of one's thoughts and actions (Zelazo, Carter, Reznick, & Frye, 1997). It includes the representation of the problem, planning the necessary actions, executing the actions, and evaluating the effects of the actions. The basic cognitive processes that appear to be necessary for effective problem solving are related to inhibition of action and memory. A number of studies with school-age children and adolescents have shown a relation between different aspects of executive functions and aggressive behavior (e.g., Cole, Usher, & Cargo, 1993; Séguin, Pihl, Harden, Tremblay, & Boulerice, 1995; Séguin, Tremblay, Boulerice, Pihl, & Harden, 1999). Deficits in executive function have also been shown for disruptive preschoolers (Hughes, Dunn, & White, 1998; Hughes, White, Sharpen, & Dunn, 2000; Speltz, DeKlyen, Calderon, Greenberg, & Fisher, 1999). Brain development during the preschool years provides children with increased ability to solve problems through a greater capacity to inhibit behavior and a greater working memory (Shonkoff & Phillips, 2000). For example, Kochanska, Murray, and Harlan (2000) showed that children were better at "effortful control" (e.g., delaying gratification, slowing down motor activity, maintaining effortful attention, lowering voice) at 33 compared to 22 months of age, and that girls had higher levels of control. The level of effortful control at 33 months was associated with the regulation of anger, and was predicted by the ability to focus attention at 9 months of age. It would be expected that children who are better at effortful control would not only better regulate their emotions, but also learn more quickly to use alternatives to physical aggressions.

## Behavioral Factors

Numerous longitudinal studies of antisocial behaviors have attempted to demonstrate that present behavioral characteristics "cause" later behavioral characteristics. In general these correlational studies have shown that the best predictors of later antisocial behavior is present antisocial behavior (e.g. Loeber, 1982; Olweus, 1979; Tremblay & LeMarquand, 2001). Other disruptive behaviors, especially hyperactivity and opposition, have also been shown to correlate positively with later antisocial behaviors (Lahey, McBurnett, & Loeber, 2000; Tremblay & LeMarquand, 2001), while anxiety and prosocial behavior are negatively correlated (Côté, Tremblay, Nagin, Zoccolillo, & Vitaro, 2002; Kerr, Tremblay, Pagani-Kurtz, & Vitaro, 1997; Tremblay et al., 1994). Personality models of antisocial behavior suggest that there are interactions among the behavioral dimensions that either increase or decrease the likelihood of antisocial behavior (e.g., Cloninger, Svrakic, & Svrakic, 1997; Eysenck & Gudjonson 1989; Lahey, Waldman, & McBurnett, 1999). The problem here is to determine whether these predictions over time reveal "causal mechanisms" or are simply an indication that such behaviors are the result of common underlying factors. One approach is to start measuring these behavioral dimensions as early as possible and examine the sequence of their appearance. Are the interactions occurring among dimensions in place during infancy, and is there a profile that facilitates learning to regulate physical aggression? For example, Tremblay and LeMarquand (2001) report a correlation of 0.29 between hyperactivity and physical aggression at 17 months of age, indicating that, if hyperactivity "causes" physical aggression, the mechanisms are in place during infancy.

There is some evidence that children learn to regulate physical aggression through the use of playful physical aggression. Rough-and-tumble play (play fighting) is a behavior found among many species (Dolhinow, 1999; Panksepp, 1998, 1999). Hamburg and van Lawick-Goodall (1974) described infant chimpanzee jumping on, hitting, and pulling the hair of their extremely tolerant mothers. Based on Harlow and Harlow's (1965) observations of play fighting in young rhesus monkeys, Blurton-Jones (1967, 1972) appears to have been the first to differentiate rough-and-tumble play from physical aggression in preschool children. Those who "play fight" are wrestling, grappling, jumping, tumbling, and running while laughing and showing a playful face. When physical aggression occurs, there is no laughing and no playful face. In the play-fighting situation children spend most of the time in close proximity. In the physical aggressive situation children come together for the aggression and then pull away.

The role of play in children's development has been repeatedly pointed out at least since Plato. The essence of early childhood is play. Children discover the world by experimenting with it, and the pleasure they get makes adults label that behavior "play." Bruner (1972) suggested that the prolonged infancy of humans relative to other species provides more time for play, and thus more time to develop sophisticated cognitive abilities. Rough-and-tumble play during early childhood may be one of the most important factors in learning to regulate aggression. Children need to learn that physical aggression is not tolerated in social interactions, but they also need to learn to express aggressive reactions in ways that are socially acceptable and even constructive. Panksepp (1999) hypothesizes that the mammalian brain is wired for rough-and-tumble play (see also Gergen, 1990).

Mothers are often the first to play fight with their infants through tickling bouts and mocked aggressions. As motor coordination develops, children become more mobile and more active, and fathers become a favorite play partner. Fathers come to be more frequently involved in rough-and-tumble play than mothers (Carson, Burks, & Parke, 1993; Roopnarine, Hooper, Ahmeduzzaman, & Pollack, 1993). The reason rough-and-tumble play may be important for learning to regulate physical aggression is that it gives children an opportunity to exercise pleasurable motor activities such as wrestling, tickling, pushing, pulling, and running in a context where they must learn a key rule, *not to hurt the partner*. Tickling is fun if you learn to tickle hard enough, but not *too* hard. Pushing and pulling is fun if you learn to push and pull hard enough, but not *too* hard. The motor behaviors involved in acts of physical aggression are motor behaviors that in and of themselves bring pleasure. Humans have invented a multitude of sports and martial arts that involve exercising these motor actions. Lorenz (1966) suggested that one of the best ways to control aggression was to create rituals. Sports involve ritualized aggression, and sports clearly have an important role in our modern societies for youth as well as for adults. Infants need to exercise these aggressive motor patterns in a context where they will learn that they give sensorimotor pleasure, and pleasure with an attachment figure, as long as there is control over the actions, that is, that the mutual pleasure rules are respected. Play fighting will sometimes degenerate into real fights. These incidents provide opportunities to learn reconciliation skills (de Wall, 1989). Furthermore, play fighting may be a precursor to make-believe aggression (Singer & Singer, 1981). Millions of peace-loving humans spend enormous amounts of money and time enjoying imaginary aggressive activities depicted in films, novels, plays, and video-computer games. Vicarious pleasure in these antisocial behaviors by adults did not appear in the 20th century with movies and computers. These pleasures were catered to by the theater during the life of Pericles, by the massacre of animals and humans in the Roman Colosseum at the time of Caligula, and by the stories of Edgar Allen Poe during the life of Abraham Lincoln. Play fighting during early childhood may be an important developmental precursor of the ability to use motor activity and make-believe to ritualize aggressive behavior.

## Environmental Factors

### Physical Capital

I include in the physical environment factors that range from perinatal complications, to food, to secondhand smoke, to availability of weapons, and to environmental toxins. Some of these environmental factors have a direct impact on genetic and physiological mechanisms that can lead to regulation or disregulation of physical aggression, others have a direct impact on psychological and behavioral mechanisms involved in aggression. Smoking is a good example of the interactions between different environmental and individual dimensions. There is increasing evidence that women who smoke during pregnancy are at higher risk of having an antisocial child (e.g., Fergusson, Woodward, & Horwood, 1998; Raine, 2002; Wakschlag et al., 1997). The mechanisms involved are not well understood. Smoking during pregnancy could be a correlate of causal factors or a causal factor in itself. The effect of nicotine on the developing nervous system could, for example, have an impact on cognitive and emotional regulation, thus on regulation of physical aggression (Fried, 1995). These effects could be increased by smoking during breastfeeding and secondhand smoke in the home. However, parents who are unable or unwilling to stop smoking during pregnancy and after the birth of a child may also have psychological and behavioral characteristics that handicap learning to regulate physical aggression (Tremblay et al., 2002; Zoccolillo et al., 2002). They may also live in environments with higher levels of toxins (Wasserman, Staghezza-Jaramillo, Shrout, Popovac, & Graziano, 1998) and lower levels of collective efficacy (Sampson, Raudenbush, & Earls, 1997), factors that also appear to have an impact on the development of antisocial behavior.

Nutrition is another good example of interactions between environmental and individual factors (Raine, 2002). Special diets are given to children born with a multitude of genetic defects (e.g., Scriver & Kaufman, 2001). The aim of these diets is to give the child proteins that are lacking because of a genetic defect. The diets may be needed throughout the individual's life or only for a limited time during a critical period for the growth of a physiological structure. Similar interventions are offered to children with nutrition deficits, such as lack of iron (Nelson et al., 2000; Wasserman et al., 1994). However, the problem will not be prevented if the parents of the child do not follow the diet, whether it be because they do not understand, or because they have problems regulating their own behavior, or because they cannot afford it. It is easy to imagine that children deprived of adequate food intake during the first few years after conception can have neurological deficits that makes it more difficult for them to learn to regulate physical aggression.

### Social Capital

I use the term "social capital" to refer to the quality of social relations in an individual's environment (Coleman, 1988). The social capital of a developing child refers to the quality of the relations established by the people he or she interacts with: caregivers (parents, extended family, parents' friends, nurses, doctors, daycare personnel, teachers, and other professionals), siblings, peers, other members of the neighborhood, and members of the extended community (e.g., through travels and the media). Much research on the development of antisocial behavior has focused on the influence of parents, siblings, peers, neighborhoods, and the media. Most of this research targeted school-age children and did not study the development of physical aggression. Lacourse et al. (2002) did show that an intensive 2-year intervention for disruptive kindergarten children, which targeted parenting skills and social skills in small groups of highly prosocial peers, apparently deflected some of them from a chronic trajectory of physical aggression. This study may be as close as we have come to showing a causal effect on CPA. There is also some evidence that parental and family characteristics are correlated with levels of physical aggression during early childhood (e.g., Keenan & Shaw, 1994; Tremblay et al., 2002). The best evidence comes from preventive intervention studies where high-risk families were given support during pregnancy and early childhood (e.g., Olds et al., 1998; Schweinhart & Weikart, 1993). These randomized control trials show a long-term impact on levels of antisocial behavior during adolescence and adulthood. However, none of these studies measured the development of physical aggression. It is thus impossible to know if they had an impact on CPA. Similarly, although there have been numerous studies on the role of peers during the school years, to my knowledge there are no studies on the role of peers in learning to regulate physical aggression during the preschool years. One would expect that the behavior of the peers one interacts with at that crucial time would play a significant role.

## A RESEARCH DESIGN TO TEST CAUSES OF CHRONIC PHYSICAL AGGRESSION

### Summary of the Developmental Model

The socialization process, which starts at conception, involves learning to regulate one's pleasure seeking to that of others. Plato writes in the *Laws* that the aim of education is to make every man as passionate and gentle as possible. We are born with the passion for living, but we learn to harmonize our passions with the passions of others. As children grow older, they generally become more and more socialized. But some do not. As their body mass increases with age, their disruptive behavior becomes more of a threat to their environment, and they are labeled "antisocial." An "antisocial," or "CD," or "delinquent" child behaves more frequently than others in an antisocial way. In essence, an antisocial individual is one who cannot or will not refrain from doing what infants do: hit because he or she is angry, take someone's belongings because he or she wants it, destroy someone's belonging because he or she is angry, or refuse to obey rules that are set for his or her and the general well-being.

Among these antisocial behaviors, physical aggression is both a natural tool for survival and the least likely to be tolerated by others. Thus there are strong internal and external pressures to learn to inhibit physical aggression. Children who learn less well than others during the preschool years are more likely to use physical aggression during the school years, and thus to be labeled "deviant" both by mental health and judicial standards. Those who maintain high levels of physical aggression from early childhood to adulthood can be considered chronic cases of physical aggression.

There are many potential "causes" of CPA, but none appear necessary or sufficient, except in extremely rare cases of serious brain damage. For example, most low-IQ, even mentally deficient, individuals are not CFA. Internal causes (genetic, physiological, psychological, behavioral) and environmental causes (physical and social) interact over time to trace developmental trajectories from which it becomes more difficult to escape as time goes by (see Figure 7.3). In some cases the factors that normally help children learn to inhibit physical aggression are not present or not powerful enough. In other cases the factors that facilitate physical aggression are exceptionally strong. The number of years it takes for an individual to reach socially acceptable regulation of physical aggression should depend on the mix of all these factors. Thus, one would expect the probability of CPA to be extremely high for a child who lacks many of the internal and external factors that inhibit physical aggression, and who also has many of the factors that facilitate physical aggression. On the other hand, a child who has many of the factors that facilitate physical aggression, but also many of the inhibiting factors, could display high levels of physical aggression during early childhood, but manage to regulate these behaviors, and eventually become a very useful member of his community, either as an aggressive tennis player, an aggressive car salesman, an aggressive politician, or an aggressive scientist! Similarly, a child who lacks many of the factors that inhibit physical aggression, but also lacks most of the factors that facilitate physical aggression, may not be at high risk of CPA.

## A General Research Strategy: Prevention Experiments

The testable hypotheses that can be generated from this theoretical framework are practically unlimited. Finding the right combination of factors, at the right time, with the adequate intensity, for each type of case, can occupy the career of many generations of investigators. The major challenge is to have large groups of competent investigators collaborate for very long periods of time.

Because of the intensity of the effort needed, and because experimental studies offer the best proofs of causal effects, I suggest the following strategy. The search for causes of CPA will be more successful if guided by a practical aim, that is, to find causal factors that can be manipulated to prevent the development of CPA. This enterprise would bring together the resources of those who are looking for causes of CPA and the resources of those who are trying to prevent the development of this problem. There is a long medical tradition of testing causal factors with pragmatic experiments (Schwartz, Flamant, & Lellouch, 1981). Preventive experiments can manipulate many putative causal factors. The effectiveness of interventions targeting different groups of putative causal factors can be compared to testing the effect of adding or subtracting causal targets. Also, the effectiveness of different interventions at different points in time during development can be compared to testing developmental hypotheses. A practical way of testing alternative hypotheses within the context of a preventive effort is to formulate alternative manipulations of putative causal factors (i.e., prevention programs) and to predict their impact. If these different programs are given to equivalent samples (randomized clinical trials), we can then compare the long-term impacts through long-term follow-ups. Not all interventions are good tests of causal hypotheses (see Rutter, Chapter 1, this volume; Tremblay & Craig, 1995; Tremblay et al., 1992), but carefully designed experimental manipulations of putative causal factors through interventions should provide better tests of causal hypotheses than correlational studies.

### Three General Hypotheses

This logic leads me to formulate three general hypotheses that I believe could, at this point in time, have the most important practical and theoretical pay-off. These three general hypotheses will then be used to generate operational hypotheses.

### The Caregiver Hypothesis

> Is thy face like thy mother's, my fair child!
> —BYRON (1816/1951, p. 710)

Whether we are considering internal or external factors facilitating or inhibiting CPA, it is difficult not to take into account the role of the caregivers, and especially the role of the primary caregiver. To be more operational, at the expense of political correctness, it is hard to imagine any successful experimental manipulation aimed at fostering the regulation of physical aggression during the preschool years that would not include mothers as a main "manipulated variable." This is true whether we want to have an impact on genes through mating, reduce the negative impact of smoking during pregnancy, examine the effect of stress on the hypothalamic–pituitary–adrenal (HPA) axis during pregnancy and infancy, provide housing in less toxic environments, test the effects of breastfeeding, provide better nutrition, increase cognitive stimulation, test the role of play fighting, facilitate secure attachment, stimulate language acquisition, examine the impact of disciplinary practices, test the impact of daycare, or foster more positive interactions with siblings and peers. Mothers come close to the criteria of a necessary and sufficient factor at least in most of our current industrialized cultures.

However, we can formulate a number of alternative hypotheses that could be tested within the same experiment or in different experiments. These will be described after the introduction to the two other general hypotheses.

## The Biological Embedding Hypothesis

The term "biological embedding" was used by Keating and Hertzman (1999) to refer to the process by which environmental factors during early childhood have an impact on brain development and how, later on in life, these biological effects become causes of different behavioral, social, and health problems. Once the effect of the early environment has become "embedded" in the biological organization, it becomes much more difficult to change the course of development. The implications from a preventive perspective are that we should modify the negative environmental conditions before they become biologically embedded. From a cost-effectiveness perspective, it is expected that interventions later on in life will be much less effective.

The alternative hypothesis, of course, is that the brain of humans remains plastic throughout most of the life course, and that the reasons for chronic behavior problems are that individuals remain in environments that continue to have a negative impact on them (e.g., Kagan, 1998). At any point during development we simply need to change the environment to change behavior. This developmental model would, for example, explain the late-onset CD phenomena. Individuals without conduct problems during childhood would suddenly start to have problems during adolescence because of changes in their environments (see Moffitt, 1993; Nagin & Tremblay, 2003).

The "biological embedding" hypothesis, and the "permanent plasticity" hypothesis are two opposites on a continuum. It is unlikely that there is rigid biological embedding or an everlasting plasticity for any social or antisocial behavior. However, these two processes could apply differently to various types of social or antisocial behavior. This is one more reason why we need to differentiate different forms of antisocial behaviors to understand their development and test their causes.

Recent work suggests that children with chronic aggression problems have disregulated HPA activity (McBurnett, Lahey, Rathouz, & Loeber, 2000; van Goozen, Matthys, Cohen-Kettenis, Thijssen, & van Engeland,

1998). One explanation for this phenomenon is that experience during infancy can cause permanent alterations to the HPA axis by its impact on steroid receptors in the hippocampus and the frontal cortex. These brain structures are, for example, related to the executive functions discussed above. Animal and human research on the impact of tactile stimulation during infancy indicates that it has an important organizing effect on different brain structures including the HPA axis (e.g., Meaney, Aitken, Van Berkel, Bhatnagar, & Sapolsky, 1988; Shonkoff & Phillips, 2000). Other studies also indicate that not only chronic, but also acute, increases in cortisol may have a deleterious effect on the hippocampus, an important physiological structure for memory (Lupien et al., 1998; Lupien, Gillin, & Hauger, 1999). Interventions during the early years, which could prevent this negative "biological embedding," could possibly prevent CPA. Alternatively, interventions that would start later, say, in first grade, would not have an impact on the HPA axis, and possibly not have an important effect on the level of physical aggression.

## The Sex-Difference Hypothesis

Because girls appear to learn more quickly to regulate their emotions and their disruptive behaviors (e.g., Côté, Vaillancourt, et al., 2002; Kochanska et al., 2000), we would expect that preventive interventions during early childhood would have a more rapid and long-lasting impact with girls than with boys. Thus preventive interventions during early childhood with boys and girls could accelerate and accentuate the difference in regulation of physical aggression between boys and girls. Such a phenomenon seems to have been observed with school performance ever since girls have been stimulated to pursue academic studies. Experimental studies could try to identify which types of environmental manipulation are more effective for each sex. It is worth noting here that girls tend to use indirect aggression earlier than boys and more frequently until adulthood (Björkqvist, Österman, & Kaukiainen, 1992; Crick, Casas, & Ku, 1999; Crick & Grotpeter, 1995; Grotpeter & Crick, 1996; Tremblay et al., 1996; Vaillancourt, Brendgen, Boivin, & Tremblay, 2002). The differential use of indirect aggression by males and females could have a causal link with the differential use of physical aggression. This should be an important area of developmental research on aggression.

## A Minor Experiment

The editors of this volume asked authors to describe how they would test their main hypotheses. I believe the field is ripe for the type of major experiments described below, but in case I am wrong I first describe a smaller study to test the following two hypotheses: (1) play fighting during early childhood has a significant impact on learning to regulate physical aggression for males; (2) development of executive functions during early childhood has a significant impact, for males, on learning to regulate physical aggression.

To test each of these hypotheses I would randomly allocate pregnant women at high risk of having children with CPA (e.g., primiparous pregnant adolescents; see Nagin & Tremblay, 2001b) to four conditions: (1) training in play-fighting games, (2) training in executive function games, (3) training in both, and (4) no training. Training should start with the mothers during pregnancy and continue with regular support until the child is 4 years of age. If the experiment is successful, other experiments could verify if a shorter intervention would have the same impact. Including female children in the experiment would help us to understand the role of play fighting and executive function in females.

The hypotheses will be disconfirmed if the experimental children, compared to the control ones, demonstrate better executive functions and better experiences of play fighting, but (1) show no differences in their trajectories of physical aggression during the school years; or (2) differences indicate that fewer experimental children are on the low-level physical aggression trajectories. The hypotheses will be supported if the differences indicate that fewer experimental children are on the high-level physical aggression trajectories. Note that such an experiment would seriously question one of my central hypotheses (i.e., males learn to use alternatives to physical aggression rather than learn to physically aggress) if males (from any of the groups) who did not use physical aggression during the preschool years increased their level of physical aggression to the point of following a chronic trajectory during their school years. The strategy could also be used to test the impact of other putative inhibitors, such as the impact of early language development on learning alternatives to physical aggression, as well as the impact of maternal responsiveness and consistent discipline.

Two important general rules concerning the manipulation of the experimental variable need to be stated here. First, regarding putative inhibitors of physical aggression, such as executive function and play fighting, we try to enhance their presence in early childhood. Second, in the case of facilitators, such as lead, nicotine, aggressive parents, and aggressive peers, we would attempt to reduce their presence. Third, to have an impact on internal factors, we need to manipulate external factors such as mother behavior. This is also true for interventions that would use medication, since medication is an external agent.

## A Major Experiment

The following experiment is labeled "major" because it attempts to test the three major hypotheses described above, and would involve the collaboration of a larger research team over a period of at least 20 years. The subjects would again be young primiparous women with a history of problem behaviors because they have more male children with a high risk of chronic physical aggression (Nagin & Tremblay, 2001b). The following five prevention programs could be given to random samples. It would be ideal to follow a random sample of the birth cohort to obtain norms on the development of physical aggression in that cohort and also a sample of at-risk families who do not participate in the experimental interventions (see Lacourse et al., 2002).

1. Support to mothers from pregnancy to 24 months after birth, of the type given in the Elmira project (Olds et al., 1998).
2. The program in 1 to which would be added components aiming at specific putative causes, such as reducing smoking and stress during pregnancy, and/or stimulating play fighting and executive functions during the first 2 years after birth.
3. A quality daycare program from birth to 24 months without support to mothers. Other components that do not try to modify mother behavior could be added in the daycare situation. Preferably, these components would target the same causal factors as those in 2 (e.g., play fighting and executive function stimulation).
4. Support to mothers from 25 to 58 months after birth, focused on parenting skills and social skills training (e.g., Lacourse et al., 2002; Patterson, 1982; Webster-Stratton, 1998), to which could be added other components such as increasing serotonin levels through diet (Moskowitz et al., 2001).
5. A quality daycare program (e.g., Schweinhart & Weikart, 1997) from 25 to 58 months without support to parents. Other components that do not try to modify mother behavior could be added in the daycare situation—for example, an enriched diet at lunch to increase serotonin levels as in 4 but given at the daycare center (Moskowitz et al., 2001).
6. No program offered, or an attention-placebo program (see Tremblay, Kurtz, Mâsse, Vitaro, & Pihl, 1995).

To test the impact of the experimental manipulation on the development of CPA, we would of course need to follow the children until the end of adolescence and measure their level of physical aggression regularly (e.g., once a year) and from different sources. To test mechanisms preventing or fostering chronic physical aggression, particularly the biological embedding hypothesis, we would need to collect regular data on biological variables such as cortisol, heart rate, testosterone, serotonin, and brain development, as well as data on executive function, anger control, language development, prosocial behavior, and the like. The development of new statistical models provides powerful means of testing hypotheses with large multisite experiments (e.g., Plewis, 2002; Raudenbush & Liu, 2000)

If results confirmed the following differences between the programs, $2 < 1 < 4 < 3 < 5 = 6$, for the proportion of children in the CPA trajectory, the proportion of children with a disregulated HPA axis, and the proportion of children with low executive function, we would conclude that the hypotheses described below are supported:

• During the preschool years mothers play a crucial role in preventing CPA.

• Smoking and stress during pregnancy, as well as lack of play fighting and executive function stimulation in the first 2 years after birth, appear to increase the likelihood of CPA. Disentangling the effect of these different factors will of course need further experiments where some components are left out.

• There is some form of biological embedding of adverse environmental conditions during the early years, which appears to have a negative impact on executive function and physical aggression. However, later mother support, between 25 and 58 months, can still have an impact on the regulation of the HPA axis. Note that further evidence of the biological embedding hypothesis from this simulation comes from the fact that a quality daycare program between birth and 24 months does have an impact on the HPA axis, while the same type of program between 25 and 58 months does not.

• The general hypothesis concerning sex differences could be tested if there were equivalent numbers of males and females in the samples and sex differences were tested. If the impact of interventions were generally better for girls than for boys, we would have an indication of a general sex effect. However, the sex effects may be interacting with the biological embedding hypothesis. Thus, if girls were doing better than boys only in the cases of a late intervention, we would have an indication that there is an early biological embedding mechanism related to the sex differences in physical aggression.

• It would also be possible to test hypotheses concerning ethnic differences, or socioeconomic differences, by comparing the effects of the programs with different ethnic groups or socioeconomic groups.

• This type of study would also permit tests of other types of developmental hypotheses. For example, to test a diathesis–stress hypothesis of CPA (Nagin & Tremblay, 2003), we can verify to what extent subjects from high-risks families who learned to regulate physical aggression in early childhood are at risk of showing increasing levels of physical aggression during adolescence, when the adolescence risk factors appear and there are no more supportive interventions (see Lacourse et al., 2002).

• Such a study would also be ideal to test to what extent the deflection from a CPA trajectory has an impact on other forms of chronic antisocial behavior. Also, some intervention programs could target other forms of antisocial behaviors, rather than physical aggression. We could then test if such programs—for example, targeting oppositional behavior—would also have an impact on the development of CPA.

• Finally, we could also contrast the early-childhood interventions with interventions that start only at school entry, or just before puberty, or even during adolescence. Evidence that interventions after early childhood can reduce the level of physical aggression comes first from the fact that the levels of physical aggression decrease during childhood, adolescence, and adulthood even for chronic cases (Brame et al., 2001; Nagin & Tremblay, 1999; White et al., 2001), and second, from preventive interventions (Lacourse et al., 2002). One of the important questions is to what extent delaying interventions reduces the returns—for example, in terms of reduction of frequency of CPA and general quality of life.

## CONCLUSIONS

I share the aim of the editors of this book to bring our field of research beyond correlational demonstrations of "causes." However, we must constantly remind ourselves that the human mind is bent on causal explanations, and tends to hurry through the required antecedents. The rush into causal explanations is probably part of the history of all sciences. In the 17th century Galileo noted that, since the time of Aristotle, the major philosophical question concerning movement was its cause, "why things move." Modern physics was born with his determination to first describe "how they moved" (Galilei, 1638/1991).

I am convinced that we will not find the causes we are looking for until we break down the field of antisocial–conduct disorder–delinquency into specific components and *describe* their development from birth to adulthood. We cannot find a cause of a phenotype that is not clearly defined. Furthermore, since we will not find *A* cause, and it is unlikely that we will find *a necessary and sufficient set of causes*, we might as well focus our efforts on finding interventions that will change the developmental course of the different types of antisocial behaviors. From this perspective, I agree with the arguments presented in Chapter 1 of this book, stating that experimental interventions are not conclusive proofs of causal effects. But, experiments are better proofs of causal factors than correlational studies, and prevention experiments can be embedded within longitudinal studies to provide the best of both worlds (see Lacourse et al., 2002; Vitaro, Brendgen, & Tremblay, 2001; Vitaro, Brendgen, Pagani, Tremblay, & McDuff, 1999). Preventive experiments also give the added advantage of providing proof of an effective or ineffective way of changing the world.

Since we would probably not earn a living doing what we are doing if our fellow citizens did not hope that we would find a way of making our societies less violent, preventing the development of CPA should be a priority. Unfortunately, even if we were successful in preventing all children from becoming CPA, there would still be much violence in our societies, since at any one point in time there appears to be more physically violent acts committed by individuals who are not CPA than by those who are CPA. This is probably due to the fact that, having all used physical aggression during early childhood, the thin veneer of self-regulation can break down under a strong environmental pressure. Situational prevention is thus essential. Paradoxically, a Nobel Prize-winning biologist came to this conclusion some years ago. Convinced that humans have an aggressive instinct that they must always keep in check, Konrad Lorenz (1966) highlighted the importance for societies to channel (socialize) competition through sports, arts, and sciences; to promote friendship among people from different ideologies and cultures; and finally to channel (socialize) militant enthusiasm.

> *Man is human, and the small amount of intelligence one*
> *may possess counts little or nothing against the rage of*
> *passion and the limits of human nature pressing upon him.*
> —GOETHE (1974, p. 62)

> *It is evident therefore that all men (since all men are born*
> *as infants) are born unfit for society; and very many*
> *(perhaps the majority) remain so throughout their lives,*
> *because of mental illness or lack of training (disciplina). . . .*
> *Therefore man is made fit for Society not by nature, but by*
> *training.*
> —HOBBES (1647/1998, p. 25)

## ACKNOWLEDGMENTS

I wish to thank the following persons for helpful comments on the chapter: Raymond Baillargeon, Sylvana Côté, Ben Lahey, Katia Maliantovitch, Terrie Moffitt, Daniel Nagin, Jean Séguin, Tracy Vaillancourt, and Frank Vitaro.

## REFERENCES

Achenbach, T. M., & Edelbrock, C. (1983). *Manual for the Child Behavior Checklist and Revised Child Behavior Profile.* Burlington: University of Vermont, Department of Psychiatry.

Anderson, C. A., & Bushman, B. J. (2002). The effects of media violence on society. *Science, 295,* 2377–2379.

Angold, A., Prendergast, M., Cox, A., Harrington, R., Simonoff, E., & Rutter, M. (1995). The Child and Adolescent Psychiatric Assessment (CAPA). *Psychological Medicine, 25*(4), 739–753.

American Psychiatric Association. (1980). *Diagnostic and statistical manual of mental disorders* (3rd ed.). Washington, DC: Author.

American Psychiatric Association. (1987). *Diagnostic and statistical manual of mental disorders* (3rd ed., rev.). Washington, DC: Author.

American Psychiatric Association. (1994). *Diagnostic and statistical manual of mental disorders* (4th ed.). Washington, DC: Author.

Archer, J. (1994). Testosterone and aggression. *Journal of Offender Rehabilitation, 21*(3–4), 3–39.

Bachevalier, J., & Hagger, C. (1991). Sex differences in the development of learning abilities in primates. *Psychoneuroendocrinology, 16*(1–3), 177–188.

Baillargeon, R., Boulerice, B., Tremblay, R. E., Zoccolillo, M., Vitaro, F., & Kohen, D. (2001). Modeling interinformant agreement in the absence of a "gold standard." *Journal of Child Psychology and Psychiatry, 42*(4), 463–473.

Björkqvist, K., Österman, K., & Kaukiainen, A. (1992). The development of direct and indirect aggressive strategies in males and females. In K. Bjoerkqvist & P. Niemelae (Eds.), *Of mice and women: Aspects of female aggression* (pp. 51–64). San Diego, CA: Academic Press.

Blackstone, W. (1857). *Commentaries on the Laws of England* (Vol. IV). London: Murray.

Blurton-Jones, N. (1967). An ethological study of some aspects of social behaviour of children in nursery school. In D. Morris (Ed.), *Primate ethology* (pp. 347–368). London: Weidenfeld & Nicolson.

Blurton-Jones, N. (1972). Characteristics of ethological studies of human behaviour. In N. Blurton Jones (Ed.), *Ethological studies of child behaviour* (pp. 3–33). New York: Cambridge University Press.

Bock, G. R., & Goode, J. A. (Eds.). (1996). *Genetics of criminal and antisocial behavior* (CIBA Foundation Symposium 1994). Toronto: Wiley.

Brame, B., Nagin, D. S., & Tremblay, R. E. (2001). Developmental trajectories of physical aggression from school entry to late adolescence. *Journal of Child Psychology and Psychiatry, 58*, 389–394.

Brendgen, M., Vitaro, F., Tremblay, R. E., & Lavoie, F. (2001). Reactive and proactive aggression: Predictions to physical violence in different contexts and moderating effects of parental monitoring and caregiving behavior. *Journal of Abnormal Child Psychology, 29*, 293–304.

Broidy, L. M., Nagin, D. S., Tremblay, R. E., Bates, J. E., Brame, B., Dodge, K., Fergusson, D., Horwood, J., Loeber, R., Laird, R., Lynam, D., Moffitt, T., Pettit, G. S., & Vitaro, F. (2003). Developmental trajectories of childhood disruptive behaviors and adolescent delinquency: A six site, cross-national study. *Developmental Psychology, 39*(2), 222–245.

Bruner, J. (1972). *Beyond the information given: Studies in the psychology of knowing.* New York: Norton.

Bushman, B. J., & Anderson, C. A. (2001). Media violence and the American public: Scientific facts versus media misinformation. *American Psychologist, 56*(6–7), 477–489.

Byron, G. G. (1816/1951). Childe Harold's Pilgrimage. In P. R. Lieder, R. M. Lovett, & R. K. Root (Eds.), *British poetry and prose. Shorter edition* (p.710). Boston: Houghton Mifflin.

Cairns, R. B., Cairns, B. D., & Neckerman, H. J. (1988). Early school dropout : Configurations and determinants. *Child Development, 60*, 1437–1452.

Cairns, R. B., Cairns, B. D., Neckerman, H. J., Ferguson, L. L., & Gariépy, J. L. (1989). Growth and aggression: 1. Childhood to early adolescence. *Developmental Psychology, 25*(2), 320–330.

Carson, J., Burks, V., & Parke, R. (1993). Parent–child physical play: Determinants and consequences. In K. MacDonald (Ed.), *Parent–child play* (pp. 197–220). Albany: State University of New York Press.

Caspi, A., McClay, J., Moffitt, T. E., Mill, J., Martin, J., Craig, I. W., Taylor, A., & Poulton, R. (2002). Role of genotype in the cycle of violence in maltreated children. *Science, 297*, 851–854.

Chamberlain, B., Ervin, F. R., Pihl, R. O., & Young, S. N. (1987). The effect of raising or lowering tryptophan levels on aggression in vervet monkeys. *Pharmacology, Biochemistry and Behavior, 28*, 503–510.

Christiansen, K., & Knussmann, R. (1987). Androgen levels and components of aggressive behavior in men. *Hormones and Behavior, 21*, 170–180.

Cloninger, C. R., Svrakic, D. M., & Svrakic, N. M. (1997). A multidimensional psychobiological model of violence. In A. Raine, D. Farrington, P. Brennan, & S. A. Mednick (Eds.), *Biosocial bases of violence* (pp. 39–54). New York: Plenum Press.

Coccaro, E. F. (1996). Understanding aggressive behavior in children. In C. F. Ferris & T. Grisso (Eds.), *Annals of the New York Academy of Sciences* (Vol. 794, pp. 82–89). New York: New York Academy of Sciences.

Coccaro, E. F., & Kavoussi, R. J. (1997). Fluoxetine and impulsive aggressive behavior in personality disordered subjects. *Archives of General Psychiatry, 54*, 1081–1088.

Coie, J. D., & Dodge, K. A. (1998). Aggression and antisocial behavior. In W. Damon (Series Ed.) & N. Eisenberg (Vol. Ed.), *Handbook of child psychology (5th ed.): Vol. 3. Social, emotional, and personality development* (pp. 779–862). New York: Wiley.

Cole, P. M., Usher, B. A., & Cargo, A. P. (1993). Cognitive risk and its association with risk for disruptive behavior disorder in preschoolers. *Journal of Clinical Child Psychology, 22*, 154–164.

Coleman, J. S. (1988). Social capital in the creation of human capital. *American Journal of Sociology, 94*, 95–120.

Constantino, J. N., Morris, J. A., & Murphy, D. L. (1997). CSF 5-HIAA and family history of antisocial personality disorder in newborns. *American Journal of Psychiatry, 154*, 1771–1773.

Constantino, J. N., & Murphy, D. L. (1996). Monoamine metabolites in "leftover" newborn human cerebrospinal fluid: A potential resource for biobehavioral research. *Psychiatry Research, 65*(3), 129–142.

Côté, S., Tremblay, R. E., Nagin, D. S., Zoccolillo, M., & Vitaro, F. (2002). Childhood behavioral profiles leading to adolescent conduct disorder: Risk trajectories for boys and girls. *Journal of the American Academy of Child and Adolescent Psychiatry, 41*(9), 1086–1094.

Côté, S., Vaillancourt, T., Farhat, A., LeBlanc, J., Nagin, D. S., & Tremblay, R. E. (2002). *The development of physical aggression during childhood.* Manuscript submitted for publication.

Crick, N. R., Casas, J. F., & Ku, H.-C. (1999). Relational and physical forms of peer victimization in preschool. *Developmental Psychology, 35*(2), 376–385.

Crick, N. R., & Grotpeter, J. K. (1995). Relational aggression, gender and social-psychological adjustment. *Child Development, 66*(3), 710–722.

Dabbs, J. M. J. (1992). Testosterone and occupational achievement. *Social Forces, 70*, 813–824.

de Waal, F. (1989). *Peacemaking among primates.* Cambridge, MA: Harvard University Press.

Did Kayla Have to Die? (2000, March 13). *Newsweek*, pp. 24–29.

Dionne, G., Tremblay, R. E., Boivin, M., Laplante, D., & Pérusse, D. (2003). Physical aggression and expressive vocabulary in 19-month-old twins. *Developmental Psychology, 39*(2), 261–273.

Dodge, K., Lochman, J. E., Harnish, J. D., Bates, J. E., & Pettit, G. S. (1997). Reactive and proactive aggression in school children and psychiatrically impaired chronically assaultive youth. *Journal of Abnormal Psychology, 106*(1), 37–51.

Dolhinow, P. (1999). Play, a critical process in the developmental system. In A. Fuentes & P. Dolhinow (Eds.), *The nonhuman primates* (pp. 231–236). Mountain View, CA: Mayfield.

Elliott, D. S. (1994). Serious violent offenders: Onset, developmental course and termination: The American Society of Criminology 1993 presidential address. *Criminology, 32*(1), 1–21.

Elliott, S., Huizinga, D., & Ménard, S. (1989). *Multiple problem youth.* New York: Springer-Verlag.

Ellis, L., & Coontz, P. D. (1990). Androgens, brain functionning, and criminality: The neurohormonal foundations of antisociality. In L. Ellis & H. Hoffman (Eds.), *Crime in biological, social and moral contexts* (pp. 162–193). New York: Praeger.

Eron, L. D. (1990). Understanding aggression. *Bulletin of the International Society for Research on Aggression, 12,* 5–9.

Eysenck, H. J., & Gudjonsson, G. H. (1989). *The causes and cures of criminality.* New York: Plenum Press.

Farrington, D. P. (1987). Epidemiology. In H. C. Quay (Ed.), *Handbook of juvenile delinquency* (pp. 33–61). New York: Wiley.

Fava, M., Nierenberg, A. A., Quitkin, F. M., Zisook, S., Pearlstein, T., Stone, A., & Rosenbaum, J. F. (1997). A preliminary study on the efficacy of setraline and imipramine on anger attacks in atypical depression and dysthymia. *Psychopharmacology Bulletin, 33,* 101–103.

Fergusson, D. M., Woodward, L. J., & Horwood, L. J. (1998). Maternal smoking during pregnancy and psychiatric adjustment in late adolescence. *Archives of General Psychiatry, 55*(8), 721–727.

Ferris, C. F. (1996). Understanding aggressive behavior in children. In C. F. Ferris & T. Grisso (Eds.), *Annals of the New York Academy of Sciences* (Vol. 794, pp. 98–103). New York: New York Academy of Sciences.

Finegan, J.-A., Niccols, G. A., & Sitarenios, G. (1992). Relations between prenatal testosterone levels and cognitive abilities at 4 years. *Developmental Psychology, 28*(6), 1075–1089.

Fried, P. A. (1995). Prenatal exposure to marihuana and tobacco during infancy, early and middle childhood: Effects and an attempt at synthesis. *Archives of Toxicology, 17,* 233–260.

Galilei, G. (1638/1991). *Dialogues concerning two new sciences.* Amherst, NY: Prometheus Books.

Gergen, M. (1990). Beyong the evil empire: Horseplay and aggression. *Aggressive Behavior, 16,* 381–398.

Goethe, J. W. (1774/1993). *The sorrows of young Werther.* New York: Modern Library.

Goodenough, F. L. (1931). *Anger in young children.* Westport, CT: Greenwood Press.

Goy, R. W., & McEwen, B. S. (1980). *Sexual differentiation of the brain.* Cambridge, MA: MIT Press.

Gray, J. A. (1971). *The psychology of fear and stress.* London: Weidenfeld & Nicolson.

Gray, J. A. (1982). *The neuropsychology of anxiety.* New York: Oxford University Press.

Grotpeter, J. K., & Crick, N. R. (1996). Relational aggression, overt aggression, and friendship. *Child Development, 67*(5), 2328–2338.

Hamburg, D. A., & van Lawick-Goodall, J. (1974). Factors facilitating development of aggressive behavior in chimpanzees and humans. In J. de Wit & W. W. Hartup (Eds.), *Origins of aggressive behavior* (pp. 59–86). The Hague, The Netherlands: Mouton.

Hampson, E., & Kimura, D. (1992). Sex differences and hormonal influences on cognitive function in humans. In J. B. Becker, S. M. Breedlove, & D. Crews (Eds.), *Behavioral endocrinology* (pp. 357–398). Cambridge, MA: MIT Press.

Harlow, H. F., & Harlow, M. H. (1965). The affectional systems. In A. N. Schrier, F. Stollnitz, & H. F. Harlow (Eds.), *Behaviour of non-human primates* (Vol. 2, pp. 287–334). London: Academic Press.

Harris, J. A., Vernon, P. A., & Boomsma, D. I. (1998). The irritability of testosterone: A study of Dutch adolescent twins and their parents. *Behavior Genetics, 28,* 165–171.

Hartup, W. W., & deWit, J. (1974). The development of aggression: Problems and perspectives. In J. deWit & W. W. Hartup (Eds.), *Determinants and origins of aggressive behavior* (pp. 595–620). The Hague, The Netherlands: Mouton.

Hay, D. F., Castle, J., & Davies, L. (2000). Toddlers' use of force against familiar peers: A precursor of serious aggression? *Child Development, 71*(2), 457–467.

Hen, R. (1996). Mean genes. *Neuron, 16,* 17–21.

Higley, J. D., Linnoila, M., & Suomi, S. J. (1994). Ethological contributions. In M. Hersen & R. T. Ammerman (Eds.), *Handbook of aggressive and destructive behavior in psychiatric patients* (pp. 17–32). New York: Plenum Press.

Higley, J. D., Mehlman, P. T., Taub, D. M., Higley, S. B., Suomi, S. J., & Linnoila, M. (1996). Stability of interindividual differences in serotonin function and its relationship to severe aggression and competent social behavior in rhesus Macaque females. *Neuropsychopharmacology, 7*, 67–76.

Hobbes, T. (1647/1998). *On the citizen.* New York: Cambridge University Press.

Huesmann, L. R., Eron, L. D., Lefkowitz, M. M., & Walder, L. O. (1984). Stability of aggression over time and generations. *Developmental Psychology, 20*(6), 1120–1134.

Huesmann, L. R., & Miller, L. S. (1994). Long-term effects of repeated exposure to media violence in childhood. In L. R. Huesmann (Ed.), *Aggressive behavior: Current perspectives* (pp. 153–186). New York: Plenum Press.

Hughes, C., Dunn, J., & White, A. (1998). Trick or treat?: Uneven understanding of mind and emotion and executive dysfunction in "hard-to-manage" preschoolers. *Journal of Child Psychology and Psychiatry, 39*, 981–994.

Hughes, C., White, A., Sharpen, J., & Dunn, J. (2000). Antisocial, angry, and unsympathetic: "Hard to manage" preschoolers' peer problems, and possible cognitive influences. *Journal of Child Psychology and Psychiatry, 41*, 169–179.

Jacklin, C. N., Wilcox, K. T., & Maccoby, E. E. (1988). Neonatal sex-steroid hormones and cognitive abilities at six years. *Developmental Psychobiology, 21*(6), 567–574.

Jessor, R., & Jessor, S. L. (1977). *Problem behaviour and psychosocial development.* New York: Academic Press.

Johnson, J. G., Cohen, P., Smailes, E. M., Kasen, S., & Brook, J. S. (2002). Television viewing and aggressive behavior during adolescence and adulthood. *Science, 295*, 2468–2471.

Kagan, J. (1974). Development and methodological considerations in the study of aggression. In J. de Wit & W. W. Hartup (Eds.), *Determinants and origins of aggressive behavior* (pp. 107–114). The Hague, The Netherlands: Mouton.

Kagan, J. (1998). *Three seductive ideas.* Cambridge, MA: Harvard University Press.

Keating, D. P., & Hertzman, C. (1999). Modernity's paradox. In D. P. Keating & C. Hertzman (Eds.), *Developmental health and the wealth of nations* (pp. 1–17). New York: Guilford Press.

Keenan, K., & Shaw, D. S. (1994). The development of aggression in toddlers: A study of low-income families. *Journal of Abnormal Child Psychology, 22*(1), 53–77.

Keenan, K., & Wakschlag, L. S. (2000). More than the terrible twos: The nature and severity of behavior problems in clinic-referred preschool children. *Journal of Abnormal Child Psychology, 28*(1), 33–46.

Kerr, M., Tremblay, R. E., Pagani-Kurtz, L., & Vitaro, F. (1997). Boys' behavioral inhibition and the risk of later delinquency. *Archives of General Psychiatry, 54*(9), 809–816.

Kimura, D., & Hampson, E. (1994). Cognitive pattern in men and women is influenced by fluctuations in sex hormones. *Current Directions in Psychological Sciences, 3*(2), 57–61.

Knutson, B., Wolkowitz, O. M., Cole, S. W., Chan, T., Moore, E. A., Johnson, R. C., Terpstra, J., Turner, R. A., & Reus, V. I. (1998). Selective alteration of personality and social behavior by serotonergic intervention. *American Journal of Psychiatry, 155*, 373–379.

Kochanska, G. (2001). Emotional development in children with different attachment histories: The first three years. *Child Development, 72*(2), 474–490.

Kochanska, G., Murray, K. T., & Harlan, E. T. (2000). Effortful control in early childhood: Continuity and change, antecedents, and implications for social development. *Developmental Psychology, 36*, 220–232.

Kraemer, H. C., Kazdin, A. E., Offord, D. R., Kessler, R. C., Jensen, P. S., & Kupser, D. J. (1997). Coming to terms with the terms of risk. *Archives of General Psychiatry, 54*, 337–343.

Lacourse, E., Côté, S., Nagin, D. S., Tremblay, R. E., Vitaro, F., & Brendgen, M. (2002). A longitudinal-experimental approach to testing theories of antisocial behavior development. *Development and Psychopathology, 14*, 909–924.

Lahey, B. B., Loeber, R., Quay, H. C., Applegate, B., Shaffer, D., Waldman, I., Hart, E. L.,

McBurnett, K., Frick, P. J., Jensen, P. S., Dulcan, M. K., Canino, G., & Bird, H. R. (1998). Validity of DSM-IV subtypes of conduct disorder based on age of onset. *Journal of the American Academy of Child and Adolescent Psychiatry, 37*(4), 435–442.

Lahey, B. B., McBurnett, K., & Loeber, R. (2000). Are attention-deficit hyperactivity disorder and oppositional defiant disorder developmental precursors to conduct disorder? In A. Sameroff, M. Lewis, & S. Miller (Eds.), *Handbook of developmental psychopathology* (pp. 431–446). New York: Plenum Press.

Lahey, B. B., Waldman, I. D., & McBurnett, K. (1999). Annotation: The development of antisocial behavior, an integrative causal model. *Journal of Child Psychology and Psychiatry, 40*(5), 669–682.

Laub, J. H., & Sampson, R. J. (2001). Understanding desistance from crime. *Crime and Justice, 28*, 1–69.

Lefkowitz, M. M., Eron, L. D., Walder, L. O., & Huesmann, L. R. (1977). *Growing up to be violent: A longitudinal study of the development of aggression.* New York: Pergamon Press.

LeMarquand, D., Benkelfat, C., Pihl, R. O., Palmour, R. M., & Young, S. N. (1999). Behavioral disinhibition induced by tryptophan depletion in nonalcoholic young men with multigenerational family histories of paternal alcoholism. *American Journal of Psychiatry, 15*, 1771–1779.

Lewis, M. (1993). The emergence of human emotions. In M. Lewis & J. M. Haviland (Eds.), *Handbook of emotions* (pp. 223–235). New York: Guilford Press.

Lewis, M., Alessandri, S. M., & Sullivan, M. W. (1990). Violation of expectancy, loss of control, and anger expressions in young infants. *Developmental Psychology, 26*, 745–751.

Lewis, M., Sullivan, M. W., Ramsay, D. S., & Alessandri, S. M. (1992). Individual differences in anger and sad expressions during extinction: Antecedents and consequences. *Infant Behavior and Development, 15*(4), 443–452.

Loeber, R. (1982). The stability of antisocial and delinquent child behaviour: A review. *Child Development, 53*, 1431–1446.

Loeber, R., & Farrington, D. P. (2001). The significance of child delinquency. In R. Loeber & D. Farrington (Eds.), *Child delinquents: Development, interventions and service needs* (pp. 1–22). Thousand Oaks, CA: Sage.

Loeber, R., Farrington, D. P., Stouthamer-Loeber, M., & Van Kammen, W. B. (1998). *Antisocial behavior and mental health problems: Explanatory factors in childhood and adolescence.* Mahwah, NJ: Erlbaum.

Loeber, R., & Stouthamer-Loeber, M. (1998). Development of juvenile aggression and violence: Some common misconceptions and controversies. *American Psychologist, 53*(2), 242–259.

Lorenz, K. (1966). *On aggression.* New York: Harcourt, Brace and World.

Lupien, S. J., deLeon, M., DeSanti, S., Convit, A., Tarshish, C., Nair, N. P. V., Thakur, M., McEwen, B. S., Hauger, R. L., & Meaney, M. J. (1998). Cortisol levels during human aging predict hippocampal atrophy and memory. *Nature Neuroscience, 1*(1), 69–73.

Lupien, S. J., Gillin, C. J., & Hauger, R. L. (1999). Working memory is more sensitive than declarative memory to the acute effects of corticosteroids: A dose–response study in humans. *Behavioral Neuroscience, 113*(3), 420–430.

Magnusson, D., & Bergman, L. R. (1990). A pattern approach to the study of pathways from childhood to adulthood. In L. N. Robins & M. Rutter (Eds.), *Straight and devious pathways from childhood to adulthood* (pp. 101–116). New York: Cambridge University Press.

Maxson, S. C. (1996). Searching for candidate genes with effects on an agonistic behavior, offense, in mice. *Behavior Genetics, 26*, 471–476.

Mazur, A., & Booth, A. (1998). Testosterone and dominance in men. *Behavioral and Brain Sciences, 21*(3), 353–397.

McBurnett, K., Lahey, B. B., Rathouz, P. J., & Loeber, R. (2000). Low salivary cortisol and persistent aggression in boys referred for disruptive behavior. *Archives of General Psychiatry,* *57*(1), 38–43.

McGrew, W. C. (1972). *An ethological study of children's behavior.* New York: Academic Press.

Meaney, M. J., Aitken, D. H., Van Berkel, C., Bhatnagar, S., & Sapolsky, R. M. (1988). Effect of neonatal handling on age-related impairments associated with the hippocampus. *Science, 239*(4841, Pt. 1), 766–768.

Meikle, A. K., Stringham, J. D., Bishop, D. T., & West, D. W. (1988). Quantitating genetic and nongenetic factors influencing androgen production and clearance rates in men. *Journal of Clinical Endocrinology and Metabolism, 67,* 104–109.

Miczek, K. A., Maxson, S. C., Fish, E. W., & Faccidomo, S. (2001). Aggressive behavioral phenotypes in mice. *Behavioural Brain Research, 125*(1–2), 167–181.

Moffitt, T. E. (1993). Adolescence-limited and life-course persistent antisocial behavior: A developmental taxonomy. *Psychological Review, 100*(4), 674–701.

Moffitt, T. E., Brammer, G. L., Caspi, A., Fawcett, J. P., Raleigh, M., Yuwiler, A., & Silva, P. (1998). Whole blood serotonin relates to violence in an epidemiological study. *Biological Psychiatry, 43*(6), 446–457.

Moffitt, T. E., Robins, R. W., & Caspi, A. (2001). A couples analysis of partner abuse with implications for abuse-prevention policy. *Criminology and Public Policy, 1,* 5–36.

Monaghan, E. P., & Glickman, S. E. (1992). Hormones and aggressive behavior. In J. B. Becker, S. M. Breedlove, & D. Crews (Eds.), *Behavioral endocrinology* (pp. 261–285). Cambridge, MA: MIT Press.

Moskowitz, D. S., Pinard, G., Zuroff, D. C., Annable, L., & Young, S. N. (2001). The effect of tryptophan on social interaction in everyday life. *Neuropsychopharmacology, 25,* 277–289.

Nagin, D., & Tremblay, R. E. (1999). Trajectories of boys' physical aggression, opposition, and hyperactivity on the path to physically violent and nonviolent juvenile delinquency. *Child Development, 70*(5), 1181–1196.

Nagin, D. S., & Tremblay, R. E. (2001a). Analyzing developmental trajectories of distinct but related behaviors: A group-based method. *Psychological Methods, 6*(1), 18–34.

Nagin, D. S., & Tremblay, R. E. (2001b). Parental and early childhood predictors of persistent physical aggression in boys from kindergarten to high school. *Archives of General Psychiatry, 58,* 389–394.

Nagin, D. S., & Tremblay, R. E. (2003). *Most fall but not all: Changes in physical aggression from childhood through adolescence.* Manuscript submitted for publication.

Nelson, C. A., Wewerka, S., Thomas, K. M., deRegnier, R.-A., Tribbey-Walbridge, S., & Georgieff, M. (2000). Neurocognitive sequelae of infants of diabetic mothers. *Behavioral Neuroscience, 114,* 950–956.

Nicolson, H. (1955). *Good behavior.* London: Constable.

Olds, D., Henderson, C. R., Cole, R., Eckenrode, J., Kitzman, H., Luckey, D., Pettitt, L., Sidora, K., Morris, P., & Powers, J. (1998). Long-term effects of nurse home visitation on children's criminal and antisocial behavior: Fifteen-year follow-up of a randomized controlled trial. *Journal of the American Medical Association, 280*(14), 1238–1244.

Olweus, D. (1979). Stability of aggressive reaction patterns in males: A review. *Psychological Bulletin, 85,* 852–875.

Panksepp, J. (1998). *Affective neuroscience: The foundations of human and animal emotions.* New York: Oxford University Press.

Panksepp, J. (1999). The perconscious substrates of conciousness: Affective states and the evolutionary origins of the self. In S. Gallagher & J. Shear (Eds.), *Models of the self* (pp. 113–130). Thorverton, UK: Imprint Academic.

Parke, R. D., & Slaby, R. G. (1983). The development of aggression. In P. H. Mussen (Ed.), *Handbook of child psychology: Vol. 4. Socialization, personality and social development* (pp. 547–641). New York: Wiley.

Patterson, G. R. (1982). *A social learning approach to family intervention: III. Coercive family process.* Eugene, OR: Castalia.

Plewis, I. (2002). Modelling impact heterogeneity. *Journal of the Royal Statistical Society, 165,* 31–38.

Poulin, F., & Boivin, M. (2000). The role of proactive aggression and reactive aggression in the formation and development of boys' friendships. *Developmental Psychology, 36*(2), 233–240.

Powers, E., & Witmer, H. (1951). *An experiment in the prevention of delinquency: The Cambridge–Somerville Youth Study.* Montclair, NJ: Columbia University Press.

Pulkkinen, L., & Tremblay, R. E. (1992). Patterns of boys' social adjustment in two cultures and at different ages: A longitudinal perspective. *International Journal of Behavioural Development, 15*(4), 527–553.

Quay, H. C. (1999). Classification of disruptive behavior disorders. In H. C. Quay & A. E. Hogan (Eds.), *Handbook of disruptive behavior disorders* (pp. 3–21). New York: Kluwer Academic/Plenum.

Quetelet, A. (1833). *Research on the propensity for crime at different ages* (2nd ed.). Brussels: M. Hayez.

Quetelet, A. (1869). *Physique sociale ou essai sur le développement des facultés de l'homme.* Bruxelles: C. Muquardt.

Raine, A. (2002). Annotation: The role of prefrontal deficits, low autonomic arousal, and early health factors in the development of antisocial and aggressive behavior in children. *Journal of Child Psychology and Psychiatry, 43,* 417–434.

Raleigh, M. J., & McGuire, M. T. (1991). Bidirectional relationships between tryptophan and social behavior in vervet monkeys. *Advances in Experimental Medicine and Biology, 294,* 289–298.

Raudenbush, S. W., & Liu, X. (2000). Statistical power and optimal design for multisite randomized trials. *Psychological Methods, 5,* 199–213.

Redl, F., & Wineman, D. (1951). *The aggressive child: Children who hate.* Glencoe, IL: Free Press.

Reiss, A. J., & Roth, J. A. (Eds.). (1993). *Understanding and preventing violence.* Washington, DC: National Academy Press.

Restoin, A., Montagner, H., Rodriguez, D., Girardot, J. J., Laurent, D., Kontar, F., Ullmann, V., Casagrande, C., & Talpain, B. (1985). Chronologie des comportements de communication et profils de comportement chez le jeune enfant. In R. E. Tremblay, M. A. Provost, & F. F. Strayer (Eds.), *Ethologie et développement de l'enfant* (pp. 93–130). Paris: Editions Stock/ Laurence Pernoud.

Robins, L. N. (1966). *Deviant children grown up.* Baltimore: Williams & Wilkins.

Roopnarine, J. L., Hooper, F. H., Ahmeduzzaman, M., & Pollack, B. (1993). Gentle play partners: Mother–child and father–child play in New Delhi, India. In K. MacDonald (Ed.), *Parent–child play: Descriptions and implications* (pp. 287–304). Albany: State University of New York Press.

Rubinow, D. R., & Schmidt, P. J. (1996). Androgens, brain, and behavior. *American Journal of Psychiatry, 153*(8), 974–984.

Sampson, R., J., Raudenbush, S. W., & Earls, F. (1997). Neighborhood and violent crime: A multilevel study of collective efficacy. *Science, 277,* 918–924.

Schaal, B., Tremblay, R. E., Soussignan, R., & Susman, E. J. (1996). Male testosterone linked to high social dominance but low physical aggression in early adolescence. *Journal of the American Academy of Child and Adolescent Psychiatry, 35*(10), 1322–1330.

Schwartz, D., Flamant, R., & Lellouch, J. (1981). *L'essai thérapeutique chez l'homme.* Paris: Flamarion Médecine-Sciences.

Schweinhart, L. J., & Weikart, D. P. (1993). Success by empowerment: The High/Scope Perry Preschool Study through age 27, Public Policy Report. *Young Children, 49*(1), 54–58.

Schweinhart, L. L., & Weikart, D. P. (1997). *Lasting differences: The High/Scope Preschool Cur-*

*riculum Comparison Study through age 23* (Monographs of the High/Scope Educational Research Foundation 12). Ypsilanti, MI: High/Scope Press.

Scriver, C. R., & Kaufman, S. (2001). Hyperphenylalaninemia: Phenylalanine hydroxylase deficiency. In C. R. Scriver, A. L. Beaudet, W. S. Sly, & D. Valle (Eds.), *The metabolic and molecular bases of inherited disease* (pp. 1667–1724). New York: McGraw-Hill.

Séguin, J. R., Pihl, R. O., Harden, P. W., Tremblay, R. E., & Boulerice, B. (1995). Cognitive and neuropsychological characteristics of physically aggressive boys. *Journal of Abnormal Psychology, 104*(4), 614–624.

Séguin, J., Tremblay, R. E., Boulerice, B., Pihl, R. O., & Harden, P. (1999). Executive functions and physical aggression after controlling for attention deficit hyperactivity disorder, general memory, and IQ. *Journal of Child Psychology and Psychiatry, 40*(8), 1197–1208.

Shaffer, D., Fisher, P., Dulcan, M. K., & Davies, M. (1996). The NIMH Diagnostic Interview Schedule for Children Version 2.3 (DISC–2.3): Description, acceptability, prevalence rates, and performance in the MECA Study. *Journal of the American Academy of Child and Adolescent Psychiatry, 35*, 865–877.

Shonkoff, J. P., & Phillips, D. A. (Eds.). (2000). *From Neurons to neighborhoods: The science of early child development*. Washington, DC: National Academy Press.

Singer, J. L., & Singer, D. G. (1981). *Television, imagination and aggression: A study of preschoolers play*. Hillsdale, NJ: Erlbaum.

Speltz, M. L., DeKlyen, M., Calderon, R., Greenberg, M. T., & Fisher, P. A. (1999). Neuropsychological characteristics and test behaviors of boys with early onset conduct problems. *Journal of Abnormal Psychology, 108*, 315–325.

Stein, N. L., & Jewett, J. L. (1986). A conceptual analysis of the meaning of negative emotions: Implications for a theory of development. In C. E. Izard & P. B. Read (Eds.), *Measuring emotions in infants and children: Vol. 2. Cambridge studies in social and emotional development* (pp. 238–267). New York: Cambridge University Press.

Stets, J. E., & Straus, M. A. (1989). The marriage license as a hitting license: A comparison of assaults in dating, cohabiting and married couples. *Journal of Family Violence, 4*(2), 161–180.

Straus, M. A. (1979). Measuring intrafamily conflict and violence: The conflict tactics (CT) scales. *Journal of Marriage and the Family, 41*, 75–88.

Suomi, S. J. (2002). Biobehavioral perspective on developmental psychopathology: Excessive aggression and serotonergic dysfunction in monkeys. In A. J. Sameroff & M. Lewis (Eds.), *Handbook of developmental psychopathology* (2nd ed., pp. 237–256). New York: Kluwer Academic/Plenum.

Tremblay, R. E. (2000a). The development of aggressive behaviour during childhood: What have we learned in the past century? *International Journal of Behavioral Development, 24*(2), 129–141.

Tremblay, R. E. (2000b, July 13). *The development of physical and indirect aggression in humans from birth to 8 years of age*. Paper presented at the 16th Biennial International Society for the Study of Behavioural Development Meetings, Beijing, China.

Tremblay, R. E., Boulerice, B., Harden, P. W., McDuff, P., Pérusse, D., Pihl, R. O., & Zoccolillo, M. (1996). Do children in Canada become more aggressive as they approach adolescence? In Human Resources Development Canada & Statistics Canada (Eds.), *Growing up in Canada: National Longitudinal Survey of Children and Youth* (pp. 127–137). Ottawa: Statistics Canada.

Tremblay, R. E., & Craig, W. (1995). Developmental crime prevention. In M. Tonry & D. P. Farrington (Eds.), *Building a safer society: Strategic approaches to crime prevention* (Vol. 19, pp. 151–236). Chicago: University of Chicago Press.

Tremblay, R. E., Japel, C., Pérusse, D., McDuff, P., Boivin, M., Zoccolillo, M., & Montplaisir, J. (1999). The search for the age of "onset" of physical aggression: Rousseau and Bandura revisited. *Criminal Behavior and Mental Health, 9*, 8–23.

Tremblay, R. E., Kurtz, L., Mâsse, L. C., Vitaro, F., & Pihl, R. O. (1995). A bimodal preventive intervention for disruptive kindergarten boys: Its impact through mid-adolescence. *Journal of Consulting and Clinical Psychology*, 63(4), 560–568.

Tremblay, R. E., & LeMarquand, D. (2001). Individual risk and protective factors. In R. Loeber & D. Farrington (Eds.), *Child delinquents: Development, interventions and service needs* (pp. 137–164). Thousand Oaks, CA: Sage.

Tremblay, R. E., Nagin, D. S., Séguin, J. R., Zoccolillo, M., Zelazo, P., Boivin, M., Pérusse, D., & Japel, C. (2002). *Predictors of high level physical aggression from 17 to 42 months after birth*. Manuscript submitted for publication.

Tremblay, R. E., Pihl, R. O., Vitaro, F., & Dobkin, P. L. (1994). Predicting early onset of male antisocial behavior from preschool behavior. *Archives of General Psychiatry*, 51, 732–738.

Tremblay, R. E., Vitaro, F., Bertrand, L., LeBlanc, M., Beauchesne, H., Boileau, H., & David, H. (1992). Parent and child training to prevent early onset of delinquency: The Montreal longitudinal-experimental study. In J. McCord & R. E. Tremblay (Eds.), *Preventing antisocial behavior: Interventions from birth through adolescence* (pp. 117–138). New York: Guilford Press.

Turiel, E. (1998). The development of morality. In W. Damon & N. Eisenberg (Eds.), *Handbook of child psychology: Social, emotional, and personality deveopment* (Vol. 3, pp. 863–932). Toronto: Wiley.

Vaillancourt, T., Brendgen, M., Boivin, M., & Tremblay R. E. (2002). *A longitudinal confirmatory factor analysis of indirect and physical aggression: Evidence of two factors over time?* Manuscript submitted for publication.

van Goozen, S. H. M., Matthys, W., Cohen-Kettenis, P. T., Thijssen, J. H. H., & van Engeland, H. (1998). Adrenal androgens and aggression in conduct disorder prepubertal boys and normal controls. *Biological Psychiatry*, 43(2), 156–158.

Vitaro, F., Brendgen, M., Pagani, L., Tremblay, R. E., & McDuff, P. (1999). Disruptive behavior, peer association, and conduct disorder: Testing the developmental links through early intervention. *Development and Psychopathology*, 11, 287–304.

Vitaro, F., Brendgen, M., & Tremblay, R. E. (2001). Preventive intervention: Assessing its effects on the trajectories of delinquency and testing for mediational processes. *Applied Developmental Science*, 5(4), 201–213.

Vitaro, F., Gendreau, P. L., Tremblay, R. E., & Oligny, P. (1998). Reactive and proactive aggression differentially predict later conduct problems. *Journal of Child Psychology and Psychiatry*, 39, 1–9.

Wakschlag, L. S., Lahey, B. B., Loeber, R., Green, S. M., Gordon, R. A., & Leventhal, B. L. (1997). Maternal smoking during pregnancy and the risk of conduct disorder in boys. *Archives of General Psychiatry*, 54(7), 670–676.

Wasserman, G. A., Graziano, J. H., Factor-Litvak, P., Popovac, D., Morina, N., Musabejovic, A., Vrenezi, N., Capuni-Paracka, S., Lekiv, V., Preteni-Redjepi, E., Hadzialjevic, S., Slavkovich, V., Kline, J., Shrout, P., & Stein, Z. (1994). Consequences of lead exposure and iron supplementation on childhood development at age 4. *Neurotoxicology and Teratology*, 16(3), 233–240.

Wasserman, G. A., Staghezza-Jaramillo, B., Shrout, P., Popovac, D., & Graziano, J. (1998). The effect of lead exposure on behavior problems in preschool children. *American Journal of Public Health*, 88, 481–486.

Webster-Stratton, C. (1998). Preventing conduct problems in Head Start children. *Journal of Consulting and Clinical Psychology*, 66(5), 715–730.

West, D. J., & Farrington, D. P. (1973). *Who becomes delinquent?* London: Heinemann.

White, H. R., Bates, M. E., & Buyske, S. (2001). Adolescence-limited versus persistent delinquency: Extending Moffitt's hypothesis into adulthood. *Journal of Abnormal Psychology*, 110(4), 600–609.

White, J. L., Moffitt, T. E., Earls, F., Robins, L., & Silva, P. A. (1990). How early can we tell?: Predictors of childhood conduct disorder and adolescent delinquency. *Criminology*, 28, 507–533.

Zelazo, P. D., Carter, A., Reznick, J. S., & Frye, D. (1997). Early development of executive function: A problem-solving framework. *Review of General Psychology, 1*, 198–226.

Zimring, F. E. (1998). *American youth violence.* New York: Oxford University Press.

Zoccolillo, M., Wakschlag, L., Baillargeon, R., Boivin, M., Pérusse, D., Vermunt, J. K., & Tremblay, R. E. (2002). *Maternal conduct problems, social disadvantage, and age at first birth in a general population.* Manuscript submitted for publication.

# *Cognitive Factors*

# 8

# An Early-Onset Model of the Role of Executive Functions and Intelligence in Conduct Disorder/Delinquency

JOEL T. NIGG
CYNTHIA L. HUANG-POLLOCK

A vast literature links cognitive deficits to antisocial behavior in children and adolescents (Loeber, Farrington, Stouthamer-Loeber, & van Kammen, 1998; Lynam & Henry, 2001; Miller, 1987).[1] If child neuropsychological vulnerabilities contribute causally to antisocial development, they probably do so in conjunction with the extensively described ecological risk factors that lead to persistent offending (Farrington & Loeber, 2000; Patterson & Capaldi, 1991). The goal of this chapter is to consider particular kinds of child cognitive vulnerabilities and how their role may develop into an antisocial pathway. Put another way, if not all children are equally vulnerable to the ecological risks, what role do child neuropsychological vulnerabilities play? The two most well-established domains are verbal and executive vulnerabilities, and they therefore comprise the focus of this chapter. Several recent scholarly reviews summarize the large literature on executive and verbal problems in antisocial development (Lynam & Henry, 2001; Moffitt, 1993; Morgan & Lilienfeld, 2000; Teichner & Golden, 2000). We therefore highlight that literature only in brief, focusing instead on developing testable causal hypotheses via an expanded integrative model of early causal contributions of these cognitive problems.

Multiple developmental pathways are evident in relation to delinquent and conduct-disordered behavior (Loeber, Farrington, Stouthamer-Loeber, Moffit, & Caspi, 1998). It is unlikely that neuropsychological weakness in verbal and executive domains are equally important in all of them. These major neuropsychological vulnerabilities appear to be most relevant for many early-onset, persistent, multiproblem delinquent youth (Donnelan, Ge, & Wenk, 2000; Elkins, Iacono, Doyle, & McGue, 1997; Kratzer & Hodgins, 1999; Loeber, Farrington, Stouthamer-Loeber, & van Kammen, 1998; Moffitt & Caspi, 2001). Other processes that have also been linked to neuropsychological perspectives, including reward response, response modulation, and others may be important for some pathways, such as psychopathy with intact executive functioning or delinquency with high IQ (Gath & Tennet, 1972). Those alternate explanations are nevertheless beyond the scope of this chapter (see Newman & Wallace, 1993; Nigg, 2000). Rather, of all the cognitive deficits that have been proposed (Nigg, 2000), verbal intelligence and executive functioning comprise our agenda here.

## WHAT ARE INTELLIGENCE AND EXECUTIVE FUNCTIONS?

### Intelligence

The performance domains under discussion here do not enjoy unitary definitions in the field. First, the operational measure of IQ refers to performance on psychometric tests purported to measure the construct of intelligence. Intelligence is subject to competing interpretations and multiple definitions (for reviews, see Kamphaus, 2001; Sattler, 2001; Sternberg & Detterman, 1986). However, most models emphasize the ability to adapt, learn, and engage in abstract thought (Sattler, 2001). Hierarchical theories posit the existence of a general "mental energy" referred to theoretically as "g," which in turn governs two or three higher order domains of ability. The latter in turn comprise several more specific skill areas (Kaufman, 1994; Sattler, 2001).

Scales that reflect this model of intelligence, in particular the Wechsler Intelligence Scale for Children (e.g., WISC-III and its precursors; Wechsler, 1991) are the most frequently used in studies of the role of intelligence in antisocial development (e.g., Cornell & Wilson, 1992; Hecht & Jurkovic, 1978; Lynam, Moffitt, & Stouthamer-Loeber, 1993; Saccuzzo & Lewandowski, 1976; White, Moffit, & Silva, 1989). Therefore, for simplicity, the current chapter will refer to "intelligence" to indicate what is measured by IQ tests such as the Wechsler scales, recognizing the theoretical debates about the nature of intelligence per se and its relation to measured IQ.

Factor analysis of the most recent Wechsler scales (WISC-III) have identified two higher order reasoning scales, Verbal Conceptualization (closely related to Verbal IQ) and (nonverbal) Perceptual Organization (closely related to Performance IQ), as well as two smaller regulation scales, Freedom from Distractibility and Processing Speed (Sattler, 2001). However, virtually the entire literature reviewed here relied on earlier versions of the Wechsler scales (e.g., WISC-R), which had two higher order factors (Verbal IQ and Performance IQ) and in some cases a third control/ speed factor that will be generally ignored in this review. Although in healthy adults Verbal and Performance IQ tend to be similar, in populations with brain injury (Lezak, 1995), as well as in children with psychopathology, divergence across skill areas may be important. In particular, conduct problems are usually related more to low verbal than to low nonverbal abilities.

## Executive Functions

Although executive function measures are well validated by linkage to frontal brain injury, executive functions still suffer from as much underspecification in their construct definition as do IQ and intelligence (Lyon & Krasnegor, 1996; Pennington, 1997). Nevertheless, tractable models of executive control are emerging (Posner & DiGirolamo, 1998), which point to an overarching emphasis on maintenance of an appropriate problemsolving mental set in pursuit of a future goal (Pennington & Ozonoff, 1996). Executive function does not comprise a known unitary process, but instead denotes multiple component operations. Component processes identified in clinical neuropsychological tasks include set shifting, interference control, inhibition, planning, and working memory (Pennington, 1997; Pennington & Ozonoff, 1996). Those traditional clinical executive function tasks (such as the Wisconsin Card Sort, Stroop, Trailmaking, Word Fluency, and the Rey–Osterrieth Complex Figure) were developed for their ability to identify brain injury in adults prior to the advent of neuroimaging technologies, and are now used clinically to assess functional deficits associated with suspected or definite injury (Lezak, 1995). They are often referred to as "molar" tasks because they are complex, such that performance may depend upon numerous executive as well as nonexecutive component operations (Pennington & Ozonoff, 1996).

In contrast, "molecular" tasks, which attempt to isolate particular component operations, are increasingly popular in neuroimaging and other studies of behavior and psychopathology (Nigg, 2000, 2001), but their clinical utility remains to be established. Executive control models based on the latter suggest a related set of components that variously includes conflict detection, sustaining working memory via control of mental interference, inhibition of competing responses, and allocation of effort (Botvinnick, Braver, Barch, Carter, & Cohen, 2001; Miller, 2000; Posner & DiGirolamo, 1998), although consensus on these components is not yet at hand.

Executive functions are often equated with the brain's frontal cortices, but in preparing to set up a causal model it is helpful to consider more precisely their neural instantiation. Brain lesion and neuroimaging data suggest that performance on various molar and componential executive tasks is supported differentially by a series of parallel neural loops that connect regions of the prefrontal cortex (dorsolateral, orbitoprefrontal, and anterior cingulate) with analogous regions in the basal ganglia (in particular, the caudate, putamen, globus pallidus, and substantia nigra) and the thalamus (Middleton & Strick, 2001). These details are notable because the subcortical connections in these networks are also involved, through their connections to the amygdala, hippocampus, and other subcortical structures, in neural circuits mediating motivational response (e.g., anxiety to possible punishment, or anger to frustration; Gray, 1991). It is thus important to note that the frontal cortices also represent emotion, and that executive processes also interact with and modulate incentive response (Davidson & Sutton, 1995; Nigg, 2000; Posner & Rothbart, 2000). In young children, component operations related to interference control or inhibition, planning, and attentional allocation, which are theorized to relate to the dorsolateral prefrontal loop and possibly to the anterior cingulate loop, appear most impaired in those with disruptive and antisocial behavior, as we detail below.

## Relation of Intelligence to Executive Functions

Both constructs refer to higher order cognitive operations and share certain important component operations (such as working memory), causing them to sometimes be placed under a unifying construct of meta-cognition (Borkowski & Burke, 1996). Also, many concepts of intelligence tend to include a component for executive operations (Sattler, 2001). Nevertheless, intelligence and executive functions are dissociable. Empirically, measures of intelligence are only weakly correlated with measures of executive function (Nigg, 2000; Nigg, Blaskey, Huang-Pollock, & Rappley, 2002; Nigg, Quamma, Greenberg, & Kusche, 1999; Pennington & Ozonoff, 1996). This is not surprising when one considers the content of the tests. For example, none of the WISC-III (Wechsler, 1991) or WISC-R subtests require suppression of a competing prepotent response, and the WISC-III subtest that most resembles planning (Mazes) is the weakest item in the WISC factor structure (Kaufman, 1994). Verbal IQ measures, in particular, rely on prior learning, whereas executive measures rely on the novelty of the problem and control of competing information. Further, whereas performance on measures of executive function is classically impaired by injury to prefrontal cortex or basal ganglia, IQ, especially Verbal IQ, is relatively insensitive to frontal brain insult (Pennington & Ozonoff, 1996, but see Thompson et al., 2001, for data that link frontal gray matter volume to IQ). We therefore might expect that low intelligence and weak executive functioning, while very often co-occurring in the most-at-risk youngsters, might also index partially dissociable processes related to antisocial development. We explore why both processes may break down in the same at-risk children in our theoretical conjectures later.

## OVERVIEW OF THE LITERATURE

We conducted computer searches in the PsychINFO and Medline databases restricted to literature published in English since 1970. The terms "conduct disorder," "delinquency," "antisocial behavior + children," and "antisocial behavior + adolescents" were combined and crossed with (1) "IQ or intelligence" (generating 817 citations), (2) "neuropsychology" (234 citations), and (3) "executive functions" (18 citations). Thus, the literature on intelligence and conduct problems/delinquency is larger and more established than the comparatively small and recent literature examining these problems in relation to executive functions. We note highlights of the literature and refer readers to extended descriptive reviews for more detail in this section.

### The Relation of Intelligence to Delinquency/Conduct Disorder

*Basic Findings*

Delinquent populations typically have Full Scale or Verbal IQs 8–10 points lower than average. Though early findings generated controversy due to serious flaws in their methods and claims (Hirschi & Hindelang, 1977; Wilson & Herrnstein, 1985), the correlation with delinquency is no longer disputed. Notably for causal theorizing, early specific weakness in verbal-learning and verbal-reasoning ability modestly but reliably predicts later persistent offending, conduct disorder, and antisocial outcomes, whereas nonverbal intelligence does not do so[2] (Elkins et al., 1997; Frost, Moffitt, & McGee, 1989; Henry, Moffitt, & Silva, 1992; White et al., 1989; for a review, see Henry & Moffitt, 1997).

Perhaps the best demonstrations come from longitudinal studies in Dunedin (New Zealand) and Pittsburgh. Moffitt (1990), using the Dunedin sample, controlled age 5 antisocial behavior in a regression model to predict age 11 antisocial behavior; Verbal IQ contributed an additional 6% of variance explained ($p = .001$), consistent with (though not demonstrative of) a causal, and not merely a correlational, role for verbal intelligence. Similar data are available for conduct disorder (Lahey et al., 1995), although the effect may be mediated by co-occurring attention-deficit/hyperactivity disorder (ADHD; see review by Hogan, 1999). The latter point is consistent with longitudinal evidence that children at highest risk for delinquency are those with both conduct disorder and comorbid ADHD

(Farrington, Loeber, & van Kammen, 1990; Hinshaw, Lahey, & Hart, 1993; Moffitt, 1990).

Thus, weakness in verbal intelligence is associated with the subgroup of delinquent youth with early onset and chronic patterns of antisocial behavior (Elkins et al., 1997; Moffitt, 1990), even though not all of those youth have antisocial outcomes (suggesting further heterogeneity). For those youth with verbal weakness and antisocial outcome, a key question has been whether verbal problems reflect an early initiating causal process or instead either a later maintaining cause or even merely an effect of the accumulation of other risk processes. Thus, how early are these effects apparent? One careful but relatively small prospective study of very-high-risk children failed to find early (preschool) differences between four groups of children classified by antisocial pathway on verbal or temperament measures, instead finding that IQ effects appeared later in childhood (Aguilar, Sroufe, Egeland, & Carlson, 2000). However, the prospective association of very early lower verbal intelligence with future conduct problems was supported in other longitudinal studies (Lipsitt, Buka, & Lipsitt, 1990; Moffitt & Caspi, 2001). Later delinquency in both boys and girls was predicted by mental abilities measured at age 4 years but not at age 8 months in one prospective study (Lipsitt et al., 1990). However, toddler language development at age 1 year predicted later delinquency for boys in another prospective effort with socioeconomic status (SES) and test motivation controlled (Stattin & Klackenberg-Larsson, 1993). Thus, early weakness in verbal development participates in the risk pathway (Loeber, Farrington, Stouthamer-Loeber, & van Kammen, 1998), but whether this may be an early *causal* effect remains to be clearly demonstrated.

## Confounds: Socioeconomic Status, Gender, Race, Test Motivation

The correlation of offending with lower intelligence cannot be explained by better detection of less bright criminals; self-report offending data still show the association with low verbal IQ (Moffitt & Silva, 1988; for a review, see Farrington, 1994). Nor is the effect simply an artifact of low SES (which correlates both with low IQ and antisocial behavior; Lynam et al., 1993; Moffitt, Gabrielli, & Mednick, 1981; for a review, see Loeber, Farrington, Stouthamer-Loeber, Moffitt, & Caspi, 1998). Efforts to measure and covary test motivation also have not accounted for the low IQ effect (Lynam et al., 1993; Stattin & Klackenberg-Larsson, 1993).

Intelligence has been a controversial construct in part because of its historical correlation with race (not fully explainable by SES). That association has led to heated disputes about the extent to which IQ scores may reflect (1) true differences in ability between racial–ethnic groups, (2) acculturation to mainstream society, or, more difficult to ascertain, (3) different constructs in different racial–ethnic groups (Prinz & Miller, 1991). Thus, the validity of the IQ–delinquency association across racial–ethnic groups is of concern. Scores on intelligence tests are correlated with measures of school achievement across racial–ethnic groups (Sattler, 2001), suggesting that these scores are valid at least for that crucial purpose. Yet the independence from race or ethnicity of IQ effects on delinquency does not enjoy consensus due to a dearth of appropriate, large, longitudinal samples. Donnellan et al. (2000) followed delinquent offenders in California from age 19 into their 30s, and found that persistence of offending was associated with lower intellectual ability in Caucasian but not in African American groups. It may be that effects do not generalize as well in that age range. The best evidence that the intelligence–delinquency effect is independent of race or ethnicity comes from children. The Pittsburgh Youth Study followed a large at-risk sample of boys from early childhood. The sample is approximately half African American and half Caucasian. In that project, early-onset and persistent delinquent youth have lower IQ than their nondelinquent peers in both ethnic groups (Loeber, Farrington, Stouthamer-Loeber, & van Kammen, 1998; Lynam et al., 1993).

A limitation on data for causal models is that the literature has heavily emphasized boys and male development. The Pittsburgh Youth Study sample, for instance, is all boys. The Dunedin sample includes both boys and girls, but many of the most important reports from that data set focused exclusively on the boys because so few girls show the early-starter, severe, persistent pathway (e.g,. Moffitt, 1990; Moffitt, Lynam, & Silva, 1994). As a result, concerns remain that the early-starter pathway may start later for many girls, which if true would alter developmental models (Silverthorn & Frick, 1999). With regard to effects of intelligence, a small number of prospective studies suggest that although the effect of Verbal IQ per se was weaker as a correlate of early-onset offending in girls than in boys, it did predict later antisocial behavior versus nonoffenders for both boys and girls (Kratzer & Hodgins, 1999; Lipsitt et al., 1990). Moffitt and Caspi (2001), revisiting this issue in the Dunedin sample, found that cognitive measures (in particular, verbal abilities) were related to girls' early problem onset also.

## Summary

Although data are mixed, the best specification of the effect of intelligence on offending may be that it applies to early-onset problems in boys, with some evidence of this effect for girls, and that the effect is most pronounced for verbal skills. For the early-onset youngsters, the effects of verbal ability *may* be causal (i.e., early verbal deficits precede serious behavior problems in most studies, and are not explained by such confounds as SES), though the evidence for that possibility is strongest for Caucasian boys in the United States, Europe, and New Zealand. Applicability to various racial–

ethnic groups requires continued scrutiny across development. Finally, the link with poor verbal or language skills is strongest for a subgroup of delinquents with a history of attentional as well as conduct problems (for reviews, see Henry & Moffitt, 1997; Hinshaw, 1992; Hogan, 1999; Quay, 1987).

## The Relation of Executive Functions to Delinquency/Conduct Disorder

Independently of intelligence, reading ability, sex effects, or earlier behavior problems, early executive neuropsychological weakness is associated with later teacher-rated externalizing behavior problems in childhood (Nigg et al., 1999) and self-reported delinquent acts in adolescence (Moffitt & Henry, 1989). Conversely, whether verbal deficits are related to conduct problems apart from executive problems is less clear (Giancola & Mezzich, 2000; Nigg et al., 1999). Thus, executive functions are important to causal models of cognitive effects. Despite the relatively smaller size of the executive function literature, several studies have replicated an association of weak executive function with conduct disorder and juvenile delinquency (see reviews by Moffitt, 1993; Morgan & Lilienfeld, 2000; Teichner & Golden, 2000). Like the IQ data, effects are not explained by a greater risk of detection for those with executive deficits (Moffit & Henry, 1989). But like studies of intelligence, evidence for executive deficits is clearest in children with comorbid attentional problems or ADHD (Aronowitz et al., 1994; Clark, Prior, & Kinsella, 2000; Moffitt & Henry, 1989; Moffit & Silva, 1988; see review by Pennington & Ozonoff, 1996).

Component operations warrant mention. Studies of preschoolers suggest that the executive domains most related to problem behaviors are inhibitory control and planning (Hughes, Dunn, & White, 1998; Hughes, White, Sharpen, & Dunn, 2000), which relate to the dorsolateral and possibly anterior cingulate prefrontal loops. Diagnostically, these key executive deficits, particularly behavioral inhibition, are specific to ADHD independently of conduct problems (Nigg, 1999, 2001; Nigg, Hinshaw, Carte, & Treuting, 1998). Whether the reverse is also true has been less clear because most studies of conduct disorder ignored ADHD status. The major executive measures specific to conduct disorder thus have been thought to be those related to verbal skills (Pennington & Ozonoff, 1996). However, global executive problems were associated with conduct disorder when ADHD was controlled in two recent studies (Giancola, Mezzich, & Tarter, 1998; Seguin, Boulerice, Harden, Tremblay, & Pihl, 1999); the former also showed effects in girls. However, other well-done studies still found that only verbal deficits were independently associated with conduct disorder (Dery, Toupin, Pauze, Mercier, & Fortin,1999; Toupin, Dery, Pauze, Mercier, & Fortin, 2000). Importantly, most data have relied on school-age children. How early can associations of executive skills and disruptive behaviors be observed? Most studies have examined schoolage children. However, Speltz, DeKlyen, Calderon, Greenberg, and Fisher (1999) found that preschoolers with oppositional behavior problems (a frequent precursor to antisocial behavior) had problems on an executive planning task, even with ADHD symptoms controlled, though children with both oppositional and ADHD symptoms had the greatest executive impairment. Hughes et al. (1998) found similar results for their difficult-to-manage preschoolers.

## Confounds: Gender, Ethnicity, Socioeconomic Status

The data on executive deficits also rely heavily on samples of boys (Nigg, 2001). The applicability of conclusions to girls is far from definitive. Girls are clearly less likely to enter the early starter pathway, but when they do, predictors may be similar to boys. Still, it remains possible that girls experience greater protective mechanisms against delinquency, and thus require more severe cognitive problems than do boys before behavioral problems emerge, or that their problems are slower to emerge despite similar cognitive deficits (Silverthorn & Frick, 1999). However, early executive problems predicted later externalizing independently of sex effects in one longitudinal study (Nigg et al., 1999), and neuropsychological effects for early-onset problems in girls have been supported when specifically examined in key studies (Giancola et al., 1998; Moffitt & Caspi, 2001). Very little research on racial–ethnic differences exists for executive functions, but effects are clearly independent of SES in virtually all studies reported (Nigg, 2001), even though children in severely adverse environments are crucially underrepresented in the major executive function studies.

## Summary

The association of poor executive function with conduct problems is to an important extent, but not entirely, attributable to (1) the very high overlap of ADHD (strongly related to executive function problems) with conduct disorder (Hinshaw et al., 1993), and (2) the verbal component of executive measures. In particular, the ADHD–executive relation may be clearer at earlier ages, whereas *unique* relations of executive control with conduct problems may be more apparent at later ages. Yet executive deficits were uniquely if modestly related to antisocial outcomes even with ADHD controlled in at least some studies. Although effects are clearest for boys, emerging data support their linkage for girls. Componentially, problems related to the dorsolateral prefrontal circuit pertaining to response suppression and planning are most salient in early childhood, but early temperament data also implicate the anterior cingulate loop. Overall, the children at highest risk for early-onset persistent offending are those with both early attentional and externalizing behavior problems (diagnostically, those with conduct disorder plus ADHD), who experience a cluster of cognitive vulnerabilities related to both executive and verbal cognitive skills. These weaknesses are apparent by preschool.

## CAUSAL MODELS AND PROCESSES

### Simple Downstream, School Mediation, Socialization, and Artifact Effects

We do not catalogue here all of the many causal hypotheses that have been proposed for these neuropsychological effects, but we note that many were not developmental or integrative (see Lynam & Henry, 2001, for a summary of different hypotheses). The simplest causal theories about the role of cognitive vulnerability in delinquency is that there is no initiating causal relation (any causal effects merely serve to maintain problems later or are merely downstream effects that play little or no causal role at any stage), or that this effect is so small compared to social–ecological processes as to be unimportant (Aguilar et al., 2000; Menard & Morse, 1984). Alternatively, effects are seen as mediated by later school-related problems, but not as early occurring. Thus, relevant processes have been variously theorized to include damaging institutional response, such as tracking low-achieving children (Menard & Morse, 1984), perhaps augmented by failure in child self-esteem or child disengagement from school due to academic frustration (followed by drift to an antisocial peer group; see Hirschi & Hindeling, 1977).

Yet it has also been suggested that early, *nonschool* socialization failures are the critical mediating process by which cognitive vulnerability may exert causal effects, if indeed it does so (Lahey, Waldman, & McBurnett, 1999; Quay, 1987). We are in sympathy with the latter models. Although school failure is surely a powerful negative mechanism for at-risk youth, it is doubtful that the only pathway for cognitive vulnerability to exert its effects is via school problems. Rather, cognitive effects, because they emerge early in development when problem behavior begins, should in theory begin prior to school age if they are causal in an important way.[3] We argue that the most interesting and likely causal role for cognitive vulnerability is through interference with extensively described socialization processes earlier in development. We therefore chose not to devote further theorizing in this chapter to middle-childhood or school socialization processes. Instead, we focus on early family socialization (Greenberg, Speltz, DeKlyen, & Jones, 2001; Stormshank, Speltz, DeKlyen, & Greenberg, 1997), which is both dependent in part on and helps support development of child cognitive and temperament characteristics. Then we turn our thoughts on causal hypotheses to two questions: (1) how do the multiple cognitive vulnerabilities themselves develop and why do they so regularly co-occur, and (2) by what specific mechanisms might early socialization break down? In keeping with the aims of this chapter, we emphasize child characteristics, which we predict are most relevant in environments that demand resilient adaptability of the child least able to muster it.

## Overarching Causal Processes: Child-by-Environment Joint Effects

Landmark family and adoption studies show that three devastating family processes involve the vulnerable child in causal antecedents of persistent antisocial development. First, a vicious family interaction process contributes to development of antisocial behavior. In this process, parents engage in greater levels of hostile, coercive behavior with children (Patterson & Capaldi, 1991). Second, this process is in part driven by the child's difficult temperament, causing a powerful genotype-to-environment correlation effect in unskilled and often unprepared parents (Ge et al., 1996). Third, the children with the vulnerable temperament are the most reactive to this negative family interaction pattern to which they themselves contribute, indicative of a harmful genotype-by-environment or child-by-environment interaction (Cadoret, Yates, Troughton, Woodworth, & Stewart, 1995). Of course, these negative effects are then later augmented through peer interactions and perhaps even through social institutional responses. But how do these early processes, especially the child's contribution to them, begin?

It has been important to note both the connection and the distinction between difficult child temperament and early neuropsychological vulnerability. Are these two levels of analysis of the same basic problems or two contributing processes (Hughes et al., 1998; Lahey et al., 1999; Moffitt, 1993)? We will suggest an integration of these processes in the early development of self-regulation shortly. The immediate point is that cognitive problems in the child may contribute to difficult interactions with caregivers, interfere with socialization, and leave the child unprepared to adapt to the greater adversity he or she faces in a high-risk environment.

Several lines of investigation suggest that child characteristics can disrupt their socialization. For example, children with executive or verbal deficits may have difficulty in foreseeing consequences of behavior and in the development of empathy (Farrington, 1994), leading to antisocial outcomes (Lahey et al., 1999). Early deficits in either reactivity (excess negative emotional response to stress or frustration) or effortful control (a temperament construct that serves as a precursor of executive control: see Nigg, 2000; Rothbart & Bates, 1998) interfere with the development of conscience or recognition of social rules in early childhood (Kochanska, 1997; Kochanska, Coy, Tjebkes, & Husarek, 1998; Kochanska, Murray, & Coy, 1997). Studies of preschoolers suggest that both executive and reactive processes contribute to breakdowns in peer socialization, further supporting this early socialization pathway as the mediator of neuropsychological vulnerability (Hughes et al., 2000).

## Toward a Testable Causal Model of Early Causal Effects of Child Cognitive Vulnerability on Later Antisocial Development

### Overview

If cognitive vulnerability plays a role in early initiation of antisocial development (not merely in maintaining problems later), how might these effects begin, what hypotheses should be tested, and how can they be tested? For both intelligence and executive functions, the early causal models that have been proposed have been united in suggesting that these cognitive vulnerabilities either weaken children's adaptive capability to adverse environments (Moffitt, 1993) or participate in the activation of negative socialization processes (Lahey et al., 1999). We agree (with minor modifications), but argue that how this might happen needs better specification so it can be more formally tested.

We attempt to articulate the outlines of a general model that emphasizes the cognitive vulnerabilities related to conduct problems in the development of self-regulation, drawing upon and extending existing interactive neural–socialization models of the early development of self-regulation (see Eisenberg et al., 1996; Posner & Rothbart, 2000; Rothbart & Bates, 1998). Because of the close neural relations between executive and motivational systems, the latter must be included for the model to be cogent, but will not be fully discussed here. We thus outline first the interdependence of the three neural systems that are related to conduct problems but that are often treated as distinct in the literature: motivational or affective response (temperamental reactivity; see Nigg, 2000; Posner & Rothbart, 2000; Rothbart & Bates, 1998), executive functioning and its precursors (specifically inhibitory and attentional control), and verbal development.

We do this in two steps: we first connect motivational and executive processes, and then link both of these to verbal development. Doing so helps clarify why these three domains are so often *all* impaired in the most at-risk groups of youngsters. Although there will inherently be some lack of precision in such an initial account, we argue that we will be further ahead by incorporating these interconnections than by treating these systems as separate domains of inquiry. We will then proceed to outline how, despite their close interconnections in development, these three processes can be distinguished to address sequence-of-development hypotheses that will enable focused tests of causal possibilities, experimental prevention trials, and computational modeling tests of specific causal hypotheses.

A developmental causal model requires recognition that the neural systems that support executive control, motivational response, and verbal learning depend for intact development on both the surrounding neural context and the social (caregiving) context. Neural development is plastic to experience, and the latter clearly supports both cognitive and language development (Posner & Rothbart, 2000), but the socialization process also depends on them. Further, during early development, these cognitive functions are supported by related but distinct neural systems that in turn support one another in yoked fashion *in a specific developmental sequence*. A corollary is that the child's ability to cope with a high-risk environment probably depends in part on the timing and duration of the environmental risks. We therefore turn to early developmental processes to seek the initial causal antecedents of early-onset antisocial behavior.

## First Basic Two-Process Component of Self-Regulation in Development

The first two processes supporting the development of self-regulation can be operationalized by their influence on the allocation of attention in infancy. First, early in development, child behavior (direction of attention) begins to be regulated by emotional *reactivity*, or the strength of negative and positive emotions in relation to immediate stimuli (Rothbart & Bates, 1998). These effects are thought to be related to ongoing development of the limbic system and to reflect that system's increased influence on behavior at about 6–8 months of age. Second, by 10–12 months of age, infants can be observed employing effortful redirection of attention to assist with the regulation of affect states (Rothbart & Bates, 1998). This effortful redirection of attention (termed "regulation" by temperament theorists) continues to develop rapidly in the second through fourth years of life. By about 30 months of age, children begin to be able to inhibit stimulus-driven motor response (Posner & Rothbart, 2000). This early regulatory process is therefore seen as a precursor to later executive control, which relies on the ability to forestall response and inhibit reflex in keeping with a goal represented in working memory (see Nigg, 2000, 2001). Effortful control, which depends in part on socialization for continued maturation, continues to develop with frontal lobe development throughout childhood and adolescence. But the "preexecutive" process is probably also related, even late in the first year of life, to ongoing development of prefrontal cortical structures.

Crucially, it is theorized that (1) frontal effortful control processes and (2) limbic-based emotional–reactivity or incentive–response processes, regulate or scaffold one another during early childhood development. Each depends on the support of the other for optimal development and for optimal self-regulation (Derryberry & Reed, 1996; Derryberry & Rothbart, 1997; Derryberry & Tucker, 1994; Nigg, 2000, 2001; Rothbart & Bates, 1998). We have illustrated this in the portion of Figure 8.1 that depicts "executive" and "motivational" interconnections. In turn, we suggest that, as the child matures in the social context, the strength of this two-component self-regulation system influences the child's capacities (1) to be normally socialized by *average expectable* parenting and peer environments and (2) to achieve adequate socialization adaptively in *adverse* caregiving environments.

Thus, the model provides the following key principles to guide our causal hypotheses: (1) Executive control and motivational strength (temperamental reactivity) are distinct but closely related to one another and both therefore partake in the socialization processes that shape risk for conduct problems. Furthermore, it suggests that (2) a developmental problem in one system could lead secondarily to problems in the other system, or that (3) interventions to strengthen one system may benefit the other system. Finally, (4) breakdown in the development of self-regulation processes *within the child* during preschool development in turn interferes with socialization, both via (4a) failure to internalize norms when the rearing envi-

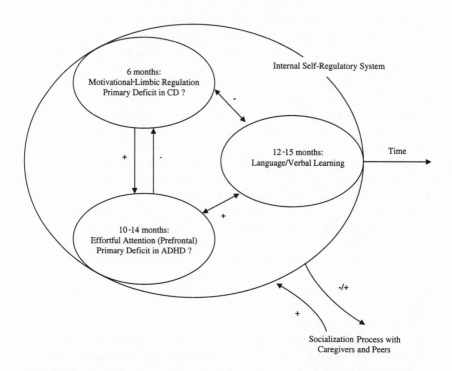

FIGURE 8.1. Schematic illustration of the processes that mutually depend on timing in development to support self-regulation, executive control, verbal learning, and socialization. Age ranges shown are intended to schematically illustrate possible earliest points at which those emerging systems can be observed to control behavior.

ronment is not well attuned to the child's vulnerable cognitive or motivational development (Kochanska, 1997) and (4b) the child's contribution to negative socialization experiences (Hughes et al., 2000). Before we elaborate on these points, how do verbal skills fit in?

### Second Synergistic Early Process

Less well worked out theoretically is how verbal learning problems, and thus language development and verbal intelligence, relate to the preceding. Instead, the verbal deficits related to externalizing behavior problems have often, in theoretical accounts of executive and motivational control, been ignored or treated as likely downstream developmental deficits. However, verbal learning problems are likely integrated in early development with the self-regulation matrix described above (as we illustrate in the remainder of Figure 8.1). In middle childhood the importance of such verbal processes as internalized speech to the development of self-regulation (i.e., executive control) has been well described (Barkley, 1997; Berk, 1996). However, how these systems may relate in very early (toddler and preschool) development has not been as well detailed.

In considering such connections, the timing of verbal development is striking. Language begins to develop from babbling to interpersonal word usage at about 10–14 months (Woodward & Markman, 1998), or around the same time that prefrontal–executive control precursors are beginning to help regulate affective response (see above). The development of verbal learning (and language learning) is related to cognitive maturation (e.g., Gopnick, 1982, 1988), and so may be related to verbal intelligence as well. Language development, of course, proceeds rapidly in the second through fourth years of life, in parallel with development of executive control.

In fact, one important support for verbal learning appears to be attention. Simply put, children learn language for that which they are attending (Hollich, Hirsh-Pasek, & Golinkoff, 2000). Yet, as we noted, the control of attention depends on differing neural structures that mature and influence behavior at different times both during infancy (Rothbart & Bates, 1998) and in childhood (Huang-Pollock, Carr, & Nigg, 2002). Word learning accelerates dramatically between 12 and 24 months of age, during the same time that effortful allocation of attention becomes a resource for the child. What follows is that the infant's ability to learn a verbal association relies on attention and intentionality (Bloom & Tinker, 2001). Whereas initial verbal learning at around 1 year of age may relate to stimulus salience (motivational response), rapid advanced learning during the second and third years of life is necessarily dependent on the ability to control attention and to inhibit immediate stimulus salience (effortful control, the precursor to executive functions).[4]

Emerging data provide empirical support for this claim. Although 13-

month-old infants cannot learn the name of a nonsalient stimulus, 19-month-old children begin to be able to orient away from the salient stimulus to locate a nonsalient named object, and 24-month-olds have mastered the ability to learn the names of nonsalient objects by deliberately directing their attention away from salient objects (Rebecca Brand, personal communication, January 25, 2002; Brand & Baldwin, 2003). The timing of these skills suggests that just as executive systems may be crucial to the development of optimal emotional and motivational self-regulation, they also support the development of verbal learning (and by extension, contribute to the precursors of verbal reasoning, and thus to verbal intelligence in early development). This latter process is also mutually reinforcing, because executive control also comes to depend on language and internalized speech (Barkley, 1997).

### Summary of Child-Locus Processes: A Three-Process Model of Timing-Dependent and Context-Dependent Development of Early Self-Regulation

Figure 8.1 represents in schematic form our integrative model of how executive control participates both in the development of (1) early verbal learning and thus language development and, indirectly, verbal intelligence; and (2) motivational regulation and reactivity. The value of such an integration is illustrated by several considerations. One can imagine, for example, that injury to the neural systems that support verbal learning would have a *later* effect on the development of executive control, while injury to systems that support emotional regulation and motivation would have an *earlier* effect on executive control. Correspondingly, injury to systems that support executive control could lead to secondary breakdowns in the development of both affective regulation and verbal learning at somewhat later points in early development; yet such secondary effects might be forestalled if those secondary systems received additional support during socialization.

One advantage of this model is that it accounts for the triad of neuropsychological vulnerabilities observed in early-onset antisocial youth: verbal learning deficits (slow early language development, later low verbal IQ), motivational deficits (e.g., excess negative affect to frustration, excess responding under conditions of cues for both punishment and reward; see Nigg, 2001), and executive control deficits. Any one of the three could be primary for a given child, but primary deficits in any one could impair the others if the injury or vulnerability occurred very early in development and compensatory processes in socialization were lacking. A second advantage of the model is that it suggests strategies for using heterogeneity among at-risk children to identify causal pathways. For example, children who have low-risk temperaments but struggle with executive deficits, or who have strong verbal skills but weak executive functions, may be important in the identification of protective mechanisms. At the same time, interventions to protect one of these three processes may enable the other two processes to catch up as well. A third point about this model is that it implies a cascade of increasing cognitive deficits through early childhood in at-risk settings; cognitive weaknesses in early-onset antisocial youth should be magnified with age relative to more normative development.

## Alternative Early Causal Pathways and Their Interaction with Socialization

Based on the model in Figure 8.1, perhaps the most likely pathway for early-onset antisocial development emanating from this model is the one that would begin earliest. That pathway would begin with vulnerability in the reactivity system (e.g., extremely strong innate reactivity), making it difficult, when appropriate caregiving compensation is lacking, for the executive control processes to develop optimally. This in turn leads to a negative feedback pattern that may be characterized by primary conduct problems and secondary ADHD in the later preschool years. This pathway is supported by evidence that in children with conduct disorder, motivational response appears to be markedly impaired, whereas executive functions appear to be only modestly affected (Nigg, 2000, 2001). Conversely, even if motivational regulation is intact, primary failure in executive systems could lead to the development of psychopathology (e.g., ADHD), with secondary weaknesses in reward response and motivational regulation of behavior. The latter is consistent with the neuropsychological literature that links ADHD primarily with substantial problems in executive control or inhibition of behavior, with smaller and thus maybe secondary effects on motivational response in ADHD (Nigg, 2001).

Consider the obstacles to socialization when this interdependent process of self-regulation begins to fall behind by either of those pathways. First, the child will be difficult to soothe due to high reactivity, taxing caregiver patience. The caregiver then may fail to provide the compensatory structuring needed to support the child's effortful control ability as it begins to influence behavior, and these forces in combination leave effortful control somewhat weaker than otherwise. Finally, as language development begins to accelerate, the expected attentional support systems are weak, and verbal learning suffers. Now, three core routes to socialization in the child are weakened: anxiety or anger response, self-soothing by effortful allocation of attention, and verbal interaction with caregivers. At that point, it is not difficult to imagine a negative socialization loop or cascade underway, which the child lacks adaptive skills to alter. The parents may also be in a weak position to alter the dynamic if they are in a high-risk environment or also lack verbal, executive, or temperamental advantages for accommodating their increasingly difficult child. By the time the child enters the peer and school socialization sequences, the likelihood of negative processes is potentially very high.

Hypotheses to Be Tested

Although the general model may appear complex, it enables us to generate a number of new testable hypotheses. Testing these hypotheses would generally either require computational models or prospective prevention experiments that feature focused early interventions on one component of the self-regulation system and/or caregiver environment. However, observational longitudinal studies could disconfirm some of these suppositions as well. Measurement of the neuropsychological systems would have to be by proxy measures of temperament (for which methodologies are well established) in the first 18 months of life. By age 3 years, adequate laboratory measures of executive control are available (Diamond, Prevor, Callender, & Druin, 1997; Hughes et al., 1998) and would ideally be incorporated, because temperament and laboratory measures of these constructs are imperfectly correlated despite their conceptual linkage (Nigg, 2000, 2001).

• *Observational longitudinal studies A: Interdependence of neural processes in development, cascade effects, and clinical pathways.* The model yields the following hypothesis for longitudinal follow-up studies of young children. (1a) Infants with a weakness in the effortful allocation of attention at 12 months of age (assessed by standard observational measures of temperamental control) will show delays in word learning at 19–20 months of age. (1b) The prediction from the cascade aspect of the model is that executive deficits will worsen relative to peers from toddler to school age in the most at-risk youngsters (cf. Aguilar et al., 2000). (1c) Conversely, parenting behavior will worsen over time from age 1 year to age 5 years in children with early problems in effortful allocation of attention. (1d) To evaluate the clinical pathways predictions, if an executive (effortful attention) deficit emerges in a child with otherwise average emotional reactivity (negative affect) and average word learning, that child will go on to develop ADHD with only mild secondary problems in motivation response or learning. However, (1e) if extreme reactivity is observed in a young child, secondary problems in executive control and in language learning will almost always co-occur, with exceptions reflecting very supportive caregiving. The children with conduct disorder with normal IQ and executive functioning will also show average reactivity levels.
    • *Observational longitudinal studies B: Experience-dependent causal effects of cognitive deficits.* (2a) To evaluate the experience-dependence component of the model, when faced with adverse environments, children who have the weakest verbal and executive skills will respond with the greatest antisocial development. (2b) Executive and verbal problems will predict later offending when parenting skills are held constant.
    • *Observational longitudinal studies C: Individual differences, heterogeneity, and compensatory processes.* These studies would have to feature

detailed videotape observations of naturalistic parent–child interactions along with temperament observations at age 1 year (or earlier), followed up by measures of cognitive and behavioral adjustment at ages 3–5 years. (3a) If young children with executive control problems are divided into those who do and do not go on to persistent offending, they will differ in prior parent responsiveness to these self-control problems. Those who do not persistently offend will have benefited from more well-prepared and well-supported parents who alter their parenting in response to child limitations during the preschool years. (3b) Successful parents will also spend more time assisting their toddlers with verbal skills. (3c) Children with reactive temperaments at age 1 year who develop normal executive and verbal skills by age 3–4 years should have had caregiving that was very attuned to language and self-control support, if the model is correct.

• *Prospective prevention experiments.* It has already been demonstrated that preschool and primary school interventions can alter antisocial trajectories (e.g., Lacourse et al., 2002). However, additional early prevention designs could further elucidate potential early causal contributors. (4a) If a child has a very reactive temperament in the first 12 months (assessed via standard observational measures of temperamental reactivity), intervention to enhance attentional control at age 10–14 months will reduce the chance of language problems and subsequently of externalizing behavior problems in early grade school. (4b) Likewise, if a child at age 18 months has difficulty with effortful control of attention, interventions to strengthen language learning at 18–24 months of age will reduce the chances of antisocial behavior in early grade school and of later offending. The logic here is that compensatory strengths can support the weaker executive system and can support self-control via other processes (such as self-talk and verbal skills) if executive control is weak early. (4c) Behavioral intervention trials that examine individual differences in neuropsychological function will find that those children with executive deficits, high reactivity, and verbal deficits will have poorer response to behavioral intervention and poorer generalization across settings than those who do not have all three deficits.

• *Computational modeling.* To date, computation models of regulatory control have emphasized component executive processes (Botvinick et al., 2001; Goela, Pullara, & Grafman, 2001; Meyer & Kieras, 1997). But other models have begun to evaluate the role of motivation and incentive response on learning and control (Aston-Jones, Rajkowski, & Cohen, 1999), as well as to model developmental sequences involving weakness in one component of a yoked system like we described (Jones, Ritter, & Wood, 2000). The present model could be evaluated by extensions of those computational models, in which the interdependence of reward and executive control processes was modeled, and then the role of language processes was also modeled, as schematized in Figure 8.1. The model would have to predict output over time in terms of either (1) replication of children's performance over time on a simple executive planning or inhibition task or (2) chances of producing an operationalized antisocial behavior (e.g., a decision to make an aggressive response to a stimulus). In principal, it would also be possible to model compensatory effects, such as whether an external output to strengthen the verbal system compensates, in performance (or behavior) over time, for a weakness in an executive component in a manner that would have to be confirmed in child studies (Erik Altman, personal communication, March 18, 2002). The logic of such models often entails the settling of response into a stable response pattern; such timetables (number of learning trials) could be mapped onto child development to evaluate whether the model replicates the stability of child antisocial behaviors. Such models could also provide additional specification with regard to inhibition, protection of working memory, and mutual influence of motivational and executive systems.

## CONCLUSION

If within-child cognitive characteristics contribute to antisocial development, it is important to evaluate their potential role early in development, at the outset of coactive parent and child contributions to the socialization process. These effects doubtless are primarily relevant in high-risk environments, in which parents are poorly equipped to provide compensatory support for emerging weakness in executive or verbal skills or for difficult temperament (reactivity). In low-risk environments, even children with self-regulation problems may not be at very high risk for conduct problems. However, in high-risk environments, children's cognitive risk may begin to be amplified rapidly and early in development. Understanding the timing and sequence by which precursors to executive and verbal skills contribute to self-regulation in toddlers and preschoolers is central to the agenda we describe. Such understanding can set the stage for identifying how child cognitive processes participate in socialization during antisocial development.

## NOTES

1. That literature variously addresses delinquency (committing illegal acts) and conduct disorder, a clinical syndrome involving a persistent pattern of violating the rights of others (American Psychiatric Association, 2000) and often a precursor to delinquency. Not all delinquents have conduct disorder and vice versa (Binder, 1988). For simplicity, we use these terms interchangeably along with "antisocial behavior" and "persistent offending," unless otherwise noted.
2. The latter point has sparked long-standing interest in a pattern of relative weak-

ness in Verbal versus Performance IQ (Cornell & Wilson, 1992; Culberton, Feral, & Gabby, 1989; Hecht & Jurkovic, 1978; Hubble & Groff, 1982; Petee & Walsh, 1988; for reviews, see Henry & Moffitt, 1997; Quay, 1987). The PIQ > VIQ sign is not without problems (e.g., by itself it does not well differentiate delinquent subgroups; see Haynes & Bensch, 1981; Hecht & Jurovic, 1978; Hubble & Groff, 1982; this holds especially for girls; see Kratzer & Hodgins, 1999) and is probably not a useful diagnostic sign of individual risk. Yet it underscores the importance of verbal weakness.

3. Multivariate analyses indicate that school performance, but not school attitudes, may mediate cognitive problems' effect on antisocial behavior (Ward & Tittle, 1994). However, Lynam et al. (1993) found that school achievement significantly attenuated the relationship between Verbal IQ and delinquency for African American (but not Caucasian) youths, while data from the Ypsilanti Perry Preschool Project, a prospective longitudinal study of 123 African American children of low SES background, indicated that low IQ predicted later delinquency independently of school achievement in that group also (Farnworth, Schweinhart, & Berrueta-Clement, 1985), all weighing against a purely school-mediated model.

4. The process of verbal learning is itself part of a complex interactive process that involves the interpersonal environment, social cues, the child's cognitive constraints and intentions, and other psychological states and attributes of the child (Bloom & Tinker, 2001; Hollich, Hirsh-Pasek, & Golinkoff, 2000). The details of that process are obviously beyond the scope of this discussion. Although speculative, the important point here is that one of these supports is likely to be the early preexecutive system. Leading theories of language development place greater emphasis on the emerging importance of social-referential and social-pragmatic processes in the second year (Hollich et al., 2000) rather than on the emerging role of effortful attention. Yet, as we note, upcoming data appear consistent with our comments, and a contribution of executive processes is not incompatible with the obvious importance of social-pragmatic processes at this age.

## REFERENCES

Aguilar, B., Sroufe, L.A., Egeland, B., & Carlson, E. (2000). Distinguishing the early-onset/persistent and adolescence-onset antisocial behavior types: From birth to 16 years. *Development and Psychopathology, 12*, 109–132.

American Psychiatric Association. (2000). *Diagnostic and statistical manual of mental disorders* (4th ed., text rev.). Washington, DC: Author.

Aronowitz, B., Liebowitz, M., Hollander, E., Fazzini, E., Durlach-Misteli, C., Frenkel, M., Mosovich, S., Garfinkel, R., Saoud, J., & DelBene, D. (1994). Neuropsychiatric and neuropsychological findings in conduct disorder and attention-deficit hyperactivity disorder. *Journal of Neuropsychiatry and Clinical Neurosciences, 6*, 245–249.

Aston-Jones, G., Rajkowski, J., & Cohen, J. (1999). Role of locus coeruleus in attention and behavioral flexibility. *Biological Psychiatry, 46*, 1309–1320.

Barkley, R. A. (1997). *ADHD and the nature of self-control.* New York: Guilford Press.

Berk, L. E. (1986). Relationship of elementary school children's private speech to behavioral accompaniment to task, attention, and task performance. *Developomental Psychology, 22,* 671–680.

Binder, A. (1988). Juvenile delinquency. *Annual Review of Psychology, 39,* 253–282.

Bloom, L., & Tinker, E. (2001). The intentionality model of language acquisition. *Monographs of the Society for Research in Child Development, 66*(4, Serial No. 267), 1–89.

Borkowski, J., & Burke, J. (1996). Theories, models, and measurements of executive functioning: An information processing perspective. In G. Lyon & N. Krasnegor (Eds.), *Attention, memory, and executive function* (pp. 235–261). Baltimore: Brookes.

Botvinick, M. M., Braver, T. S., Barch, D. M., Carter, C. S., & Cohen, J. D. (2001). Conflict monitoring and cognitive control. *Psychological Review, 108,* 624–652.

Brand, R. J., & Baldwin, D. A. (2003, April). *Inhibitory control, temperament, and vocabulary in 13- to 17-month-old infants.* Poster presented at the annual meeting of the Society for Research in Child Development, Tampa, FL.

Cadoret, R. J., Yates, W. R., Troughton, E., Woodworth, G., & Stewart, M. A. (1995). Genetic–environmental interaction in the genesis of aggressivity and conduct disorders. *Archives of General Psychiatry, 52,* 916–924.

Clark, C., Prior, M., & Kinsella, G. (2000). Do executive function deficits differentiate between adolescents with ADHD and oppositional defiant/conduct disorder?: A neuropsychological study using the Six Elements Test and Hayling Sentence Completion Test. *Journal of Abnormal Child Psychology, 28,* 403–414.

Cornell, D., & Wilson, L. (1992). The PIQ greater than VIQ discrepancy in violent and nonviolent delinquents. *Journal of Clinical Psychology, 48,* 256–261.

Culberton, F., Feral, C., & Gabby, S. (1989). Pattern analysis of Wechsler Intelligence Scale for Children—Revised profiles of delinquent boys. *Journal of Clinical Psychology, 45,* 651–660.

Davidson, R. J., & Sutton, S. K. (1995). Affective neuroscience: The emergence of a discipline. *Current Opinions in Neurobiology, 5,* 217–222.

Dery, M., Toupin, J., Pauze, R., Mercier, H., & Fortin, L. (1999). Neuropsychological characteristics of adolescents with conduct disorder: Association with attention-deficit-hyperactivity and aggression. *Journal of Abnormal Child Psychology, 27,* 225–236.

Derryberry, D., & Reed, M. A. (1996). Regulatory processes and the development of cognitive representations. *Development and Psychopathology, 8,* 215–234.

Derryberry, D., & Rothbart, M. K. (1997). Reactive and effortful processes in the organization of temperament. *Development and Psychopathology, 9,* 633–652.

Derryberry, D., & Tucker, D. M. (1994). Motivating the focus of attention. In P. Niedentha & S. Kiayama (Eds.), *The heart's eye: Emotional influences on perception and attention* (pp. 167–196). San Diego: Academic Press.

Diamond, A., Prevor, M. B., Callender, G., & Druin, D. P. (1997). Prefrontal cortex cognitive deficits in children treated early and continuously for PKU. *Monographs of the Society for Research in Child Development, 62*(4, Serial No. 252), 1–205.

Donnellan, M., Ge, X., & Wenk, E. (2000). Cognitive abilities in adolescent-limited and life-course-persistent criminal offenders. *Journal of Abnormal Psychology, 109,* 396–402.

Eisenberg, N., Fabes, R. A., Guthrie, I. K., Murphy, B. C., Maszk, P., Holmgren, R., & Suh, K. (1996). The relations of regulation and emotionality to problem behavior in elementary school children. *Development and Psychopathology, 8,* 141–162.

Elkins, I., Iacono, W., Doyle, A., & McGue, M. (1997). Characteristics associated with the persistence of antisocial behavior: Results from recent longitudinal research. *Aggression and Violent Behavior, 2,* 101–124.

Farnworth, M., Schweinhart, L., & Berrueta-Clement, J. (1985). Preschool intervention, school success, and delinquency in a high-risk sample of youth. *American Educational Research Journal, 22,* 445–464.

Farrington, D. (1994). Early developmental prevention of juvenile delinquency. *Criminal Behaviour and Mental Health, 4,* 209–227.

Farrington, D. P., & Loeber, R. (2000). Epidemiology of juvenile violence. *Juvenile Violence, 9,* 733–748.

Farrington, D. P., Loeber, R., & van Kammen, W. B. (1990). Long term criminal outcomes of hyperactivity–impulsivity–attention deficit and conduct problems in childhood. In L. Robins & M. Rutter (Eds.), *Straight and devious pathways from childhood to adulthood* (pp. 62–81). New York: Cambridge University Press.

Frost, L., Moffitt, T., & McGee, R. (1989). Neuropsychological function and psychopathology in an unselected cohort of young adolescents. *Journal of Abnormal Psychology, 98,* 307–313.

Gath, D., & Tennent, G. (1972). High intelligence and delinquency: A review. *British Journal of Sociology, 12,* 174–181.

Ge, X., Conger, R. R., Cadoret, R. J., Neiderhiser, J. M., Yates, W., Troughton, E., & Stewart, M. A. (1996). The developmental interface between nature and nurture: A mutual influence model of child antisocial behavior and parent behaviors. *Developmental Psychology, 32,* 574–589.

Giancola, P., & Mezzich, A. (2000). Executive cognitive function mediates the relation between language competence and antisocial behavior in conduct-disordered adolescent females. *Aggressive Behavior, 26,* 359–375.

Giancola, P., Mezzich, A., & Tarter, R. (1998). Executive cognitive functioning, temperament, and antisocial behavior in conduct-disordered adolescent females. *Journal of Abnormal Psychology, 107,* 629–641.

Goela, V., Pullara, S. D., & Grafman, J. (2001). A computational model of frontal lobe dysfunction: Working memory and the Tower of Hanoi task. *Cognitive Science, 25,* 287–313.

Gopnick, A. (1982). Words and plans: Early language and the development of intelligent action. *Journal of Child Language, 9,* 303–318.

Gopnick, A. (1988). Three types of early word: The emergence of social words, names, and cognitive-relational words in the one-word stage and their relation to cognitive development. *First Language, 8,* 49–70.

Gray, J. A. (1991). Neural systems, emotion, and personality. In J. Madden (Ed.), *Neurobiology of learning, emotion, and affect* (pp. 273–306). New York: Raven Press.

Greenberg, M., Speltz, M., DeKlyen, M., & Jones, K. (2001). Correlates of clinic referral for early conduct problems: Variable and person-oriented approaches. *Development and Psychopathology, 13,* 255–276.

Haynes, J., & Bensch, M. (1981). The P > V sign on the WISC-R and recidivism in delinquents. *Journal of Consulting and Clinical Psychology, 49,* 480–481.

Hecht, I., & Jurkovic, G. (1978). The Performance–Verbal IQ discrepancy in differentiated subgroups of delinquent adolescent boys. *Journal of Youth and Adolescence, 7,* 197–201.

Henry, B., & Moffitt, T. (1997). Neuropsychological and neuroimagining studies of juvenile delinquency and adult criminal behavior. In D. Stoff & J. Breiling (Eds.), *Handbook of antisocial behavior* (pp. 280–288). New York: Wiley.

Henry, B., Moffitt, T., & Silva, P. (1992). Disentangling delinquency and learning disability: Neuropsychological function and social support. *International Journal of Clinical Neuropsychology, 13,* 1–6.

Hinshaw, S. P. (1992). Externalizing behavior problems and academic underachievement in childhood and adolescence: Causal relationships and underlying mechanisms. *Psychological Bulletin, 111,* 127–155.

Hinshaw, S. P., Lahey, B. B., & Hart, E. L. (1993). Issues of taxonomy and comorbidity in the development of conduct disorder. *Development and Psychopathology, 5,* 31–50.

Hirschi, T., & Hindelang, M. (1977). Intelligence and delinquency: A revisionist review. *American Sociological Review, 42,* 571–587.

Hogan, A. (1999). Cognitive functioning in children with oppositional defiant disorder and conduct disorder. In H. C. Quay & A. E. Hogan (Eds.), *Handbook of disruptive behavior disorders* (pp. 317–335). New York: Kluwer Academic Press.

Hollich, G. J., Hirsh-Pasek, K., & Golinkoff, R. M. (2000). Breaking the language barrier: An emergenist coalition model for the origins of word learning. *Monographs of the Society for Research in Child Development, 65*(3, Serial No. 262), 1–135.

Huang-Pollock, C. L., Carr, T. H., & Nigg, J. T. (2002). Perceptual load influences late versus early selection in child and adult selective attention. *Developmental Psychology, 38*, 363–375.

Hubble, L., & Groff, M. (1982). Magnitude and direction of WISC-R Verbal–Performance IQ discrepancies among adjudicated male delinquents. *Journal of Youth and Adolescence, 10*, 179–184.

Hughes, C., Dunn, J., & White, A. (1998). Trick or treat?: Patterns of cognitive performance and executive function among "hard-to-manage" preschoolers. *Journal of Child Psychology and Psychiatry, 39*, 981–994.

Hughes, C., White, A., Sharpen, J., & Dunn, J. (2000). Antisocial, angry, and unsympathetic: "Hard to manage" preschoolers' peer problems and possible cognitive influences. *Journal of Chld Psychology and Psychiatry, 41*, 169–179.

Jones, G., Ritter, F. E., & Wood, D. J. (2000). Using a cognitive architecture to examine what develops. *Psychological Science, 11*, 93–100.

Kamphaus, R. W. (2001). *Clinical assessment of child and adolescent intelligence* (2nd ed.). Boston: Allyn & Bacon.

Kaufman, A. S. (1994). *Intelligent testing with the WISC-III.* New York: Wiley.

Kochanska, G. (1997). Multiple pathways to conscience for children with different temperaments: From toddlerhood to age 5. *Developmental Psychology, 33*, 228–240.

Kochanska, G., Coy, K. C., Tjebkes, T. L., & Husarek, S. J. (1998). Individual differences in emotionality in infancy. *Child Development, 69*, 375–390.

Kochanska, G., Murray, K., & Coy, K. C. (1997). Inhibitory control as a contributor to conscience in early childhood: From toddler to early school age. *Child Development, 68*, 263–277.

Kratzer, L., & Hodgins, S. (1999). A typology of offenders: A test of Moffitt's theory among males and females from childhood to age 30. *Criminal Behaviour and Mental Health, 9*, 57–73.

Lacourse, E., Cote, S., Nagin, D. S., Vitaro, E., Brendgen, M.B., & Tremblay, R. E. (2002). A longitudinal–experimental approach to testing theories of antisocial development. *Development and Psychopathology, 14*, 909–924.

Lahey, B. B., Loeber, R., Hart, E. L., Frick, P. J., Applegate, B., Zhang, Q., Green, S. M., & Russo, M. F. (1995). Four-year longitudinal study of conduct disorder in boys: Patterns and predictors of persistence. *Journal of Abnormal Psychology, 104*, 83–93.

Lahey, B. B., Waldman, I. D., & McBurnett, K. (1999). The development of antisocial behavior: An integrative causal model. *Journal of Child Psychology and Psychiatry, 40*, 669–682.

Lezak, M. (1995). *Neuropsychological assessment* (3rd ed.). New York: Oxford University Press.

Lipsitt, P., Buka, S., & Lipsitt, L. (1990). Early intelligence scores and subsequent delinquency: A prospective study. *American Journal of Family Therapy, 18*, 197–208.

Loeber, R., Farrington, D., Stouthamer-Loeber, M., Moffitt, T., & Caspi, A. (1998). The development of male offending: Key findings from the first decade of the Pittsburgh Youth Study. *Studies on Crime and Prevention, 7*, 141–171.

Loeber, R., Farrington, D. P., Stouthamer-Loeber, M., & van Kammen, W. B. (1998). *Antisocial behavior and mental health problems: Explanatory factors in childhood and adolescence.* Mahwah, NJ: Erlbaum.

Lynam, D., & Henry, B. (2001). The role of neuropsychological deficits in conduct disorders. In J. Hill & B. Maughan (Eds.), *Conduct problems in childhood and adolescence* (pp. 235–263). New York: Cambridge University Press.

Lynam, D., Moffit, T., & Stouthamer-Loeber, M. (1993). Explaining the relation between IQ and delinquency: Class, race, test motivation, school-failure, or self-control? *Journal of Abnormal Psychology, 102,* 187–196.

Lyon, G. R., & Krasnegor, N. A. (1996). *Attention, memory and executive function.* Baltimore: Brookes.

Menard, S., & Morse, B. J. (1984). A structuralist critique of the IQ–delinquency hypothesis: Theory and evidence. *American Journal of Sociology, 89,* 1347–1378.

Meyer, D. E., & Kieras, D. E. (1997). EPIC—A computational theory of executive cognitive processes and multiple-task performance: Part 1. Basic mechanisms. *Psychological Review, 104,* 3–64.

Middleton, F. A., & Strick, P. L. (2001). A revised neuroanatomy of frontal–subcortical circuits. In D. G. Lichter & J. L. Cummings (Eds.), *Frontal–subcortical circuits in psychiatric and neurological disorders* (pp. 44–58). New York: Guilford Press.

Miller, E. K. (2000). The prefrontal cortex and cognitive control. *Nature Reviews: Neuroscience, 1,* 59–65.

Miller, L. (1987). Neuropsychology of the aggressive psychopath: An integrative review. *Aggressive Behavior, 13,* 119–140.

Moffitt, T. (1990). Juvenile delinquency and attention deficit disorder: Boys' developmental trajectories from age 3 to age 15. *Child Development, 61,* 893–910.

Moffitt, T. (1993). The neuropsychology of conduct disorder. *Development and Psychopathology, 5,* 135–151.

Moffitt, T., & Caspi, A. (2001). Childhood predictors differentiate life-course persistent and adolescence-limited antisocial pathways among males and females. *Development and Psychopathology, 13,* 355–375.

Moffitt, T., Gabrielli, W., & Mednick, S. (1981). Socioeconomic status, IQ, and delinquency. *Journal of Abnormal Psychology, 90,* 152–156.

Moffitt, T., & Henry, B. (1989). Neuropsychological assessment of executive functions in self-reported delinquents. *Development and Psychopathology, 1,* 105–118.

Moffitt, T., Lynam, D., & Silva, P. (1994). Neuropsychological tests predict persistent male delinquency. *Criminology, 32,* 101–124.

Moffitt, T., & Silva, P. (1988). IQ and delinquency: A direct test of the differential detection hypothesis. *Journal of Abnormal Psychology, 97,* 330–333.

Morgan, A. B., & Lilienfeld, S. O. (2000). A meta-analytic review of the relation between antisocial behavior and neuropsychological measures of executive functions. *Clinical Psychology Review, 20,* 113–136.

Newman, J. P., & Wallace, J. F. (1993). Diverse pathways to deficient self-regulation: Implications for disinhibitory psychopathology in children. *Clinical Psychology Review, 13,* 690–720.

Nigg, J. T. (1999). The ADHD response inhibition deficit as measured by the stop task: Replication with DSM-IV combined type, extension, and qualification. *Journal of Abnormal Child Psychology, 27,* 393–402.

Nigg, J. T. (2000). On inhibition/disinhibition in developmental psychopathology: View from cognitive and personality psychology and a working inhibition taxonomy. *Psychological Bulletin, 126,* 220–246.

Nigg, J. T. (2001). Is ADHD an inhibitory disorder? *Psychological Bulletin, 127,* 571–598.

Nigg, J. T., Blaskey, L. G., Huang-Pollock, C. L., & Rappley, M. D. (2002). Neuropsychological executive functions and DSM-IV ADHD subtypes. *Journal of the American Academy of Child and Adolescent Psychiatry, 41,* 59–66.

Nigg, J. T., Hinshaw, S. P., Carte, E. T., & Treuting, J. J. (1998). Neuropsychological correlates of childhood attention-deficit hyperactivity disorder: Explainable by comorbid disruptive behavior or reading problems? *Journal of Abnormal Psychology, 107,* 468–480.

Nigg, J. T., Quamma, J. P., Greenberg, M. T., & Kusche, C. A. (1999). A two-year longitudinal study of neuropsychological and cognitive performance in relation to behavioral problems and competencies in elementary school children. *Journal of Abnormal Child Psychology*, 27, 51–63.

Patterson, G. R., & Capaldi, D. M. (1991). Antisocial parents: Unskilled and vulnerable. In P. A. Cowan & M. Hetherington (Eds.), *Family transitions* (pp. 195–218). Hillsdale, NJ: Erlbaum.

Pennington, B. (1997). Dimensions of executive functions in normal and abnormal development. In N. A. Krasnegor, G. R. Lyon, & P. S. Goldman-Rakic (Eds.), *Development of the prefrontal cortex: Evolution, neurobiology, and behavior* (pp. 265–281). Baltimore: Brookes.

Pennington, B., & Ozonoff, S. (1996). Executive functions and developmental psychopathology. *Journal of Child Psychology and Psychiatry*, 37, 51–87.

Petee, T., & Walsh, A. (1988). Violent delinquency, race, and the Wechsler Performance > Verbal discrepancy. *Journal of Social Psychology*, 127, 353–354.

Posner, M. I., & DiGirolamo, G. J. (1998). Executive attention: Conflict, target detection, and cognitive control. In R. Parasuraman (Ed.), *The attentive brain* (pp. 401–423). Cambridge, MA: MIT Press.

Posner, M. I., & Rothbart, M. K. (2000). Developing mechanisms of self-regulation. *Development and Psychopathology*, 12, 427–441.

Prinz, R. J., & Miller, G. E. (1991). Issues in understanding and treating childhood conduct problems in disadvantaged populations. *Journal of Clinical Child Psychology*, 20, 279–385.

Quay, H. (1987b). Intelligence. In H. Quay (Ed.), *Handbook of juvenile delinquency* (pp. 106–117). New York: Wiley.

Rothbart, M. K., & Bates, J. E. (1998). Temperament. In W. Damon (Series Ed.) and N. Eisenberg (Vol. Ed.), *Handbook of child psychology: Vol 3. Social, emotional, and personality development* (pp. 105–176). New York: Wiley.

Saccuzzo, D., & Lewandowski, D. (1976). The WISC as a diagnostic tool. *Journal of Clinical Psychology*, 32, 115–124.

Sattler, J. M. (2001). *Assessment of children: Cognitive applications* (4th ed.). San Diego, CA: Sattler.

Seguin, J. R., Boulerice, B., Harden, P. W., Tremblay, R. E., & Pihl, R. O. (1999). Executive functions and physical aggression after controlling for attention deficit hyperactivity disorder, general memory, and IQ. *Journal of Child Psychology and Psychiatry*, 40, 1197–1208.

Silverthorn, P., & Frick, P. (1999). Developmental pathways to antisocial behavior: The delayed-onset pathway in girls. *Development and Psychopathology*, 11, 101–126.

Speltz, M. L., DeKlyen, M., Calderon, R., Greenberg, M. T., & Fisher, P. A. (1999). Neuropsychological characteristics and test behaviors of boys with early onset conduct problems. *Journal of Abnormal Psychology*, 108, 315–325.

Stattin, H., & Klackenberg-Larsson, I. (1993). Early language and intelligence development and their relationship to future criminal behavior. *Journal of Abnormal Psychology*, 102, 369–378.

Sternberg, R. J., & Detterman, D. K. (Eds.). (1986). *What is intelligence?: Contemporary viewpoints on its nature and definition.* Norwood, NJ: Ablex.

Stormshank, E., Speltz, M., DeKlyen, M., & Greenberg, M. (1997). Observed family interaction during clinical interviews: A comparison of families containing preschool boys with and without disruptive behavior. *Journal of Abnormal Child Psychology*, 25, 345–357.

Teichner, G., & Golden, C. (2000). The relationship of neuropsychological impairment to conduct disorder in adolescence: A conceptual review. *Aggression and Violent Behavior*, 5, 509–528.

Thompson, P. M., Cannon, T. D., Narr, K. I., van Erp, T., Poutanen, V., Huttunen, M., Lonnqvist, J., Standertskjol-Nordenstam, C. G., Kaprio, J., Khaledy, M., Dail, R., Zoumalan, C. I., & Toga, A. W. (2001). Genetic influences on brain structure. *Nature Neuroscience*, 4, 1253–1258.

Toupin, J., Dery, M., Pauze, R., Mercier, H., & Fortin, L. (2000). Cognitive and familial contributors to conduct disorder in children. *Journal of Child Psychology and Psychiatry, 41*, 333–344.

Ward, D., & Tittle, C. (1994). IQ and delinquency: A test of two competing explanations. *Journal of Quantitative Criminology, 10*, 189–212.

Wechsler, D. (1991). *Wechsler Intelligence Scale for Children—3rd edition manual*. San Antonio, TX: Harcourt Brace.

White, J., Moffitt, T., & Silva, P. (1989). A prospective replication of the protective effects of IQ in subjects at high risk for juvenile delinquency. *Journal of Consulting and Clinical Psychology, 57*, 719–724.

Wilson, J., & Herrnstein, R. (1985). *Crime and human nature*. New York: Simon & Schuster.

Woodward, A., & Markman, E. (1998). Early word learning. In W. Damon (Series Ed.) & D. Kuhn & R. Siegler (Vol. Eds.), *Handbook of child psychology: Vol. II. Cognition, perception, and language* (pp. 371–420). New York: Wiley.

# 9

# Do Social Information-Processing Patterns Mediate Aggressive Behavior?

KENNETH A. DODGE

The notion that the manner in which a person routinely processes situational stimuli has a dramatic impact on that person's production of aggressive behavior is intuitively appealing and has guided numerous intervention attempts to treat children with conduct disorder (e.g., Conduct Problems Prevention Research Group, 1999; Hudley & Graham, 1993; Kazdin, Siegel, & Bass, 1992; Lochman & Lenhart, 1995). The underlying premise is that psychotherapeutic intervention might directly change how a person thinks and feels, and therefore indirectly alter how that person behaves. These interventions are based on the hypothesis that one's stylistic pattern of processing social information causes one's display of aggressive behavior. But what is the scientific status of this hypothesis? The current chapter addresses this question.

Although intuitively appealing, the hypothesis that processing patterns cause aggressive behavior is extraordinarily difficult to prove with reasonable scientific rigor. Problems arise in finding a valid "window" into mental processes, in experimentally manipulating those processes, and in rebutting alternate explanations for any empirical correlation between mental processes and behavioral output. The purposes of this chapter are to pose testable hypotheses and to evaluate existing empirical findings that address those hypotheses. Finally, future studies are proposed that could refine the state of knowledge in this area.

## THE HYPOTHESIS THAT MENTAL PROCESSES GUIDE AGGRESSIVE BEHAVIOR

Consider an adolescent boy who is talking with a group of peers, one of whom "disses" him by repeatedly joking about his poor taste in clothes and girlfriends. Imagine that the peer group laughs and jointly belittles the boy. What behavioral response is made by the boy? Does the boy avoid a conflict by deflecting attention to a different topic, by shrugging off the provocation, or by joining in the laughter? Or does the boy escalate the conflict by retaliating with hostile comments or even by impulsively pulling a knife on his tormenters? Of course, the answer is that "it depends," not only on the features of the social context but on the characteristics of the boy. It is easy to surmise that individual differences would be found in the propensity of a boy to respond to this stimulus with violence; indeed, individual differences in aggressive behavior, even considering similar stimulus circumstances, are among the most robust in all of personality and developmental psychology (Coie & Dodge, 1998).

What determines individual differences in the boy's behavioral response in this circumstance? The major concept of problem-solving and information-processing theories (Newell & Simon, 1972) is that humans have evolved a sophisticated information-processing system that consists of attending to important stimuli, interpreting those stimuli in meaningful ways, associating that interpretation in memory with possible behavioral responses, evaluating those responses, and then deciding to act on a particular response alternative. During any single event, these mental processes can be described through methods such as "think-aloud" directives and protocol analysis and used to predict that individual's behavioral response. Social information-processing (SIP) theory (Dodge, 1993; Huesmann, 1988; McFall, 1982) further posits that children develop routinized patterns of processing cues, which form personality-like traits, and that these patterns predict individual differences in conduct problems. Although this theory is difficult to refute or to support in its whole, it suggests testable hypotheses of great importance to the field of developmental psychopathology. Three hypotheses are posed and evaluated in this chapter:

1. It is hypothesized that across middle childhood children develop multidimensional, stable, and unique patterns of processing social stimuli, which form the working components of personality.
2. It is hypothesized that these personality-like (SIP) patterns predict the likelihood of aggressive behavior problems, including growth in such problems over time, which cannot be accounted for by third-variable confounds.
3. It is hypothesized that SIP patterns mediate the relation between early environmental experiences, such as child abuse and peer social rejection, and the development of conduct problems and chronic violence.

## SOCIAL INFORMATION-PROCESSING THEORY

In responding to a social cue such as the provocation described above, it is posited that individuals perform several mental operations in sequence (Dodge, 1986, 1993). It is further posited that individual differences develop during middle childhood in how children perform these operations.

The first action is to receive stimulus information through attention and sensation. This informational cue set includes both environmental stimuli and internal thoughts, feelings, and scripts. Because the possible cue set is too large for any individual to process fully in real time, it is posited that individuals learn to attend selectively to specific portions of the stimulus array over others. The adolescent in the scenario above might attend to the peers laughing, to the emotional pain that he feels, to the presence of authorities in the distance who will intervene if a fight ensues, or to the internal script of maintaining a supportive peer group. Within categories of stimuli, such as (1) provocations, (2) opportunities for social initiation, (3) failures, or (4) adult-initiated directives (Dodge, McClaskey, & Feldman, 1985), individual differences develop in attention patterns, such that some children acquire hypervigilance to threat cues, whereas other children come to attend to possible mitigating factors. Both skill (perhaps related to intelligence, practice, or neurally mediated attention deficits) and heuristically based biases contribute to a child's pattern of attention to cues. Temporary factors such as fatigue and alcohol ingestion can alter responding as well.

The plausible antecedents and outcomes of these individual differences form important hypotheses. It is posited that children who are routinely hypervigilant to threatening cues will be relatively likely to behave aggressively in response to provocations, whereas children who attend to mitigating features will be likely to withhold aggressive retaliatory responses. The antecedents of attention patterns may involve a combination of constitutional and socialization factors. It is hypothesized that hypervigilance may emerge at least partially as an adaptive mental response to past life experiences of actual threat, such as physical abuse and peer victimization.

As cues are received, they are interpreted and stored in memory. In circumstances of stimulus clarity, little variation in interpretation is likely, but many stimuli involve ambiguity and a wide range of possible interpretations. The hypothetical boy named above might interpret the "dissing" as a hostile act designed to belittle the boy or as a benign act of harmless fun. *Hostile attributional bias* is the term first used by Nasby, Hayden, and DePaulo (1979) to describe the tendency of some children to routinely make attributions of hostile intent. As with patterns of selective attention, attributional patterns involve a combination of skill and heuristic bias; they may predict aggressive behavioral responding; and they may have antecedents in a combination of constitutional and life experience factors.

Once a cue is interpreted and given meaning, it is associated in memory with one or more potential behavioral responses. These behavioral responses are "called to mind" for consideration. For example, if the hypothetical boy interprets the provocation cue as an intentional hostile threat, that boy might access from memory the potential responses of retaliating aggressively, leaving the scene, deflecting group attention in a different direction, or making a direct confrontation. As with previous processing steps, it is posited that regular patterns of response access develop, have implications for actual behavioral responding, and are acquired through life experiences. Both the rules guiding association in memory and the repertoire of possible response alternatives may develop at least partially through life experiences and socialization.

The next step of processing is response decision making. Each of the behavioral responses that has been called to mind is evaluated and either enacted or rejected. A rejected response is phenomenologically experienced as a withheld impulse (as in, "I could have killed him but thought better of it"), whereas an accepted response is enacted in behavior. The rules guiding decision making involve multiple domains that include evaluation of the likely interpersonal, intrapersonal, and instrumental consequences of a behavior, as well as the valuation of those consequences (Fontaine, Burks, & Dodge, 2002). In some cases, multiple responses might be evaluated *serially* until a response above a threshold level of acceptability is reached or *simultaneously* until the best alternative is reached. As with previous steps, decision-making responses are patterned, predict behavior, and have antecedents in life experiences.

Details of SIP theory vary across theorists (e.g., Huesmann, 1988, emphasizes cognitive schema stored in memory, but Crick and Dodge, 1994, distinguish the processing steps of goal formulation from response generation), but three hypotheses are common to this perspective. These hypotheses are articulated and evaluated next.

## HYPOTHESIS 1: PATTERNS OF SOCIAL INFORMATION PROCESSING BECOME MULTIDIMENSIONAL, STABLE, AND UNIQUE COMPONENTS OF PERSONALITY

Cervone (1999) has argued that trait theories of personality lack causal power. Traits are often offered as tautological explanations of outcomes that are measured by the trait itself. "Aggressiveness" is hardly a causal explanation for "aggressive behavior." In contrast, Zelli and Dodge (1999) have proposed that domain-specific patterns of processing information, following from the model outlined above, constitute the building blocks for the development of personality from the bottom up rather than from the top down.

The first methodological issue to be addressed concerns the measurement of processing patterns. Dodge, Pettit, McClasky, and Brown (1986) solved this problem by creating videorecorded stimuli depicting social situations that children frequently encounter. They asked children to observe these stimuli and to imagine being the protagonist who encounters a provocation or is rebuffed from peer group entry. At that point, they stopped the video and asked the child questions that were designed to measure the child's selective attention, intent attributions, response generation, and response evaluation patterns. By presenting 36 scenarios to children (12 in each of the situations of peer provocation, rebuff from peer entry, and authority directive), Dodge and Price (1994) were able to demonstrate reasonable within-construct reliability in responding across items, as indicated by coefficient alphas that range from .6 to .9.

Three subhypotheses regarding the structure of processing patterns can be evaluated empirically. First, it is hypothesized that patterns of SIP are multidimensional and cannot be explained as indicators of a single underlying construct. Findings that support this hypothesis come from many sources. For example, Fontaine et al. (2002) found that assessments of two subaspects of decision-making processes, response valuation, and outcome expectancy, in a sample of 14 ninth-grade boys and girls load on to two separate factors in a standard factor analysis. Likewise, Hubbard, Dodge, Cillessen, Coie, & Schwartz (2001) found that assessments of attribution biases and response evaluations load on to distinct factors.

Most findings evaluating this hypothesis come from studies that have tested whether multiple measures of processing patterns provide unique increments in predicting aggressive behavior outcomes, as operationalized by significant increments in multiple regression analyses. Fontaine et al. (2002) found that measures of response generation and response valuation provide unique increments in predicting parent- and self-reported externalizing problems among ninth-graders. Dodge et al. (1986) found that measures of selective attention, hostile attributional bias, response generation, and response evaluation each provided a significant and unique contribution to the prediction of individual differences in aggressive behavior in both provocation and rebuff from peer group entry situations among elementary school-age boys and girls. Individually, these measures predicted aggressive behavior to a modest degree, but together the multiple correlations reached .75. Slaby and Guerra (1988) found that these measures predicted aggressive behavior in an adolescent population in a similar manner, with individual correlations being modest but the multiple correlation ranging up to .89.

The most direct test of this hypothesis has been made by Dodge, Laird, Lochman, Zelli, and Conduct Problems Prevention Research Group (2002), who used recent advancements in multidimensional latent-construct analysis

(Arbuckle & Wothke, 1999) to test the hypothesis that the between-construct variance in measurement would be greater than the within-construct measurement. Their subjects were 332 7-year-old boys and girls from four geographic sites. Using multiple-item responses within the four constructs of intent attribution, goal orientation, response generation, and response evaluation, they found that a structural equation model that included four latent constructs provided a significantly better fit to the data than did a model that included only one latent construct. Furthermore, the four-construct model fit better than did the best three-factor model, suggesting that these four constructs are measured as distinct from each other. In an even more differentiated analysis, they found empirical support for a two-dimensional model, in which the four processing constructs were evaluated within each of two types of situations (responding to a peer provocation and responding to a peer group entry challenge). It appears that children's processing patterns vary systematically across the component of processing as well as across situations.

The second aspect of structure that can be evaluated is the stability of these processing patterns. In order to function as personality building blocks, processing patterns must display not only within-time coherence but also cross-time stability. Dodge and Price (1994) assessed processing patterns in 259 boys and girls across multiple years in elementary school. They found both that multi-item within-construct scores are moderately stable across 12 months and that the degree of cross-time stability increases across the elementary school years. That is, they found evidence for emergent stability in processing patterns, as if children are acquiring characteristic patterns of processing the social world that become more stable with advancing age.

The third question regarding structure that can be evaluated is whether these processing patterns are distinct from measures of intelligence and measures of different kinds of mental structures such as beliefs and emotion knowledge. Waldman (1996) measured both processing patterns and intelligence and found that even after statistically controlling for intelligence, processing patterns provided a significant increment in the prediction of aggressive behavior. Zelli, Dodge, Lochman, and Conduct Problems Prevention Research Group (1999) found that processing patterns provide a significant increment even after controlling for Huesmann and Guerra's (1997) measure of beliefs about the legitimacy of aggressing. Dodge et al. (2002) found that processing patterns provide a significant increment after controlling for children's knowledge about emotions.

These findings are consistent with the hypothesis that SIP patterns emerge across middle childhood to become stable multidimensional personality-like characteristics that operate within situations in a manner that is distinct from intelligence, beliefs, and knowledge.

## HYPOTHESIS 2: PATTERNS OF SOCIAL INFORMATION PROCESSING PREDICT GROWTH IN AGGRESSIVE BEHAVIOR

Over 100 studies have reported significant correlations between one or more processing patterns and measures of aggressive behavior problems (reviewed by Coie & Dodge, 1998; Crick & Dodge, 1994; Gifford-Smith & Rabiner, in press). Aggressive behavior problems have been found to be correlated with various aspects of children's encoding of social cues, including selective attention to relevant cues (Dodge, Pettit, Bates, & Valente, 1995), total attention to cues (Slaby & Guerra, 1988), selective recall of hostile cues (Milich & Dodge, 1984), and recall of relevant cues (Lochman & Dodge, 1994). Aggressive behavior problems have also been correlated with hostile attributional biases concerning peers' intent (Bickett, Milich, & Brown, 1996; Dodge, 1980), attributions of anger in teachers (Trachtenberg & Viken, 1994), and accuracy of interpretations of others' intent (Dodge, Murphy, & Buchsbaum, 1984). Children's social problem-solving patterns have been related to aggressive behavior, including the overall number of solutions that they are able to generate (Rabiner, Lenhart, & Lochman, 1990), as well as the failure to generate competent-assertive solutions (Quiggle, Panak, Garber, & Dodge, 1992) and the tendency to generate numerous different aggressive responses (Waldman, 1996). Aggressive behavior has been correlated with children's response-decision processes, including their evaluation of the consequences of aggressive behavior as being favorable (Boldizar, Perry, & Perry, 1989), their judgments of aggressive responses as being "good" (Astor, 1994), their perceptions of the suffering that victims experience from aggression (Perry, Williard, & Perry, 1990), their positive valuing of the outcomes that accrue to aggressive behavior (Fontaine et al., 2002), and their evaluations of their own efficacy in being able to enact aggressive responses but not competent responses (Perry, Perry, & Rasmussen, 1986).

Findings hold using diverse measures of aggressive behavior, including teacher reports of classroom aggression and externalizing problems (Astor, 1994), parent reports of externalizing problems at home (Weiss, Dodge, Bates, & Pettit, 1992), peer reports of aggression (Hughes, Robinson, & Moore, 1991), direct observations of aggressive behavior toward peers in laboratory-contrived play groups (Dodge & Coie, 1987), psychiatric records (Milich & Dodge, 1984), social service records (Slaby & Guerra, 1988), and official records of arrests and crimes (Dodge, Price, Bachorowski, & Newman, 1990). Findings hold across diverse groups of children, including African Americans (Graham & Hudley, 1994), white European Americans (Dodge et al., 1986), girls (Crick, 1995), boys (Waas, 1988), young children (Spetter, LaGreca, Hogan, & Vaughn, 1992), middle schoolers (Lochman & Dodge, 1994), and adolescents (Lochman, Wayland, & White, 1993).

The relation between children's patterns of processing social information and their aggressive behavior is exquisitely precise. Processing patterns in response to ambiguous provocations are correlated with aggressive behavior in the same type of situation, but less so in response to a peer group entry situation; in contrast, their processing of peer group entry information is correlated with their aggressive behavior in that situation but less so in response to provocations (Dodge et al., 1986). Children's attributions of hostile intent by peers are positively correlated with their aggressive behavior toward those very peers (Lochman & Dodge, 1994). Furthermore, within-child correlational analyses reveal that the extent to which a child makes attributions of hostile intent toward a particular peer is correlated with that child's directly observed rate of aggressive behavior toward that same peer, even controlling for that child's more general tendency to display aggressive behavior toward other peers (Hubbard, Schwartz, Dodge, & Coie, 1999).

An obvious problem with contemporaneous correlations between processing patterns and conduct problem behavior is the ambiguity with regard to the direction of effect. The hypothesis under consideration is that processing patterns cause behavior problems, but it is also plausible (and not mutually exclusive) that behavior problems could lead a child to display processing biases and deficits. A child who is aggressive toward peers is likely to become the object of negative peer evaluation and aggressive retaliation, factors that have been posed as antecedents to hypervigilance to hostile cues and hostile attributional biases (Dodge, 1993). Likewise, if a child's aggressive behavior leads to favorable outcomes, that child might well learn to evaluate aggression favorably and to access aggressive responses in similar future situations.

Longitudinal studies that statistically control for prior levels of aggressive behavior provide a stronger test of the hypothesis. These studies typically find lower magnitude effects but nonetheless continue to provide support for the basic hypothesis. Several independent samples have been followed to evaluate this hypothesis. Fontaine et al. (2002) followed 100 boys and girls from grade seven through grade 11. Measures of response selection, response evaluation, and outcome expectancy assessed at grade nine were found to predict parent- and self-reports of externalizing problems in grades 10 and 11 even after controlling for externalizing problems in grades seven and eight. Zelli et al. (1999) followed 386 boys and girls from grade one through grade five and found that measures of response generation and response evaluation assessed at grade three predicted teacher-rated aggressive behavior problems in grades four and five even after controlling for behavior problems in grades one and two. Weiss et al. (1992) followed 585 boys and girls from prekindergarten through second grade and found that measures of selective attention to relevant cues, hostile attributional biases, response generation, and response evaluation predicted growth in aggressive behavior as rated by teachers, parents, and peers even after controlling for initial levels of aggression. Follow-ups of the same sample through fifth grade revealed that the effect continues to hold over time (Dodge et al., 1995). Follow-ups through 11th grade found that this effect continues to hold into adolescence and applies to serious violent behaviors (Dodge, Crozier, & Lansford, 2001). Similar findings of processing patterns predicting growth and change in aggression over time have been reported by Egan, Monson, and Perry (1998).

In addition to controlling for initial levels of aggressive behavior, various studies have controlled for other factors that might be correlated with both processing patterns and aggressive behavior. Waldman (1996) controlled for children's intelligence scores and found that the unique correlation between hostile attributional biases and aggressive behavior continued to hold. Dodge, Bates, and Pettit (1990) controlled for various aspects of the family environment, including marital violence and family stress, and found that the relation still held. Dodge et al. (2002) controlled for children's more general understanding of emotions and found that processing patterns continued to predict growth in aggressive behavior from kindergarten through third grade.

A lingering problem with longitudinal studies is that no matter how much attention is devoted to controlling for prior measures of aggressive behavior or correlated factors, the possibility will always exist that an unknown variable is correlated with, and responsible for, the association between processing patterns and aggressive behavior. The most rigorous test of the hypothesis that a processing response causes growth in aggressive behavior is the experiment in which the child's processing is manipulated externally and the effects on that child's behavior are observed directly. Rabiner and Coie (1989) conducted one of the very few such studies. In a laboratory setting, an experimenter induced child subjects to believe that a peer liked the subject and held no ill will toward that subject. In contrast with children who had not received this induction, these children subsequently behaved in ways that indeed led peers to like the child. This study is as close to a direct test of the effect of the attribution of hostile intent on a child's behavior as exists in the field; however, Rabiner and Coie were unable to identify which aspect of the child's behavior directly accounted for the effect on peers. Their conclusion of an effect is based on the peer's ultimate rating of the child, which presumably is based on some undetected aspect of the child's behavior.

Another form of experiment is the clinical intervention. Several scholars have developed interventions to change children's patterns of processing social information as an indirect way to reduce their aggressive behavior. Hudley and Graham (1993) developed an intervention to reduce hostile attributional biases in African American adolescent boys and successfully reduced their reported aggressive behavior, including juvenile delinquency.

In this well-conducted study, however, it is unclear whether the aggressive behavior change was due to changes in children's hostile attributional biases or some other unmeasured process that changed as a function of the intervention. The Conduct Problems Prevention Research Group (2002) implemented a comprehensive intervention for aggressive children called "Fast Track." Among other goals, the intervention includes attempts to alter children's processing of cues through structured peer group interactions that involve didactic instruction and positive social experiences. Evaluations of this randomized experiment indicate that children assigned to this intervention indeed demonstrate lower rates of aggressive problem behavior and interaction with deviant peers. Furthermore, structural equation model analyses revealed that the effect of the intervention on these outcomes can be explained statistically by changes in children's attributions of hostile intent by peers, rather than by changes in other targets of intervention (such as parenting). Although not conclusive, this evidence brings scholars one step closer to concluding that these cognitive–emotional processes play a causal role in the activation of aggressive behavior.

## HYPOTHESIS 3: PATTERNS OF SOCIAL INFORMATION PROCESSING MEDIATE THE EFFECT OF EARLY EXPERIENCE ON THE DEVELOPMENT OF AGGRESSIVE BEHAVIOR

The power of SIP theory comes from its ability to explain how early life experiences exert an enduring effect on children's later aggressive behavior. Two assertions have been articulated in SIP theory. First, it is hypothesized that adverse early life experiences (notably, the experience of physical abuse and the experience of social rejection by peers) lead children to process social information in biased ways, such as becoming hypervigilant to hostile cues and evaluating aggressive behavior as an acceptable and successful way to defend oneself. Second, it is hypothesized that the effect of these adverse life experiences on children's aggressive behavior is directly accounted for by the extent to which the experiences lead children to develop biased processing patterns. Two recent studies have evaluated this hypothesis.

### Peer Rejection and Growth in Aggressive Behavior

One of the major predictors of later growth in aggressive behavior is early rejection by the peer group (Parker & Asher, 1987). Although it is debated whether peer rejection is merely a marker or a causal factor in this growth, numerous intervention programs have been created to help children become more accepted by the peer group (e.g., Bierman, Miller, & Stabb, 1987). In many ways, these interventions have preceded the rigorous evaluation of whether peer rejection plays a causal role in aggressive growth and the likely mechanisms through which this growth might occur.

A recent study by Dodge et al. (in press) was intended to answer these questions. They followed the 259 boys and girls in the Social Development Project (SDP) from grades one, two, and three through grades five, six, and seven. They found that early peer social rejection increased the prediction of later Teacher Rating Form (TRF) Aggression scale scores even after controlling for early teacher- and peer-rated aggression and other problem behaviors. Children who had been rejected in year 1 had raw TRF Aggression scores in year 5 that were almost twice as high as children who had not been rejected in year 1 (M's = 11.3 and 6.6, respectively). Children who had been rejected in year 2 had scores in year 5 that were almost three times as high as those of children who had not been rejected in year 2 (M's = 17.5 and 6.0, respectively). Children who had been rejected in both years 1 and 2 had a mean year 5 TRF Aggression score of 22.2. The question to be considered here is how to explain this effect.

Dodge et al. (in press) hypothesized two ways that rejection may lead to growth in aggressive behavior. First, being rejected by peers denies a child important opportunities for social growth and the development of social-cognitive skills. Piaget (1932/1965), Hartup (1983), and Youniss (1980) all posit that these skills develop during free exchange with an accepting peer group. A child who is denied access to this group will have difficulty developing these skills. When confronted with challenging social situations in the future, that child may be ill-equipped to respond competently and may be much more likely to resort to aggressive behavior. Second, peer rejection may have a stressful effect on children. Rejecting peers can be awfully cruel to a child. Being rejected by peers may lead a child to feel angry, lonely, and socially alienated. These emotions may dispose a child to become defensive, leading the child to become hypervigilant to hostile cues and to attribute hostile intent to the rejecting peers and, soon, to all peers in future social interactions. This child might also feel inefficacious in resolving social problems peacefully and may instead develop a repertoire of aggressive responses that are self-evaluated as morally justified and instrumentally effective in solving problems.

To test this hypothesis, Dodge et al. (in press) assessed key components of SIP patterns in their sample in year 4 of this study. As they hypothesized, peer rejection in year 1 was significantly correlated with three of five SIP scores in year 4. Furthermore, peer rejection predicted growth in biased SIP patterns, as tested by controlling for year 1 SIP patterns. Next, three SIP scores in year 4 were significantly correlated with TRF Aggression scores in year 5. Mediation was tested following the criteria defined by Baron and Kenny (1986) and a series of path analyses. Using the Amos computer program (Arbuckle & Wothke, 1999), 39% of the total effect of early peer rejection on later aggressive behavior was statistically accounted for by the intervening development of biased SIP patterns.

Dodge et al. (in press) next sought to replicate these findings with a larger sample of 585 boys and girls in the Child Development Project (CDP) followed from kindergarten to grade three. Consistent with the SDP sample findings, children who had been socially rejected by peers in kindergarten had mean TRF Aggression scores in grade three that were almost three times higher than those of nonrejected children, and children who had been continuously rejected in kindergarten, grade one, and grade two had TRF Aggression scores in grade three that were five times higher. This pattern held even when other factors in kindergarten were controlled for, including kindergarten TRF Aggression, School Performance, and Internalizing scores and peer-nominated aggression scores.

Again consistent with the SDP sample findings, kindergarten peer rejection significantly predicted SIP patterns in grade two, and grade two SIP patterns predicted TRF Aggression scores in grade three. Finally, contrasts among path models indicated that a significant 16% of the total effect of kindergarten peer rejection on grade three TRF Aggression scores was accounted for by the intervening development of biased SIP patterns.

The findings of these two samples provide replicated support for the dual hypotheses that biased SIP patterns grow out of the experience of social rejection by peers and that these biased SIP patterns partially mediate the effect of peer rejection on growth in aggressive behavior. The finding is remarkably specific and cannot be accounted for by preexisting patterns in aggression, other problem behaviors, or SIP patterns.

One problem with these findings is that the magnitude of the mediation effect is relatively small. SIP patterns were found to account for between 16 and 39% of the effect of peer rejection on later aggression. Mediation is partial at best. What remains for future research is to determine whether improved conceptualization and measurement of acquired SIP patterns could account for a higher proportion of the mediation effect or a different mechanism must be posited to account for the remainder of the effect.

## Child Maltreatment and Growth in Aggressive Behavior

The experience of physical maltreatment in early life has been recognized as a major predictor of serious conduct problems in adolescence, whether measured by restrospective accounts from adolescents (Simons, Whitbeck, Conger, & Wu, 1991) or prospective follow-ups of children identified by social service agencies as maltreated (Widom, 1989). A major problem with this literature, however, is that virtually all studies consider children who have been identified as abused by social service agencies; thus, it is not clear whether the conduct problem outcomes are due to the child's maltreatment or to the treatment of that child by the social service system. Although the intent of that treatment is ameliorative, it often involves public labeling, removal from the home, and other possibly iatrogenic actions.

Recent studies of the CDP sample were intended to determine whether early physical maltreatment that is not necessarily detected by social service agencies is predictive of serious adolescence aggressive behavior and the likely mechanisms of this effect. In the first year of this project, mothers were interviewed regarding the child's life history of discipline, especially the experience of physical harm. Of the 585 preschool boys and girls, 69 (11.8%) met criteria as having experienced physical maltreatment. At grade 11, deviant outcomes were assessed through mother reports on the Child Behavior Checklist (CBCL); adolescent reports of trouble with the police, illicit drug use, gang membership, and aggressive behavior; and review of archival records. Lansford et al. (2002) found that adolescents who had been physically maltreated in early life were at risk for a variety of conduct problems in adolescence, including school suspensions and absenteeism; mother-reported CBCL, Delinquency, and Social Problems scores; and adolescent-reported serious behavior and adjustment problems. Most of these effects remained statistically significant even after controlling for risk factors that are associated with maltreatment, including socioeconomic status, single-parent status, early-life family stress, maternal social support, the child's exposure to marital and neighborhood violence, child temperament, child health, and even harsh parenting in adolescence.

Dodge et al. (2001) tested the effect of early physical maltreatment on the child's development of biased SIP patterns and the mediating role of SIP patterns in accounting for long-term outcomes in conduct problems. Previously reported findings with this sample had established the effect of early physical maltreatment on biased SIP patterns in kindergarten (Dodge, Bates, & Pettit, 1990). Dodge et al. (2001) found that early maltreatment continued to exert a significant effect on biased SIP patterns as measured in grade eight and again in grade 11. Early maltreatment predicted later hypervigilance to social cues, hostile attributional biases, aggressive response generation, and favorable evaluations of the consequences of aggressing at one or more later time points.

Mediation tests were conducted by contrasting structural equation models that did or did not include a path from the acquired SIP patterns to a latent construct of grade 11 aggressive conduct problems. Analyses indicated that SIP patterns at each time point (including kindergarten, grade eight, and grade 11) significantly mediated part of the effect of early physical maltreatment on grade 11 aggressive behavior, accounting for up to 46% of the total effect.

It thus appears that biased SIP patterns grow out of early adverse life experiences such as peer social rejection and physical maltreatment by adults. The acquisition of biased SIP patterns, in turn, appears to predict growth in the child's aggressive behavior problems across childhood and into adolescence. Furthermore, these acquired biased SIP patterns provide a partial explanation for the effect of early adversity on later aggressive behavior, and therefore constitute one mechanism for the development of aggressive conduct problems.

## SOCIAL INFORMATION PROCESSING AND EPIDEMIOLOGY

One task for any comprehensive model in developmental psychopathology is to explain differences in the prevalence of a disorder that occur across major demographic groups (e.g., ethnicity, gender, age, socioeconomic status). In conduct disorder and antisocial personality disorder, group differences are huge. Aggressive behavior rates decrease markedly across childhood, although the rate of serious violence increases dramatically and peaks in adolescence (Coie & Dodge, 1998). Males are much more likely than females to be diagnosed with these disorders (Coie & Dodge, 1998) and to be identified early in life as showing signs of aggressive behavior problems (Lochman & Conduct Problems Prevention Research Group, 1995). In the United States, African Americans are several times more likely than white European Americans to be arrested for violent crimes, although the differences in confidential self-reports of aggressive behaviors are smaller and the degree to which these differences can be attributed to socioeconomic confounds remains under debate (Elliott, 1994). These group variations challenge any explanatory theory.

An SIP model offers a strong, though largely untested, hypothesis to explain these epidemiological variations. On the one hand, the decline in aggressive behavior between age 3 and age 7 can be hypothesized to be due to the child's social-cognitive development, especially in the skills of interpreting others' intentions (and thus understanding the concept of an "accident" or benign intent) and generating alternative solutions to interpersonal dilemmas. On the other hand, the skills of anticipating the consequences of one's own actions (and mentally contemplating hypothetical scenarios, as in formal operations) grow during adolescence, leading one to expect declines in self-defeating aggressive behaviors, but epidemiological data indicate otherwise.

Gender differences in aggressive behavior, which surely have biological correlates (Hill, 2002), might also be explained by gender differences in SIP. Relative to girls, boys demonstrate stronger hostile attributional biases, more aggressive response-generation patterns, and greater confidence in aggressing and its consequences (Coie & Dodge, 1998). These gender-based processing differences might explain at least some of the gender differences in aggressive behavior. Furthermore, it is plausible that some of the origins of SIP patterns may lie in the same biological or neuropsychological factors that underlie aggressive behaviors (e.g., neurally based impulsivity, inability to delay gratification, attentional limits).

Examining the empirical ability of processing measures to explain patterns in the epidemiology of aggressive behavior remains a major task for future scholars. The findings of these studies will strongly influence the status of SIP models in this field.

## HOW TO DISCONFIRM THE SOCIAL INFORMATION-PROCESSING MODEL

Science proceeds both by efforts to support a theory and skeptical attempts to refute that theory. Although the overall SIP framework is not likely to be confirmed or disconfirmed by empirical studies of the sort described in this chapter, specific hypotheses can be disconfirmed by more rigorous scrutiny than the field has enjoyed to date. The following examples represent possible ways of refuting the major hypotheses of the SIP model.

Meta-analyses of findings from multiple studies can be used to summarize the empirical status of major hypotheses. de Castro, Veerman, Koops, Bosch, and Manshouwer (2002) recently completed a meta-analysis of the studies of the correlation between hostile attributional bias and aggressive behavior. Based on 41 studies with 6,017 participants, a robust significant association was found between the tendency to display a hostile attributional bias and aggressive behavior. Effect sizes ranged from small to large, and these differences could be accounted for by moderators such as the severity of aggression and the method of assessment.

Although meta-analyses can provide a control on the tendency to ignore disconfirming findings, the causal status of these correlations is far more problematic. Future studies of three kinds can provide more rigorous tests of the direction and explanation of effects. First, longitudinal studies can include more comprehensive assessment of third variables that might explain both processing patterns and aggressive behavior. A fundamental problem with descriptive longitudinal data is that it is *always* possible that an unmeasured third variable could account for the correlation between two variables. Past studies of the correlation between processing patterns and growth in aggressive behavior have controlled for prior levels of aggressive behavior (e.g., Fontaine et al., 2002), intelligence (Waldman, 1996), and demographic factors (e.g., Dodge et al., 1995). Future studies might include measures of other plausible explanatory factors, such as biological systems (e.g., brainwave activity) and psychosocial environments (e.g., neighborhood violence). Of course, even if these factors empirically account for the correlation between SIP and aggressive behavior, it remains possible that SIP is merely the proximal mechanism that relates biological and psychosocial–environment systems to aggressive behavior.

A second kind of study that should be encouraged is the experimental manipulation of children's SIP as a way of evaluating its effect on subsequent aggressive behavior. Rabiner and Coie (1989) have provided a splendid example of the laboratory manipulation of children's expectancies about interactions with peers. Future studies might attempt to manipulate other aspects of SIP, such as children's attributions of peers' intent, goals for social interaction, accessibility of possible solutions to interpersonal problems, and evaluations of the consequences of aggressing. Manipulation might occur through exposure to stimuli, verbal persuasion, or incentives. A major advantage of this kind of study is the potential for manipulating a child's SIP without simultaneously altering other factors that are usually confounded with processing (e.g., parenting, child's interactions with others). Thus, an important issue in these studies is the preciseness of the manipulation. The advantages would be lost if the manipulation were too broad or if it inadvertently confounded another factor.

Yet another kind of study that should be encouraged is the intervention experiment. Clinical interventions are not only the outcome of basic scientific research; they offer an important method for testing hypotheses about development and basic processes. The Fast Track Project (Conduct Problems Prevention Research Group, 1999) is one example of a randomized trial that tests important hypotheses from developmental theory. Unfortunately, that intervention involves numerous targets (including SIP, but also parenting, peer relations, and academic skills); thus, the effects of the intervention cannot be attributed to children's SIP in any precise way.

In sum, science will proceed best if scholars utilize multiple methods to test the hypotheses articulated here, including good-faith attempts to disconfirm the hypotheses.

## SUMMARY AND FUTURE DIRECTIONS

The literature reviewed here largely supports the three hypotheses posed at the outset of the chapter. First, children's patterns of processing social information can be measured reliably in multiple discrete processing constructs that are distinguishable from intelligence and other cognitive and emotional constructs. Furthermore, these SIP constructs grow in middle childhood and remain constant across time. Second, SIP patterns have been found to predict growth in aggressive behavior by a child, even after controlling for previous aggressive behavior and when other risk factors are correlated with SIP patterns and aggressive outcomes. Third, SIP patterns have been found to grow out of early adverse life experiences and to account for at least some of the effect of those experiences on the child's development of aggressive behavior problems.

Although the findings reported here are compelling, at least three problems remain for future inquiry. First, the measurement of SIP patterns must be improved. Measurement has been based largely on the child's verbal responses to a variety of challenging hypothetical social problems presented via cartoons, stories, or videorecorded means. Although the child's perceptions of these stimuli constitute the SIP phenomena, the child's verbal report represents the output of SIP rather than an SIP action per se. Innovative methods for assessing children's SIP are needed. These methods can be adapted from work in cognitive science and might include measurement of eye movements during presentation of visual stimuli, response times (in milliseconds) to key questions, and brain activity during SIP tasks. Crozier et al. (2002) have recently measured autonomic nervous system activity during SIP tasks as yet another window on the child's response to challenging social situations. Improved measurement of SIP actions can refine our understanding of how processing occurs as well as test alternate explanations of findings.

Second, an explanation for the relatively small proportion of variance that has been accounted for by SIP measures must be found. The hypotheses guiding SIP studies have been articulated in a strong fashion, as if these measures should account for all of the variance in aggressive behavior and all of the effect of adverse life experiences on aggressive outcomes. The empirical findings repeatedly support statistically significant effects but effect sizes that are not as large as the hypotheses would suggest. It is not clear whether this pattern is due to inadequate and incomplete measurement of SIP patterns or to other factors playing important roles in aggressive behavioral development. The former possibility is that the measurement of SIP patterns to date is insufficiently reliable and valid. Perhaps better means can be found to measure SIP patterns, as noted in the first point above, or perhaps refinements in SIP theory itself will lead to new processing constructs for measurement. The second possibility is that some aggressive behavior problems may be mediated by means other than SIP. For example, it is plausible that children who display identical SIP patterns in response to challenging social stimuli may vary in their aggressive behavior problem outcomes because of differential exposure to those challenging stimuli. Perhaps a child who would display problematic SIP in response to a provocation by peers can avoid aggressive behavior outcomes by avoiding contact with peer provocations. A comprehensive theory of individual differences in aggressive behavior problems must account for exposure to ecological circumstances that afford aggressive behavior as well as SIP responses to those circumstances. Other components of a comprehensive theory (such as biased diagnostic and adjudication practices) must also be articulated.

Finally, although some intervention experiments have tested and supported the role of SIP patterns in aggressive behavior outcomes, this literature is far from compelling. The interventions themselves have had multiple components beyond the changing of SIP patterns that reduce the precise conclusion that change in SIP is responsible for preventing aggressive behavior. Furthermore, no study has tested the hypothesis that intervention in SIP can mitigate risk that is related to a specific early life experience, such as physical maltreatment or peer social rejection. The further development of these interventions and the testing of hypotheses in intervention experiments that parse out intervention in SIP from other components of intervention await future inquiry.

## REFERENCES

Arbuckle, J. L., & Wothke, W. (1999). *AMOS 4.0 user's guide*. Chicago: Small Waters Group.

Astor, R. A. (1994). Children's moral reasoning about family and peer violence: The role of provocation and retribution. *Child Development, 65*, 1054–1067.

Baron, R. M., & Kenny, D. A. (1986). The moderator–mediator variable distinction in social psychological research: Conceptual, strategic, and statistical considerations. *Journal of Personality and Social Psychology, 51*, 1173–1182.

Bickett, L. R., Milich, R., & Brown, R. T. (1996). Attributional styles of aggressive boys and their mothers. *Journal of Abnormal Child Psychology, 24*, 457–472.

Bierman, K. L., Miller, C. L., & Stabb, S. D. (1987). Improving the social behavior and peer acceptance of rejected boys: Effects of social skill training with instructions and prohibitions. *Journal of Consulting and Clinical Psychology, 55*, 194–200.

Boldizar, J. P., Perry, D. G., & Perry, L. C. (1989). Outcome values and aggression. *Child Development, 60*, 571–579.

Cervone, D. (1999). Bottom-up explanation in personality psychology: The case of cross-situational coherence. In D. Cervone & Y. Shoda (Eds.), *The coherence of personality: Social-cognitive bases of personality consistency, variability, and organization* (pp. 303–344). New York: Guilford Press.

Coie, J. D., & Dodge, K. A. (1998). Aggression and antisocial behavior. In W. Damon (Series Ed.) & N. Eisenberg (Vol. Ed.), *Handbook of child psychology (5th ed.): Vol. 3. Social, emotional, and personality development* (pp. 779–862). New York: Wiley.

Conduct Problems Prevention Research Group. (1999). Initial impact of the Fast Track Prevention Trial for Conduct Problems: I. The high-risk sample. *Journal of Consulting and Clinical Psychology, 67*, 631–647.

Conduct Problems Prevention Research Group. (2002). Mediators of the impact of the Fast Track Prevention Program on children's adjustment outcomes. *Development and Psychopathology, 14*, 925–943.

Crick, N. R. (1995). Relational aggression: The role of intent attributions, feelings of distress, and provocation type. *Development and Psychopathology, 7*, 313–322.

Crick, N. R., & Dodge, K. A. (1994). A review and reformulation of social information-processing mechanisms in children's social adjustment. *Psychological Bulletin, 115*, 74–101.

Crozier, J., Dodge, K. A., Lansford, J. E., Pettit, G. S., Bates, J. E., Levenson, R. E., & Fontaine, R. (2002). *Autonomic nervous system and social information processing correlates of aggressive behavior in adolescence.* Manuscript submitted for publication.

de Castro, B. O., Veerman, J. W., Koops, W., Bosch, J. D., & Manshouwer, H. J. (2002). Hostile attribution of intent and aggressive behavior: A meta-analysis. *Child Development, 73*, 916–934.

Dodge, K. A. (1980). Social cognition and children's aggressive behavior. *Child Development, 51*, 162–170.

Dodge, K. A. (1986). A social information-processing model of science competence in children. In M. Perlmutter (Ed.), *Minnesota symposium in child psychology* (pp. 77–125). Hillsdale, NJ: Erlbaum.

Dodge, K. A. (1993). Social-cognitive mrechanisms in the development of conduct disorder and depression. *Annual Review of Psychology, 44*, 559–584.

Dodge, K. A., Bates, J. E., & Pettit, G. S. (1990). Mechanisms in the cycle of violence. *Science, 250*, 1678–1683.

Dodge, K. A., & Coie, J. D. (1987). Social information-processing factors in reactive and proactive aggression in children's peer groups. *Journal of Personality and Social Psychology, 53*, 1146–1158.

Dodge, K. A., Crozier, J., & Lansford, J. E. (2001). *Social information processing mediators of the effect of early physical maltreatment on the development of aggressive behavior.* Paper presented at the biennial meeting of the Society for Research in Child Development, Minneapolis, MN.

Dodge, K. A., Laird, R., Lochman, J. E., Zelli, A., & Conduct Problems Prevention Research Group. (2002). Multi-dimensional latent construct analysis of children's social information-processing patterns: Correlations with aggressive behavior problems. *Psychological Assessment.*

Dodge, K. A., Lansford, J. E., Burks, V. S., Bates, J. E., Pettit, G. S., Fontaine, R., & Price, J. M. (in press). Peer rejection and social information processing factors in the development of aggressive behavior problems in children. *Child Development.*

Dodge, K. A., McClaskey, C. L., & Feldman, E. (1985). A situational approach to the assessment of social competence in children. *Journal of Consulting and Clinical Psychology, 53*, 334–353.

Dodge, K. A., Murphy, R. R., & Buchsbaum, K. (1984). The assessment of intention-cue detection skills in children: Implications for developmental psychopathology. *Child Development, 55*, 163–173.

Dodge, K. A., Pettit, G. S., Bates, J. E., & Valente, E. (1995). Social information-processing patterns partially mediate the effect of early physical abuse on later conduct problems. *Journal of Abnormal Psychology, 104*, 632–643.

Dodge, K. A., Pettit, G. S., McClaskey, C. L., & Brown, M. (1986). Social competence in children. *Monographs of the Society for Research in Child Development, 51*(2), Serial No. 213).

Dodge, K. A., & Price, J. M. (1994). On the relation between social information processing and socially competent behavior in early school-aged children. *Child Development, 65*, 1385–1397.

Dodge, K. A., Price, J. M., Bachorowski, J. A., & Newman, J. P. (1990). Hostile attributional biases in severely aggressive adolescents. *Journal of Abnormal Psychology, 99*, 385–392.

Egan, S., Monson, T., & Perry, D. (1998). Social-cognitive influences on change in aggression over time. *Developmental Psychology, 34*, 996–1006.

Elliott, D. S. (1994). Serious violent offenders: Onset, developmental course, and termination—The American Society of Criminology 1993 presidential address. *Criminology, 32*, 1–21.

Fontaine, R. G., Burks, V. S., & Dodge, K. A. (2002). Response decision processes and externalizing behavior problems in adolescents. *Development and Psychopathology, 14*, 107–122.

Gifford-Smith, M. E., & Rabiner, D. L. (in press). Social information processing and children's social adjustment. In J. Kupersmidt & K. A. Dodge (Eds.), *Children's peer relations: From development to intervention to policy.* Washington, DC: American Psychological Association.

Graham, S., & Hudley, C. (1994). Attributions of aggressive and nonaggressive African-American male early adolescents: A study of construct accessibility. *Developmental Psychology, 30*, 365–373.

Hartup, W. W. (1983). Peer relations. In P. H. Mussen (Series Ed.) & E. M. Hetherington (Vol. Ed.), *Handbook of child psychology (4th ed.): Vol. 4. Socialization, personality, and social development* (pp. 103–196). New York: Wiley.

Hill, J. (2002). Biological, psychological and social processes in the conduct disorders. *Journal of Child Psychology and Psychiatry, 43*, 133–164.

Hubbard, J. A., Dodge, K. A., Cillessen, A. H. N., Coie, J. D., & Schwartz, D. (2001). The dyadic nature of social information processing in boys' reactive and proactive aggression. *Journal of Personality and Social Psychology, 80*(2), 268–280.

Hudley, C. A., & Graham, S. (1993). An attributional intervention to reduce peer-directed aggression among African-American boys. *Child Development, 64*, 124–138.

Huesmann, L. R. (1988). An information-processing model for the development of aggression. *Aggressive Behavior, 14*, 13–24.

Huesmann, L. R., & Guerra, N. G. (1997). Children's normative beliefs about aggression and aggressive behavior. *Journal of Personality and Social Psychology, 72*, 408–419.

Hughes, J. N., Robinson, M. S., & Moore, L. A. (1991). Children's attributions for peers' positive behaviors. *Journal of Abnormal Child Psychology, 19*, 645–657.

Kazdin, A. E., Siegel, T. C., & Bass, D. (1992). Cognitive problem-solving skills training and parent management training in the treatment of antisocial behavior in children. *Journal of Consulting and Clinical Psychology, 60*, 733–747.

Lansford, J. E., Dodge, K. A., Pettit, G. S., Bates, J. E., Crozier, J., & Kaplow, J. (2002). A 12-year prospective study of the long-term effects of early child physical maltreatment on psychological, behavioral, and academic problems in adolescence. *Archives of Pediatrics and Adolescent Medicine, 156*, 824–830.

Lochman, J. E., & Conduct Problems Prevention Research Group. (1995). Screening of child behavior problems for prevention programs at school entry. *Journal of Consulting and Clinical Psychology, 63*, 549–559.

Lochman, J. E., & Dodge, K. A. (1994). Social-cognitive processes of severely violent, moderately aggressive, and nonaggressive boys. *Journal of Consulting and Clinical Psychology, 62*, 366–374.

Lochman, J. E., & Dodge, K. A. (1998). Distorted perceptions in dyadic interactions of aggressive and nonaggressive boys: Effect of prior expectations, context, and boys' age. *Development and Psychopathology, 10*, 495–512.

Lochman, J. E., & Lenhart, L. (1995). Cognitive behavior therapy of aggressive children: Effects of schemas. In H. van Bilsen (Ed.), *Behavioral approaches for children and adolescents* (pp. 145–166). New York: Plenum Press.

Lochman, J. E., Wayland, K., & White, K. (1993). Social goals: Relationship to adolescent adjustment and to social problem solving. *Journal of Abnormal Child Psychology, 21*, 135–151.

McFall, R. M. (1982). A review and reformulation of the concept of social skills. *Behavioral Assessment, 4*, 1–33.

Milich, R., & Dodge, K. A. (1984). Social information processing patterns in child psychiatric populations. *Journal Abnormal Child Psychology, 12*, 471–490.

Nasby, W., Hayden, B., & DePaulo, B. M. (1979). Attributional bias among aggressive boys to interpret unambiguous social stimuli as displays of hostility. *Journal of Abnormal Psychology, 89*, 459–468.

Newell, A., & Simon, H. A. (1972). *Human problem solving.* Englewood Cliffs, NJ: Prentice-Hall.

Parker, J. G., & Asher, S. R. (1987). Peer relations and later personal adjustment: Are low-accepted children at risk? *Psychological Bulletin, 102*, 357–389.

Perry, D. G., Perry, L. C., & Rasmussen, P. (1986). Cognitive social learning mediators of aggression. *Child Development, 57*, 700–711.

Perry, D. G., Williard, J. C., & Perry, L. C. (1990). Peers' perceptions of the consequences that victimized children provide aggressors. *Child Development, 61*, 1310–1325.

Piaget, J. (1932/1965). *The moral judgment of the child.* New York: Free Press.

Quiggle, N., Panak, W. F., Garber, J., & Dodge, K. A. (1992). Social information processing in aggressive and depressed children. *Child Development, 63*, 1305–1320.

Rabiner, D. L., & Coie, J. D. (1989). The effect of expectancy inductions on rejected children's acceptance by unfamiliar peers. *Developmental Psychology, 25*, 450–457.

Rabiner, D. L. Lenhart, L., & Lochman, J. E. (1990). Automatic versus reflective social problem solving in relation to children's sociometric status. *Developmental Psychology, 26,* 1010–1016.

Simons, R. L., Whitbeck, L. B., Conger, R. D., & Wu, C. (1991). Intergenerational transmission of harsh parenting. *Developmental Psychology, 27,* 159–171.

Slaby, R. G., & Guerra, N. G. (1988). Cognitive mediators of aggression in adolescent offenders: I. Assessment. *Developmental Psychology, 24,* 580–588.

Spetter, D. S., LaGreca, A. M., Hogan, A., & Vaugh, S. (1992). Subgroups of rejected boys: Aggressive responses to peer conflict situations. *Journal of Clinical Child Psychology, 21,* 20–26.

Trachtenberg, S., & Viken, R. J. (1994). Aggressive boys in the classroom: Biased attributions or shared perceptions? *Child Development, 65,* 829–835.

Waas, G. A. (1988). Social attributional biases of peer-rejected and aggressive children. *Child Development, 59,* 969–992.

Waldman, I. D. (1996). Aggressive boys' hostile perceptual and response biases: The role of attention and impulsivity. *Child Development, 67,* 1015–1033.

Weiss, B., Dodge, K. A., Bates, J. E., & Pettit, G. S. (1992). Some consequences of early harsh discipline: Child aggression and a maladaptive social information processing style. *Child Development, 63,* 1321–1335.

Widom, C. S. (1989). Does violence beget violence?: A critical examination of the literature. *Psychological Bulletin, 106,* 3–28.

Youniss, J. (1980). *Parents and peers in social development.* Chicago: University of Chicago Press.

Zelli, A., & Dodge, K. A. (1999). Personality development from the bottom up. In D. Cervone & Y. Shoda (Eds.), *The coherence of personality: Social-cognitive bases of personality consistency, variability, and organization* (pp. 94–126). New York: Guilford Press.

Zelli, A., Dodge, K. A., Lochman, J. E., Laird, R. D., & Conduct Problems Prevention Research Group. (1999). The distinction between beliefs legitimizing aggression and deviant processing of social cues: Testing measurement validity and the hypothesis that biased processing mediates the effects of beliefs on aggression. *Journal of Personality and Social Psychology, 77,* 150–166.

# Genetic, Environmental, and Biological Influences

# 10

# Prefrontal Deficits
# and Antisocial Behavior
## A Causal Model

SHARON S. ISHIKAWA
ADRIAN RAINE

One fateful day in 1848, a bizarre work accident changed a man's life and ultimately—albeit belatedly—provided the inspiration for exploring the neural basis of decision making and social behavior (Damasio, Grabowski, Frank, Galaburda, & Damasio, 1994). In this well-known neurological case, Phineas Gage suffered profound personality and behavioral changes following a construction accident in which a tamping iron exploded out of a rock and pierced his brain, completely passing through his skull. The injury to the frontal region of his brain (particularly the ventromedial prefrontal cortex) transformed Gage from a responsible, intelligent, well-liked, and sociable man into someone who was markedly irresponsible, unreliable, vagrant, and prone toward excessive profanity, despite the retention of his intellect and ability to learn new information (Damasio et al., 1994).

Since that time, empirical research and detailed neurological case studies have confirmed the importance of the frontal lobes in one's ability to organize, execute, and inhibit behavior; engage in socially appropriate behavior; regulate emotions; and experience empathy (Damasio, 1994). Not surprisingly, then, disruptions of the frontal lobe—particularly the prefrontal area and its neural circuitry—have been linked to antisocial and aggressive behavior.

The current chapter posits a model implicating prefrontal structural and functional deficits as a causal mechanism of chronically dysregulated and antisocial behavior. To begin with, a brief overview of the frontal lobe and its associated functions is presented, followed by relevant research on antisocial behavior from neuropsychological testing, lesion studies, and brain imaging in both children and adults. The chapter concludes with a preliminary model of conduct problems beginning in childhood and persisting through adulthood. Although this chapter centers exclusively on the functions of the prefrontal region, several limits should be stated up front. First, it is recognized that the prefrontal region is not the sole neuroanatomical area implicated in antisocial behavior. Second, all studies on the prefrontal region and antisocial behavior conducted to date have been cross-sectional. Thus, it is recognized that the developmental model of antisocial behavior presented here is highly speculative.

## INTRODUCTION TO THE PREFRONTAL REGIONS OF THE FRONTAL LOBE

When referring to location and directionality within the brain, standard nomenclature is used. The terms "dorsal" and "ventral" represent location along a vertical axis, with *dorsal* referring to "superior or toward the top of the head" and *ventral* referring to "inferior or down toward the jaw." The terms "medial" and "lateral" represent location along a horizontal axis extending between the ears, with *lateral* referring to the sides or surface of the brain and *medial* referring to the middle portion deep within the brain. The terms "rostral" and "caudal" are also located on a horizontal axis, although this axis extends from the front to the back of the head (i.e., *rostral* = front, or toward the nose; *caudal* = toward the back of the head).

The frontal lobe encompasses approximately one-third of the human brain and supports many complex cognitive functions. It is located rostral to the central sulcus and dorsal to the lateral sulcus (see Figure 10.1A). Parcellation of the functional regions of the frontal lobe can be done in one of two ways: cytoarchitectonic (i.e., based on cellular structure) and topographical (i.e., based on physical landmarks). Using cytoarchitectonic features, the frontal lobe can be functionally segmented into motor, premotor, prefrontal, and paralimbic areas (see Figure 10.1A and 10.1B). The first three areas are delineated on the surface of, and extend into the medial portion of, the frontal lobe. In contrast, the paralimbic area is located solely within the medial portion of the frontal lobe.

Although cytoarchitectonic typing methods offer more precision, they are highly invasive. Thus, parcellation of the frontal lobe in living human subjects is usually based on topographical landmarks. Based on this segmentation method, the prefrontal area is typically separated into the dorsolateral prefrontal, orbitofrontal, and medial cortices (defined below). These three cortices are part of frontal–subcortical circuits that integrate information from throughout the brain to organize behavior (Cummings,

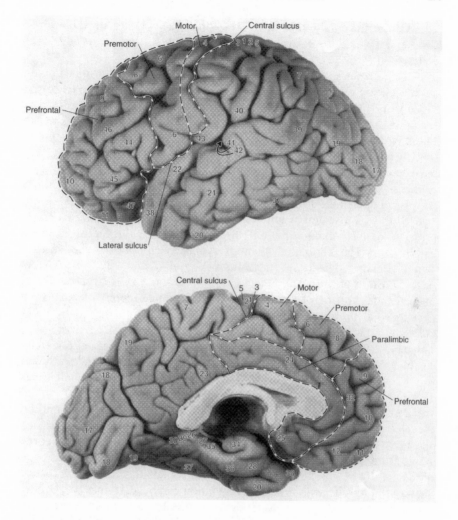

FIGURE 10.1. Delineation of subdivisions of the human frontal lobe as seen in left lateral (A) and right medial (B) views. Numbers indicate the approximate location of Brodmann's areas. From Kaufer and Lewis (1999). Copyright 1999 by The Guilford Press. Reprinted by permission.

1995). When the studies cited below segmented the prefrontal area, they generally used this classification system. One should note, however, that in contrast to the term "dorsolateral prefrontal cortex," which is restricted solely to the lateral convexity (i.e., Brodmann's area 46 and part of area 9; see Figure 10.1A; Kaufer & Lewis, 1999), the more general term "prefrontal cortex" refers to a larger area including the dorsolateral prefrontal cortex, ventrolateral prefrontal cortex (i.e., Brodmann's area 44; see Figure

10.1A), and the contiguous medial prefrontal regions (i.e., Brodmann's areas 9 and 10, and the rostral portion of area 32; see Figure 10.1B; Kaufer & Lewis, 1999).

The *dorsolateral prefrontal* cortex (DLPFC) is located in the superior, lateral portion of the prefrontal area (Brodmann's area 46 and part of area 9; see Figure 10.1A), and is extensively interconnected with the cortical association areas and the orbitofrontal cortex. It has traditionally been associated with information-processing skills such as working memory and executive functions (Cummings, 1995; Damasio & Anderson, 1993). With regard to specific working memory processes, functional brain imaging studies have found that the DLPFC appears to be necessary for the manipulation and encoding of information (D'Esposito, Postle, & Rypma, 2000). The DLPFC is also important for the maintenance of information in the presence of distracting stimuli (D'Esposito et al., 2000; Stern, Sherman, Kirchhoff, & Hasselmo, 2001), and is hypothesized to be involved in emotion processing (Davidson, Jackson, & Kalin, 2000). The *medial* (i.e., rostral portion of the paralimbic area) prefrontal cortex is largely made up of the caudal portion of Brodmann's area 32 (which represents part of the ventromedial prefrontal cortex) and extends back into the anterior cingulate (i.e., Brodmann's area 24; see Figure 10.1B; Kaufer & Lewis, 1999). The medial prefrontal cortex interconnects with the dorsolateral prefrontal cortex and posteriorly projects to the hypothalamus and amygdala. It subserves motivational processes and maintenance of activity (Cummings, 1995). The *orbitofrontal* cortex is located just above the orbits, or eye sockets, and extends along the ventral portion of the prefrontal region into the ventral/caudal portion of the paralimbic region (i.e., Brodmann's areas 11, 12, 47, and 25; see Figure 10.1A and 10.1B). The orbitofrontal cortex significantly interconnects with the temporal pole (i.e., Brodmann's area 38 on Figure 10.1A and 10.1B) and amygdala. It regulates autonomic reactivity, social and self-awareness, and regulation of affect (Damasio & Anderson, 1993; LaPierre, Braun, & Hodgins, 1995). It also contains the remaining part of the ventromedial prefrontal cortex, which is implicated in risk-related and emotion-based decision making (Bechara, Damasio, Damasio, & Lee, 1999). Although response inhibition has traditionally been ascribed to the orbitofrontal cortex, recent imaging research has found that this executive function is subserved by a wide frontal neural network where the dorsal anterior cingulate is responsible for monitoring and decision formation, and the lateral prefrontal cortex (i.e., dorso- and ventrolateral PFC) is responsible for actual response inhibition (Elliot, Rubinsztein, Sahakian, & Dolan, 2000; Liddle, Kiehl, & Smith, 2001).

Although much remains to be learned about its developmental course, the human brain appears to go through an extensive period of maturation beginning *in utero* and extending into at least early adulthood. At the simplest level, the brain consists of gray and white matter. *Gray matter* refers to neurons and unmyelinated fibers (i.e., cell body, dendrites, presynaptic terminals) that, in response to environmental stimulation, either initiate or conduct electrical signals. *White matter* refers to the myelinated axons that project out of neurons and connect different regions of the cerebral cortex to each other, to other parts of the brain, and to the spinal cord. *Myelin*, or the fatty sheath surrounding the axon, serves to increase the speed at which the electrical signals from the cell body are conducted. White matter increases steadily from early childhood through early adulthood (i.e., ages 4–22; Giedd et al., 1999), with some indication that the frontal lobes generally complete myelination last (Sowell, Thompson, Holmes, Jernigan, & Toga, 1999). In contrast, recent research indicates that frontal gray matter shows a growth spurt during the first 2 years of life (Matsuzawa et al., 2001) and again in preadolescence (Giedd et al., 1999), but then decreases between adolescence and early adulthood as white matter significantly increases (Giedd et al., 1999; Sowell et al., 1999). It has been speculated that the structural changes in frontal gray and white matter improve efficiency of frontal lobe function by selectively pruning away unused synapses and by improving the conductance of electrical signals among active neurons, respectively (Giedd et al., 1999).

Human brain structure and function has been assessed via direct and indirect methods. Historically, neuropsychological testing has been used to infer frontal dysfunction. The sensitivity of the tests (e.g., Wisconsin Card Sorting Test) to frontal dysfunction has typically been validated in studies comparing test performance of selective brain lesion patients to that of normal controls and/or nonfrontal brain lesion patients. Nevertheless, performance on these neuropsychological tests can still be significantly affected by impairment of other brain regions. Conversely, adequate test performance may be achieved despite frontal damage. Recently, more direct measures of human frontal structure and function have been possible through neuroimaging. Techniques such as magnetic resonance imaging (MRI), functional MRI (fMRI), and positron emission technology (PET) allow one to directly assess the structure and function of specific brain regions, which has revolutionized the study of human behavior.

## EMPIRICAL SUPPORT FOR A PREFRONTAL DYSFUNCTION–ANTISOCIAL BEHAVIOR ASSOCIATION

### Executive Function Deficits

*Executive functions* refer to a cluster of higher order cognitive processes involving initiation, planning, cognitive flexibility, abstraction, and decision making that together allow the execution of contextually appropriate behavior (Spreen & Strauss, 1998). When executive dysfunction is observed, the prefrontal cortex is traditionally thought to be involved, although dysfunction may reflect some abnormality in one or more of the neural pathways connected to the prefrontal cortex (Lezak, 1995). In addition, executive function deficits are not always accompanied by measurable frontal neuroanatomical deficits.

Reviews of research on child and adolescent samples suggest that antisocial behavior is characterized by neuropsychological impairments (Moffitt, 1993; Raine, 1993), with some arguing that antisocial children and delinquents have a specific deficit in executive functions (Lueger & Gill, 1990; Moffitt, 1993). Executive dysfunction is hypothesized to relate to antisocial and/or aggressive behavior by decreasing behavioral inhibition and impairing one's ability to generate socially acceptable responses in challenging situations (Giancola, 1995). Despite a strong theoretical base for postulating frontal dysfunction in antisocial persons, a qualitative review of executive function deficits in antisocial children determined that findings across studies are inconsistent (Teicher & Golden, 2000). A recent meta-analysis of executive dysfunction and antisocial behavior, however, found that overall effect sizes for conduct disorder and juvenile delinquency were small to medium and large in magnitude, respectively (i.e., Cohen's $d$ = 0.40 and 0.86) and statistically significant (Morgan & Lilienfeld, 2000). Nevertheless, the magnitude of association between the constructs (i.e., executive dysfunction and antisocial behavior subtypes) suggests that other factors affect and/or account for this relationship, particularly with regard to conduct disorder.

In particular, debate has emerged as to whether the association between conduct problems and executive dysfunction is attributable to attention-deficit disorder (ADD; e.g., Clark, Prior, & Kinsella, 2000), which is frequently comorbid in antisocial children. There is clearly strong evidence linking ADD to executive deficits and attention-deficit/hyperactivity disorder (ADHD; Barkley, 2000). Nevertheless, recent studies controlling for diagnostic comorbidity and other methodological issues generally support the executive dysfunction hypothesis in aggressive antisocial individuals. Poorer executive functions are correlated with increased antisocial aggressive behavior in preschoolers (Hughes, White, Sharpen, & Dunn, 2000), and differentiate children with conduct disorder or aggressive children from nonaggressive controls (Seguin, Pihl, Harden, Tremblay, & Boulerice, 1995; Seguin, Boulerice, Harden, Tremblay, & Pihl, 1999; Toupin, Dery, Pauze, Mercier, & Fortin, 2000). Although the majority of studies using child samples only look at boys, similar findings of executive dysfunction have been observed in aggressive girls (Giancola, Mezzich, & Tarter, 1998a, Giancola, Mezzich, & Tarter, 1998b).

Because earlier studies on executive function are limited by their failure to account for third variable effects, it is important to note that the executive dysfunction in these studies was observed after controlling for potential confounds such as ADHD (Seguin et al., 1999; Toupin et al., 2000), family socioeconomie status (SES; Toupin et al., 2000), hard-to-manage temperament (Hughes et al., 2000), IQ (Krakowski et al., 1997; Seguin et al., 1995; Seguin et al., 1999), early family psychosocial adversity (Seguin et al., 1995; Seguin et al., 1999), and age, race, gender, and other measures of neurocognitive function (Krakowski et al., 1997; Seguin et al., 1995; Seguin et al., 1999). Nevertheless, it is also important to note that executive dysfunction in children still appears to be strongest in those with ADHD or with ADHD and conduct disorder rather than in those with conduct disorder alone (Speltz, DeKlyen, Calderon, Greenberg, & Fisher, 1999).

Among adults, executive dysfunction is also related to antisocial behavior, again with the most consistent findings observed for aggressive forms of antisocial behavior. Neuropsychological (and neurological) assessments of frontal dysfunction relate fairly consistently to the commission of violent crimes by adult males (e.g., Blake, Pincus, & Buckner, 1995; Langevin, Ben-Aron, Wortzman, Dickey, & Handy, 1987). Adult psychiatric inpatients with a history of community violence exhibit significantly greater executive and psychomotor dysfunction than inpatients without such a history (Krakowski et al., 1997). Similarly, poor executive functioning in males drawn from the community is correlated with aggressive behavior (Giancola & Zeichner, 1994) and with DSM-III criteria for antisocial personality disorder (Deckel, Hesselbrock, & Bauer, 1996). Although executive dysfunction has been inconsistently observed in psychopathic males (see Schalling & Rosen, 1968, and Gorenstein, 1982, for significant effects, and Hare, 1984, and Hoffman, Hall, & Bartsch, 1987, for null findings), there is some suggestion that executive dysfunction in psychopaths may be specific to neuropsychological tests theoretically linked to orbitofrontal–ventromedial function (Lapierre et al., 1995).

The observation that antisocial children and adults often suffer from executive dysfunction as measured by traditional neuropsychological tests may be attributable, at least in part, to dysfunction in the prefrontal regions that subserve these cognitive processes. The performance of antisocial individuals on various neuropsychological tests suggests that they suffer from response disinhibition, an impaired ability to organize behavior and/or integrate information on complex tasks, and difficulty with adapting to changing environmental contingencies. These results may provide an experimental correlate for the recidivistic criminal behavior and impulsivity that is characteristic of chronically antisocial individuals. However, one should keep in mind that executive function measures are subserved by multiple prefrontal as well as nonfrontal brain regions. Thus, demonstration of prefrontal dysfunction cannot necessarily be determined by poor neuropsychological test performance alone.

## Clinical Evidence: Head Injury and Lesion Studies

In addition to the neuropsychological studies described above, research looking at behavioral changes in individuals who have experienced head injuries or frontal brain lesions provides evidence that frontal damage can cause antisocial behavior. Studies with children generally find an onset of conduct disorder and externalizing behavior problems following head trauma (Butler, Rourke, Fuerst, & Fisk, 1997; Hux, Bond, Skinner, Belau, & Sanger, 1998; Max et al., 1998; Mittenberg, Wittner, & Miller, 1997). However, a few studies have also found an increased likelihood of internalizing behavior problems (e.g., Max et al., 1998), and at least one other has found that delinquents are not statistically more likely to suffer from head injury than are nondelinquents (Hux et al., 1998). Thus, a clear relationship between the occurrence of head injury and externalizing behavior problems has not been established. It should be noted, however, that head injury does not always result in frontal damage. As such, contradictory findings do not necessarily attenuate a prefrontal dysfunction hypothesis of antisocial behavior. Interestingly, parents of delinquent children are also much more likely to report that behavior problems began after head trauma compared to parents of nondelinquents (Hux et al., 1998). However, it is unclear whether this finding was the result of reporting bias on the part of the parents or other intervening variables (e.g., unstructured home environment or poorer medical care or rehabilitation services for families whose children developed problems).

Consistent with the head injury literature, case studies of individuals suffering lesions to the prefrontal cortex indicate that such damage causes long-term deleterious alterations in behavior. In a report on nine children who suffered frontal lesions within the first 10 years of life, seven were diagnosed with conduct disorder and the remaining two exhibited significantly impulsive, labile, and/or uncontrollable behavior post-lesion onset (Pennington & Bennetto, 1993). Two healthy toddlers who suffered selective lesions to the prefrontal cortex in the first 16 months of life (i.e., bilateral polar–ventromedial, right polar–medial–dorsal) initially displayed minor disruptive and impulsively aggressive behavior within a few years post-lesion onset that eventually escalated into severe antisocial and irresponsible behavior by early adulthood (Anderson, Bechara, Damasio, Tranel, & Damasio, 1999; Anderson, Damasio, Tranel, & Damasio, 2000). At a follow-up in their early 20s, both subjects exhibited impaired autonomic functioning in risky situations, executive functions, emotion regulation, decision making, and feedback learning (Anderson et al., 1999), all of which have been linked to orbitofrontal–ventromedial damage (Damasio, 1994). This is not to say, however, that all frontal lesions inevitably result in antisocial behavior. Although a socially and academically well-adjusted 7-year-old boy who suffered a lesion to his right dorsolateral prefrontal cortex began to experience social and academic problems, at 4 years postonset he exhibited no specific problems with anger or hostility (Eslinger, Biddle, Pennington, & Page, 1999).

Similarly, lesion research with adults demonstrates that significant damage to both gray and white matter within the prefrontal region can result in the development of an antisocial, pseudopsychopathic personality (Giancola, 1995) or aggressive behavioral changes (Anderson et al., 1999; Blair & Cipolotti, 2000). In addition to these changes in antisocial behavior, when the damage is localized to the orbitofrontal and/or ventromedial sectors of the frontal lobe, patients also exhibit disinhibition (Blair & Cipolotti, 2000; Dimitrov, Phipps, Zahn, & Grafman, 1999; Mataro et al., 2001), as well as attention deficits and/or autonomic hyporesponsivity to socially meaningful events (Blair & Cipolotti, 2000; Damasio, 1994; Damasio, Tranel, & Damasio, 1990; Dimitrov et al., 1999). A quasi-experimental group study found that ventromedial patients exhibit significantly greater aggressive, violent, and/or antisocial behavior than do nonfrontal brain lesion patients and nonlesion controls (Grafman et al., 1996). Of these ventromedial patients, those with focal frontal medial lesions are generally aware of and able to self-report the increase in their own aggressive behavior (as reported by a family member), whereas those with focal orbitofrontal lesions are unaware of the behavioral change reported by a family member. It should be noted, however, that despite the onset of socially inappropriate behavior, not all adult frontal lesion patients have demonstrated a specific increase in aggressive antisocial behavior (i.e., Phineas Gage; patient MGS as reported by Dimitrov et al., 1999). Interestingly, however, both of these individuals suffered from the frontal lesions in early adulthood and MGS, in particular, was rehabilitated and cared for in a structured supportive environment.

Overall, then, clinically based research provides support for the notion that brain damage, particularly to the polar, orbitofrontal, and/or medial cortices of the frontal lobes, contributes to the development of antisocial behavior. In addition, inferences drawn from the above studies tentatively suggest that biological and social risk factors may interact in the development of antisocial behavior. That is, head injury may be more likely to result in antisocial behavior when the injury occurs in an environment that is less equipped to medically, behaviorally, and/or socially rehabilitate the injured child. Similarly, the small sample of lesion studies tentatively suggest that damage to the prefrontal cortex—particularly the polar, orbital frontal, and ventromedial cortices—is more likely to result in antisocial and/or aggressive behavior when the damage (1) occurs very early in life before social and moral behavior has had an opportunity to be internalized, and/or (2) when the injured individual does not have a social and instrumental support system to provide structure following the frontal lesion. Obviously, however, these are speculations based on extremely small, specialized samples of neurological patients that require more systematic evaluation in future research.

## Frontal Deficits in Adults: Evidence from Neuroimaging Studies

The advent of noninvasive brain imaging has revolutionized the study of brain–behavior relationships by making it possible to examine brain structure and function directly in developmentally antisocial individuals. Reviews of imaging studies conducted through 1994—while showing variability in findings—concur that violent offenders have functional deficits to the anterior regions of the brain, particularly the frontal region (Henry & Moffitt, 1997; Raine, 1993; Raine & Buchsbaum, 1996). Since then, research utilizing a variety of imaging techniques has continued to find frontal deficits in various classes of antisocial individuals. Alcoholics with antisocial personality disorder (APD) show significantly reduced frontal regional cerebral blood flow (rCBF) compared to alcoholics with non-APD personality disorders and nonalcoholic controls (Kuruoglu et al., 1996). Compared to healthy controls, pretrial forensic patients arrested for impulsive violent offenses exhibit reduced cerebral blood flow in the frontal and temporal lobes (Soderstrom, Tullberg, Wikkelsoe, Ekholm, & Forsman, 2000). Similarly, impulsive, affective murderers show reduced glucose metabolism in the prefrontal cortex relative to predatory, instrumental murderers (Raine et al., 1998).

Consistent with the implication that prefrontal deficits may particularly characterize impulsive behavior, research has found that—compared to normal controls—repetitively violent psychiatric inpatients have reduced neuronal density and abnormal phosphate metabolism in the prefrontal cortex (Critcheley et al., 2000), and reduced glucose metabolism in bilateral prefrontal and medial temporal regions (Volkow et al., 1995). The frequency of aggressive, impulsive acts is also associated with reduced glucose metabolism in the frontal cortex of personality-disordered patients (Goyer et al., 1994). In addition, reduced prefrontal metabolic activity has been observed when violent psychiatric patients are compared to nonviolent psychiatric controls (Amen, Stubblefield, Carmichael, & Thisted, 1996). Thus, these frontal and frontotemporal deficits do not simply appear to be an artifact of comparing patients to normal controls.

In addition to findings with criminal offenders and psychiatric patients, evidence for frontal dysfunction has been observed in neurological patients after controlling for a variety of demographic and premorbid functioning factors (e.g., age, gender, SES, premorbid education, Mini Mental Status Exam (MMSE) score, severity of cognitive impairment, current medication use; Hirono, Mega, Dinov, Mishkin, & Cummings, 2000; Miller, Darby, Benson, & Cummings, 1998). For example, repetitive violence in patients with temporal lobe epilepsy is related to frontal abnormalities

(Woermann et al., 2000). Patients diagnosed with frontotemporal dementia are significantly more likely to engage in inappropriate aggressive, sexual, and antisocial behavior than are patients diagnosed with nonfrontal forms of dementia (Miller et al., 1998). Similarly, aggressive dementia patients show significant hypoperfusion in the left and right dorsolateral frontal areas (as well as in the left anterior temporal cortex and the right superior parietal areas) compared to nonaggressive dementia patients (Hirono et al., 2000).

Contrary to expectation, atypical frontal function in antisocial populations has sometimes been characterized by *excessive* rather than *reduced* frontal activation. Drug-abusing psychopaths—compared to nonpsychopaths—show increased regional cerebral blood flow bilaterally in frontotemporal regions during the processing of emotional words (Intrator et al., 1997). In addition, during the acquisition phase of an aversive conditioning paradigm, antisocial individuals—relative to nonantisocial controls—show atypical signal increases in the dorsolateral prefrontal cortex and amygdala (Schneider et al., 2000). Interestingly, the antisocial groups do not differ from controls on behavioral measures of either task. Thus, it is speculated that the increased frontal activity reflects burdensome task demands resulting from the antisocial individuals' impairment in automatically processing the socially relevant stimuli employed as activation tasks in these studies (i.e., emotional cues, aversive smells). Prefrontal dysfunction that is associated with deficits in emotion recognition/responsivity or aversive conditioning may contribute to the development of antisocial behavior by interfering with the socialization process. In contrast, the hypoactivity that was observed at rest or during cognitive tasks in the other imaging studies cited above may represent an alternative neurobiological pathway underpinning antisocial behavior. There has been extensive support for an autonomic underarousal hypothesis of antisocial behavior (Raine, 1993) that may reflect central nervous system functioning (i.e., autonomic underarousal and antisocial behavior have each been linked to deficits in the orbitofrontal cortex, dorsolateral prefrontal cortex, anterior cingulate, hypothalamus, and amygdala; Ishikawa & Raine, 2002). It has been hypothesized that underarousal is an uncomfortable psychophysiological state that predisposes to antisocial behavior by encouraging the individual to seek out stimulation in an effort to boost psychophysiological arousal (Raine, Venables, & Mednick, 1997).

In addition to the body of functional imaging studies that utilize hospitalized or incarcerated subjects, initial research provides evidence that antisocial individuals from the community exhibit structural prefrontal deficits. Males who meet DSM-IV criteria for APD demonstrate significantly reduced prefrontal gray matter volume compared to healthy controls, substance-dependent non-APD controls, and psychiatric controls matched on affective and schizophrenia-spectrum disorders (Raine, Lencz, Bihrle,

LaCasse, & Colletti, 2000). Thus, prefrontal deficits observed in the above studies should not automatically be dismissed as an artifact of institutionalization or substance abuse, either of which may adversely affect brain structure and/or function.

Finally, a small body of brain imaging research suggests that the prefrontal deficit–antisocial behavior link may depend on social factors. Specifically, prefrontal deficits may be most pronounced in violent individuals who have been spared exposure to significant psychosocial stress. When Raine and colleagues divided a psychiatric forensic sample into subjects who had and who had not experienced early psychosocial deprivation, the authors found that nondeprived murderers show significantly reduced right orbitofrontal functioning relative to deprived murderers (Raine, Stoddard, Bihrle, & Buchsbaum, 1998). They speculated that individuals without a psychosocial "push" toward violence require a greater neurobiological "push." This is not to say, however, that violent individuals who suffer early trauma do not show brain deficits. Other research from the same laboratory found that violent offenders who were severely abused in childhood showed greater abnormality in their overall (i.e., not specifically prefrontal) brain activation patterns than did nonabused violent offenders (Raine et al., 2001). Thus, prefrontal deficits and physical abuse may independently and additively relate to later aggressive behavior. Future research should attempt to elucidate the circumstances in which biological and social factors interact with each other to elicit chronic antisocial behavior problems and those circumstances in which they exert independent influences on its development.

## THEORIES THAT ACCOUNT FOR THE RELATIONSHIP BETWEEN SPECIFIC PREFRONTAL CORTICAL AREAS AND ANTISOCIAL BEHAVIOR

Although the overall body of research has implicated prefrontal damage or dysfunction in antisocial behavior, what remains to be elucidated are the mechanisms and processes through which such dysfunction predisposes to significant forms of antisocial behavior. Within the past few years, at least two mechanisms have been delineated. First, the dorsolateral prefrontal cortex is thought to play a significant role in antisocial behavior. This prefrontal region was initially thought to contribute to antisocial behavior in one of two ways. On the one hand, it was speculated that the dorsolateral prefrontal cortex specifically subserves aggressive antisocial behavior, whereas the orbitofrontal cortex underpins nonaggressive antisocial behavior (Giancola, 1995). However, subsequent frontal lesion studies failed to confirm this hypothesis (e.g., Eslinger et al., 1999), and more recent functional imaging studies have observed that the orbitofrontal cortex is involved in angry affect (Pietrini, Guazzelli, Basso, Jaffe, & Grafman,

2000). On the other hand, damage to the dorsolateral prefrontal cortex—which would theoretically account for the executive dysfunction observed in antisocial populations—is thought to play a role in the maintenance of recidivistic antisocial behavior, which could be regarded as perseverative behavior (Raine, 2002). In addition, the prefrontal cortex is part of a neural circuit that plays a central role in fear conditioning and stress responsivity (Hugdahl, 1998; Frysztak & Neafsey, 1991), and a recent human fMRI study has identified the dorsolateral prefrontal cortex as an important component in the neural circuitry underlying aversive conditioning (Schneider et al., 2000). A number of psychophysiological experiments have repeatedly confirmed that antisocial groups show poor fear conditioning (Raine, 1993), which, in turn, is thought to result in poor conscience development (Raine, 1993). Thus, individuals with prefrontal dysfunction resulting in poor autonomic responsiveness would be less susceptible to socializing punishments, thus predisposing them to engage in antisocial behavior.

Alternatively, Damasio has presented a theory that integrates neuroanatomy with psychophysiological functioning (Damasio et al., 2000). He posits that the prefrontal cortex regulates behavior, in part, through the generation of somatic markers (i.e., skin conductance and other autonomic responses to aversive stimuli). Somatic markers, in turn, alert individuals to risky or threatening situations, thus allowing them to maintain homeostasis by intuitively guiding their behavior toward advantageous decision making (Damasio, 1994; Damasio et al., 2000). The original model, based on patients with selective lesions (Bechara et al., 1999; Bechara, Damasio, & Damasio, 2000; Bechara, Tranel, Damasio, & Damasio, 1996), placed primary emphasis on the ventromedial prefrontal cortex. However, subsequent research has implicated the amygdala, which is interconnected with the orbitofrontal and ventromedial prefrontal cortices (Bechara et al., 1999), as well as the connections between the ventromedial prefrontal cortex and other subcortical structures involved in emotion and homeostasis regulation (e.g., cingulate, hypothalamus, motor cortex, dorsal pons, midbrain, insula, cerebellum; Damasio et al., 2000; Davidson, Putnam, & Larson, 2000).

Drawing upon this theory and other related research, scientists have postulated that the risk for antisocial behavior may be elevated when an individual is unable to generate or appreciate the significance of somatic markers due to prefrontal abnormalities (i.e., skin conductance is related to the orbitofrontal and ventromedial prefrontal cortex; Critchley, Elliott, Mathias, & Dolan, 2000; Damasio, 1994). The resulting impairment in being able to exercise sound judgment and make appropriate decisions in risky situations would likely contribute to the impulsivity, rule breaking, recklessness, and irresponsibility characteristic of APD. In support of this theory, studies have not only found that pseudopsychopathic patients with ventromedial and/or subcortical damage fail to give anticipatory autonomic responses when selecting risky choice options (Bechara et al., 1999), but that they continue to perseverate with bad choices even after being able to articulate the more advantageous response option (Bechara et al., 1997). Developmentally, psychopathic boys have shown similar impairment in risk-related decision making compared to nonpsychopathic controls (Blair, Colledge, & Mitchell, 2001; although see Schmitt, Brinkley, & Newman, 1999, for failure to find an effect in psychopathic adults). Orbitofrontal functioning has also been associated with various aspects of addictive behavior and impaired decision making in substance abusers, many of whom met diagnostic criteria for APD (London, Ernst, Grant, Bonson, & Weinstein, 2000).

In all likelihood, however, both prefrontal cortices play a role in the onset and persistence of antisocial behavior. Their impact on antisocial behavior may occur on a relatively independent basis (e.g., orbitofrontal dysfunction decreases inhibition of aggressive or hostile impulses generated by limbic dysfunction and/or environmental triggers, whereas dorsolateral dysfunction contributes to perseveration of previously punished behavior). In addition, dysfunction in one or both of these cortices may interact and disrupt a complex cognitive function that is subserved by both prefrontal sectors. It has been suggested, for example, that dysfunction in either the dorsolateral or the orbitofrontal cortex may render one unable to utilize affective information by interfering with *affective working memory*, or the ability to use emotional memory to guide current behavior based on anticipation of future consequences (Damasio, 1994; Davidson et al., 2000; London et al., 2000). Such impairment could result in chronic antisocial behavior or repetitive violence by impeding the development of a social conscience.

## EARLY HEALTH FACTORS HYPOTHESIZED TO CONTRIBUTE TO PREFRONTAL DAMAGE

Although there are discrepant findings, the overall research to date can leave little doubt that—at least in some circumstances—damage to the prefrontal cortex can result in antisocial behavior and pseudopsychopathic personality changes. The lesion studies cited above clearly demonstrate that focal neurological insult may cause such deleterious changes. In addition, a growing body of research suggests that other, relatively more common early health factors may increase the risk of brain damage or maturational delays. Three common factors (i.e., birth complications, minor physical anomalies [MPAs], prenatal nicotine exposure) are briefly reviewed below.

Several studies have shown that the combination of birth complications—which significantly increase the risk of brain damage—and psychosocial deficits such as maternal rejection within the first year of life (Raine,

Brennan, & Mednick, 1994), a disadvantaged family environment (Piquero & Tibbetts, 1999), or poor parenting (Hodgins, Kratzer, & McNeil, 2001) significantly increase the risk for developing serious delinquent, criminal, or violent behavior in adulthood (although see Laucht et al., 2000, for failure to replicate this biosocial interaction). Birth complications such as anoxia (i.e., lack of oxygen), pre-eclampsia (i.e., hypertension leading to anoxia), and forceps delivery may be one of several early sources of brain dysfunction observed in antisocial groups. When combined with a risky environment that fails to foster socialization through appropriate attachment or parenting and disciplinary practices, the predisposition toward engaging in later crime and violence may be substantially elevated. It should be noted, however, that birth complications would not necessarily specifically affect the prefrontal cortex but would involve multiple brain sites.

In addition to birth complications, MPAs are considered indicators of fetal neural maldevelopment toward the end of the first 3 months of pregnancy. As such, they may be viewed as an indirect marker of abnormal brain development. Although MPAs such as low-seated ears, adherent ear lobes, and a furrowed tongue may, in part, have a genetic basis, they may also be caused by environmental factors such as anoxia, bleeding, and infection that adversely affect the fetus (Guy, Majorski, Wallace, & Guy, 1983).

MPAs are associated with heightened antisocial behavior, increased aggression, and/or difficult temperament in preschool-age boys (Paulus & Martin, 1986; Waldrop, Bell, McLaughlin, & Halverson, 1978), elementary-school-age boys (Halverston & Victor, 1976), and 17-year-old males (Arseneault, Tremblay, Boulerice, Seguin, & Saucier, 2000). As with the findings for birth complications, several studies have also found that MPAs interact with the presence of a negative psychosocial factor (e.g., family adversity, unstable home) in order to elicit criminal behavior (Brennan, Mednick, & Raine, 1997; Pine et al., 1996). An issue that remains to be clarified is whether MPAs are particularly likely to lead to conduct problems or whether they reflect a risk factor for disruptive behavior in general. Although MPAs have generally been associated with behavior disorders in children drawn from the normal population (Pomeroy, Sprafkin, & Gadow, 1988), at least one study failed to observe a link between MPAs and conduct disorder within a larger group of emotionally disturbed children (Pomeroy et al., 1988).

Finally, a series of recent methodologically strong studies has established that individuals who experience prenatal exposure to cigarette smoke are at increased risk for developing later conduct problems. Children of mothers who smoked while pregnant were twice as likely to have a criminal record by young adulthood (Rantakallio, Laara, Isohanni, & Moilanen, 1992), with some suggestion that the increased risk may be specific to violent offending (Brennan, Gerkin, & Mednick, 1999; Rasanen et al., 1999). Similarly, at least three studies have found a two- to fourfold increase risk for conduct disorder in the children of mothers who smoked during pregnancy (Fergusson, Woodward, & Horwood, 1998; Wakschlag et al., 1997; Weissman, Warner, Wickramaratne, & Kandel, 1999). As with the other health concerns reported above, interaction effects have been observed between prenatal cigarette exposure and factors such as delivery complications (Brennan et al., 1999), teenage pregnancy, single-parent family, unwanted pregnancy, and/or developmental motor lags (Rasanen et al., 1999).

The link between maternal smoking during pregnancy and antisocial behavior may be mediated by brain deficits resulting from prenatal nicotine exposure. Animal research has clearly demonstrated the neurotoxic effects of carbon monoxide and nicotine, both of which are contained in cigarette smoke (Olds, 1997). Prenatal nicotine exposure, even at relatively low levels, disrupts the development of the noradrenergic neurotransmitter system (Levin, Wilkerson, Jones, Christopher, & Briggs, 1996). The majority of norandrenergic neurons are located in the brainstem, which densely project to the prefrontal cortex and facilitate enhanced alertness and performance of executive functions (Feifel, 1999). Thus, prenatal exposure to smoking may indirectly and deleteriously affect the functioning of the child's developing prefrontal cortex. When further compounded by a chaotic or deprived environment that is unable to facilitate compensatory neuronal organization and functional skills, the risk for antisocial behavior problems is likely to be exacerbated.

## FRONTAL FUNCTIONS AND ANTISOCIAL BEHAVIOR: A DEVELOPMENTAL MODEL

As the above review demonstrates, several sources of data (i.e., neuropsychology, lesion studies, imaging) link prefrontal damage to antisocial behavior. Although each source suffers from certain methodological limitations, the fact that all three fields converge on the same conclusion provides compelling support for a prefrontal dysfunction hypothesis of antisocial behavior. In addition, imaging research has begun to delineate the normal maturation process of the human brain. When this evidence is considered together, the opportunity arises to generate a preliminary model that incorporates neuroanatomical and social maturational processes in relation to antisocial behavior subtypes. Although a number of different classifications of antisocial behavior have been put forth, one particularly useful distinction has been that of "life-course-persistent" versus "adolescent-limited" antisocial individuals (Moffitt, 1993). Life-course-persistent antisocial behavior is stable across the lifespan and typically begins in childhood or early adolescence. In contrast, adolescent-limited antisocial behavior refers to "typical" delinquent acts limited to the adolescent developmental period. Moffitt argues that life-course-persistent antisocials, who engage in more serious delinquent and antisocial activities, have a biological basis to their behavior, whereas their adolescent-limited counterparts experience more of a social push into delinquency.

Up through adolescence, children live in a relatively structured environment where complex life-changing plans and decisions are left to the responsibility of their caretakers. Toddlers—who are at the stage in life when the developmental norm is to engage in aggressive behavior such as hitting, biting, and excessive temper tantrums (Tremblay, 2001)—begin to learn to inhibit aggression and engage in more prosocial behavior that eventually facilitates peer interactions and the development of friendships. During this stage, the environment at home and at school generally continues to be structured. In contrast, late adolescence is characterized by enormous social demands. As part of this developmental stage, adolescents must learn to deal with challenges and social pressures that arise within their peer groups, focus on school performance in order to maximize career prospects, and regulate a growing sex drive. Those leaving school at 18 to either enter the work force or college lose the social structure and support systems to which they have grown accustomed. Instead, they must independently adapt their behavior to, and make decisions based on, the relatively more variable contingencies that drive adult life. In addition, they likely will be concerned with attracting a partner (or choosing between possible partners), and may need to make early parenting decisions. Throughout this period, they must evaluate and assess competing life-course strategies and engage in complex decision making. Thus, the normative rebellious spirit and antisocial behavior that characterized most of adolescence (Moffitt, 1993) must be inhibited and suppressed in order to develop new, more adaptive, behavioral strategies.

Interestingly, significant changes in frontal structure are occurring at around the same time of these social developmental stages (i.e., up through age 2, preadolescence, postadolescence). It is likely that the prefrontal cortex, in part, subserves these behavioral and cognitive demands (e.g., aggression inhibition, delay of gratification, complex decision making, multiple executive functions such as sustained attention, behavioral flexibility to changing contingencies, working memory, planning, organization). Drawing upon Moffitt's (1993) theory, it is speculated here that life-course-persistent antisocial individuals suffer from an interaction of early health and family environment risk factors (e.g., head injury, prenatal nicotine exposure, ADHD, genetic predisposition to delayed frontal maturation, social adversity, chaotic family environment, physical child abuse) that disrupts both the socialization process and the maturation of frontal gray and white matter. More specifically, delayed or disrupted frontal maturation—combined with poor parenting or an otherwise chaotic home life—may contribute to the child's failure to learn to inhibit impulses (including aggression) and/or a decreased responsiveness to discipline. In turn, this failure to internalize and act according to social norms may lead to peer rejection, foster the development of friendships with delinquent peer groups, adversely affect school performance, and result in disregard for authority and socially normative behavior.

As this child grows older, it is hypothesized that the increased social and executive function demands of late adolescence place an additional burden on the prefrontal cortex. If earlier health and family experiences delayed prefrontal maturation or resulted in abnormal development, then the expected increase in frontal gray matter at this developmental stage that helps accommodate the increased executive demands may not occur, thereby contributing to poor inhibition over antisocial aggressive behavior. Furthermore, it is hypothesized that the reduction of frontal gray matter during postadolescence is selective rather than random, and is guided by the adolescent's environment and activities (Giedd et al., 1999). Thus, under circumstances where the individual is repetitively engaging in antisocial behavior with little consequence, the postadolescent decrease in gray matter and increase in white matter may actually facilitate the persistence of antisocial behavior into adulthood by strengthening the neural connections subserving such behavior.

Amplified executive demands on the prefrontal cortex in adolescence may also contribute to the more normative, adolescent-limited antisocial behavior in a number of ways. As with the life-course-persistent individuals, the overload on executive functions at a time when the frontal lobe is still developing and reorganizing may predispose adolescents—even those without risk factors such as birth complications, head injury, or psychosocial stressors—to engage in impulsive behavior, act without thought for the future, and make careless decisions. However, such individuals would be likely to discontinue their antisocial behavior as the frontal lobes mature and allow them to manage such cognitive and behavior challenges. Alternatively, others may have frontal dysfunction resulting from earlier health complications but may be protected from persistent antisocial behavior by living in a supportive rearing environment that helps guide behavior and choices and/or places fewer social-transitional demands on them.

Obviously, the above model is speculative and will need to be revised based on exploration of several intermediary hypotheses. Such testing would ideally take place in a longitudinal study with twins who undergo repeated structural MRI scans (and fMRI scans once they are old enough to lie still for longer periods of time); behavioral assessments by parents, teachers, and self-report; search of medical records for pregnancy and delivery complications; observations and family reports on home life and conditions; neuropsychological testing; collection of DNA; and a search of juvenile and adult criminal records. The study should target children who are at high and low risk for conduct disorder, preferably beginning when they are toddlers (although various considerations may preclude initial brain imaging at such a young age). Finally, with regard to the research program, the following hypotheses are suggested as places to begin an exploration of the causal factors in the onset of life-course-persistent antisocial behavior:

- *Research Aim 1*: To determine whether prefrontal structural deficits identified using MRI at various points in the lifespan are associated with persistent elevations in later antisocial behavior.

  Hypothesis 1a: Structural prefrontal deficits characterized by decreased prefrontal gray matter are associated with the onset of antisocial behavior.

  Hypothesis 1b: Structural prefrontal deficits characterized by decreased white matter within the prefrontal cortex are associated with the onset of antisocial behavior.

  Hypothesis 1c: The prefrontal deficits associated with antisocial behavior are most pronounced at key developmental stages (i.e., up to and around age 2, preadolescence, postadolescence).

  Hypothesis 1d: Antisocial behavior associated with a maturational lag in an otherwise normally developing prefrontal cortex will dissipate as the prefrontal cortex matures.

  Hypothesis 1e: Prefrontal deficits associated with antisocial behavior are most likely to involve the orbitofrontal and ventromedial cortices relative to other prefrontal cortices.

- *Research Aim 2*: To determine whether prefrontal structural deficits in antisocial individuals are associated with functional prefrontal deficits.

  Hypothesis 2a: Antisocial individuals, relative to controls, will show impaired performance on neuropsychological tests of executive function involving response inhibition and emotion-based decision making.

  Hypothesis 2b: Antisocial individuals, relative to controls, will show impaired activation during fMRI brain imaging using activation tasks such as response inhibition, decision making, emotional cues, and aversive conditioning.

  Hypothesis 2c: The presence of prefrontal structural deficits will be associated with an increased likelihood of prefrontal functional deficits among antisocial individuals.

- *Research Aim 3*: To determine the extent to which genetic and environmental factors contribute to decreased prefrontal gray volume (if support for Hypothesis 1a is found).

  Hypothesis 3a: Decreased prefrontal gray matter is an inherited characteristic.

  Hypothesis 3b: Decreased prefrontal gray matter is associated with—and preceded by—environmental risk factors such as the indirect consequences of child abuse (e.g., poor attachment and bonding experiences; erratic, inconsistent, and/or inappropriately harsh disciplining practices) and/or child neglect (e.g., environment that provides inadequate stimulation; lack of attachment and bonding).

Hypothesis 3c: Decreased prefrontal gray matter is associated with—and preceded by—nongenetic biological factors such as birth complications, MPAs, prenatal nicotine (and other drug) exposure, head injury from accidents or physical child abuse, and poor nutrition (particularly at key stages in brain development) resulting from poverty or child neglect.

Hypothesis 3d: The relationship between prenatal nicotine exposure and antisocial behavior, in particular, is accounted for by disrupted attention and arousal processes mediated by the prefrontal cortex.

- *Research Aim 4*: To determine whether prefrontal deficits, in combination with other risk factors, are more strongly associated with antisocial behavior than a single risk factor.

Hypothesis 4a: The interaction of prefrontal deficits and other environmental/nongenetic biological risk factors (i.e., listed in Research Aim 3) is more strongly associated with later antisocial behavior than either prefrontal deficits or the other risk factor(s) alone.

Hypothesis 4b: This interaction effect is most strongly related to antisocial behavior if the risk factors occur at key brain and social development stages (i.e., up to and around age 2, preadolescence, postadolescence).

Hypothesis 4c: Despite the occurrence of one risk factor (e.g., slowly maturing prefrontal cortex), the risk of persistent antisocial behavior is attenuated in the presence of a protective factor (i.e., well-structured and supportive home environment).

- *Research Aim 5*: To determine whether the association between the interaction in Research Aim 4 (if supported) and persistent antisocial behavior is mediated, in part, by poor fear conditioning.

Hypothesis 5a: Children with prefrontal deficits and environmental risk factors exhibit poor fear conditioning, and

Hypothesis 5b: Children with poor fear conditioning exhibit increased antisocial behavior, and

Hypothesis 5c: Children with prefrontal deficits and environmental risk factors exhibit increased antisocial behavior (i.e., Hypothesis 4a).

Hypothesis 5d (independent of tests of mediation): There is a positive correlation between parental reports of decreased responsiveness to discipline and laboratory measures of poor fear conditioning.

- *Research Aim 6*: To determine whether the association between early structural prefrontal deficits and persistent antisocial behavior is mediated, in part, by childhood adjustment problems (i.e., social, academic).

    Hypothesis 6a: Structural prefrontal deficits are associated with later academic failure, peer rejection, and/or affiliation with delinquent peers, and

    Hypothesis 6b: Structural prefrontal deficits are associated with later antisocial behavior (i.e., Research Aim 1), and

    Hypothesis 6c: Academic failure, peer rejection, and affiliation with delinquent peers are associated with antisocial behavior.

## LIMITATIONS OF THE PROPOSED MODEL AND DIRECTIONS FOR FUTURE RESEARCH

The model suggested above was developed by pulling together findings and trends from generally disconnected fields of research. Obviously, statements regarding its applicability cannot be made until studies designed to address its related components are conducted. Testing of these intermediary components will inevitably result in multiple revisions of the model. Moreover, research has identified subtypes of antisocial behavior (e.g., adolescent-limited vs. life-course-persistent; impulsive vs. predatory/proactive aggression; hyperactive vs. nonhyperactive) and begun to generate models that account for a particular behavioral expression (e.g., impulsive aggression; Davidson, Putnam, & Larson, 2000). Thus, different operationalizations of antisocial behavior will necessitate different causal models. For example, the model proposed here might apply to chronic antisocial behavior associated with executive dysfunction, but would not account for the fact that psychopathic criminals who evade legal conviction actually exhibit superior executive functions as measured by the Wisconsin Card Sorting Test (Ishikawa, Raine, Lencz, Bihrle, & LaCasse, 2001).

The above model also does not fully and adequately take into account the different prefrontal cortices, which may provide slightly different contributions to the development and manifestation of antisocial behavior. Thus, imaging studies with nonneurological antisocial populations that more thoroughly test competing models of orbitofrontal and dorsolateral function (as well as their interconnected subcortical structures) would help elucidate the neurobiological underpinnings of antisocial behavior. Fortunately, the current knowledge base of antisocial behavior and the technological advances in neuroimaging have poised themselves so that multifaceted issues such as these can now be tackled. While much work remains to be done, it nevertheless represents the beginning of a complex yet exciting field of study that perhaps one day may inform public policy in a meaningful and constructive way.

## ACKNOWLEDGMENTS

This research was conducted with the support of a National Research Service Award (1 F32 MH12951-01) to Sharon S. Ishikawa and an Independent Scientist Award (K02 MH01114) to Adrian Raine.

## REFERENCES

Amen, D. G., Stubblefield, M., Carmichael, B., & Thisted, R. (1996). Brain SPECT findings and aggressiveness. *Annals of Clinical Psychiatry, 8*(3), 129–137.

Anderson, S. W., Bechara, A., Damasio, H., Tranel, D., & Damasio, A. R. (1999). Impairment of social and moral behavior related to early damage in human prefrontal cortex. *Nature Neuroscience, 2*, 1032–1037.

Anderson, S. W., Damasio, H., Tranel, D., & Damasio, A. R. (2000). Long-term sequelae of prefrontal cortex damage acquired in early childhood. *Developmental Neuropsychology, 18*(3), 281–296.

Arseneault, L., Tremblay, R. E., Boulerice, J. R., Seguin, J. R., & Saucier, J. F. (2000). Minor physical anomalies and family adversity as risk factors for violent delinquency in adolescence. *American Journal of Psychiatry, 157*, 917–923.

Barkley, R. A. (2000). Genetics of childhood disorders: XVII. ADHD, Part I: The executive functions and ADHD. *Journal of the American Academy of Child and Adolescent Psychiatry, 39*(8), 1064–1068.

Bechara, A., Damasio, H., Damasio, A. R., & Lee, G. P. (1999). Different contributions of the human amygdala and ventromedial prefrontal cortex to decision-making. *Journal of Neuroscience, 19*, 5473–5481.

Bechara, A., Damasio, H., Tranel, D., & Damasio, A. R. (1997). Deciding advantageously before knowing the advantageous strategy. *Science, 275*(5304), 1293–1295.

Bechara, A., Tranel, D., & Damasio, H. (2000). Characterization of the decision-making deficit of patients with ventromedial prefrontal cortex lesions. *Brain, 123*, 2189–2202.

Bechara, A., Tranel, D., Damasio, H., & Damasio, A. R. (1996). Failure to respond autonomically to anticipated future outcomes following damage to prefrontal cortex. *Cerebral Cortex, 6*, 215–225.

Blair, R. J. R., & Cipolotti, L. (2000). Impaired social response reversal: A case of "acquired sociopathy." *Brain, 123*, 1122–1141.

Blair, R. J. R., Colledge, E., & Mitchell, D. G. V. (2001). Somatic markers and response reversal: Is there orbitofrontal cortex dysfunction in boys with psychopathic tendencies? *Journal of Abnormal Child Psychology, 29*(6), 499–511.

Blake, P. Y., Pincus, J. H., & Buckner, C. (1995). Neurologic abnormalities in murderers. *Neurology, 45*(9), 1641–1647.

Brennan, P. A., Grekin, E. R., & Mednick, S. A. (1999). Maternal smoking during pregnancy and adult male criminal outcomes. *Archives of General Psychiatry, 56*, 215–219.

Brennan, P., Mednick, S. A., & Raine, A. (1997). Biosocial interactions and violence: A focus on perinatal factors. In A. Raine, P. Brennan, D. P. Farrington, & S. A. Mednick (Eds.), *Biosocial bases of violence* (pp. 163–174). New York: Plenum Press.

Butler, K., Rourke, B. P., Fuerst, D. R., & Fisk, J. L. (1997). A typology of psychosocial functioning in pediatric closed-head injury. *Child Neuropsychology, 3*, 98–133.

Clark, C., Prior, M., & Kinsella, G. J. (2000). Do executive function deficits differentiate between adolescents with ADHD and oppositional defiant/conduct disorder?: A neuropsychological study using the Six Elements Test and Hayling Sentence Completion Test. *Journal of Abnormal Psychology, 28*(5), 403–414.

Critchley, H. D., Elliott, R., Mathias, C. J., & Dolan, R. J. (2000). Neural activity relating to generation and representation of galvanic skin conductance responses: A functional magnetic resonance imaging study. *Journal of Neuroscience, 20*(8), 3033–3040.

Critchley, H. D., Simmons, A., Daly, E. M., Russell, A., van Amelsvoort, T., Robertson, D. M., Glover, A., & Murphy, D. G. M. (2000). Prefrontal and medial temporal correlates of repetitive violence to self and others. *Biological Psychiatry, 47*, 928–934.

Cummings, J. L. (1995). Anatomic and behavioral aspects of frontal–subcortical circuits. In J. Grafman, K. J. Holyoak, & F. Boller (Eds.), *Structure and functions of the human prefrontal cortex: Annals of the New York Academy of Sciences, 769*, pp. 1–13.

Damasio, A. R. (1994). *Descartes' error: Emotion, reason, and the human brain.* New York: Grosset/Putnam.

Damasio, A. R., & Anderson, S. W. (1993). The frontal lobes. In K. M. Heilman & E. Valenstein (Eds.), *Clinical neuropsychology* (3rd ed., pp. 409–460). New York: Oxford University Press.

Damasio, A. R., Grabowski, T. J., Bechara, A., Damasio, H., Ponto, L. L., Parvizi, J., & Hichwa, R. D. (2000). Subcortical and cortical brain activity during the feeling of self-generated emotions. *Nature Neuroscience, 3*(10), 1049–1056.

Damasio, H., Grabowski, T., Frank, R., Galaburda, A. M., & Damasio, A. R. (1994). The return of Phineas Gage: Clues about the brain from the skull of a famous patient. *Science, 264*, 1102–1105.

Damasio, A. R., Tranel, D., & Damasio, H. (1990). Individuals with psychopathic behavior caused by frontal damage fail to respond autonomically to social stimuli. *Behavioral and Brain Research, 41*, 81– 94.

Davidson, R. J., Jackson, D. C., & Kalin, N. H. (2000). Emotion, plasticity, context and regulation: Perspectives from affective neuroscience. *Psychological Bulletin, 126*, 890–909.

Davidson, R. J., Putnam, K. M., & Larson, C. L. (2000). Dysfunction in the neural circuitry of emotion regulation: A possible prelude to violence. *Science, 289*, 591–594.

Deckel, A. W., Hesselbrock, V., & Bauer, L. (1996). Antisocial personality disorder, delinquency, and frontal brain dysfunction: EEG and neuropsychological findings. *Journal of Clinical Psychology, 52*(6), 639–650.

D'Esposito, M., Postle, B. R., & Rypma, B. (2000). Prefrontal cortical contributions to working memory: Evidence from event-related fMRI studies. *Experimental Brain Research, 133*, 3–11.

Dimitrov, M., Phipps, M., Zahn, T. P., & Grafman, J. (1999). A thoroughly modern Gage. *Neurocase, 5*, 345–354.

Elliott, R., Rubinsztein, J. S., Sahakian, B. J., & Dolan, R. J. (2000). Selective attention to emotional stimuli in a verbal go/no-go task: An fMRI study. *Brain Imaging, 11*(8), 1739–1744.

Eslinger, P. J., Biddle, K., Pennington, B., & Page, R. B. (1999). Cognitive and behavioral development up to 4 years after early right frontal lobe lesion. *Developmental Neuropsychology, 15*(2), 157–191.

Feifel, D. (1999). Neurotransmitters and neuromodulators in frontal–subcortical circuits. In B. L. Miller & J. L. Cummings (Eds.), *The human frontal lobes* (pp. 174–186). New York: Guilford Press.

Fergusson, D. M., Woodward, L. J., & Horwood, J. (1998). Maternal smoking during pregnancy and psychiatric adjustment in late adolescence. *Archives of General Psychiatry, 55*, 721–727.

Frysztak, R. J., & Neafsey, E. J. (1991). The effect of medial frontal cortex lesions on respiration, "freezing," and ultrasonic vocalizations during conditioned emotional responses in rats. *Cerebral Cortex*, 1(5), 418–425.

Giancola, P. R. (1995). Evidence for dorsolateral and orbital prefrontal cortical involvement in the expression of aggressive behavior. *Aggressive Behavior*, 21, 431–450.

Giancola, P. R., Mezzich, A. C., & Tarter, R. E. (1998a). Executive cognitive functioning, temperament, and antisocial behavior in conduct-disordered adolescent females. *Journal of Abnormal Psychology*, 107(4), 629–641.

Giancola, P. R., Mezzich, A. C., & Tarter, R. E. (1998b). Disruptive, delinquent and aggressive behavior in female adolescents with a psychoactive substance use disorder: Relation to executive cognitive functioning. *Journal of Studies on Alcohol*, 59, 560–567.

Giancola, P. R., & Zeichner, A. (1994). Neuropsychological performance on tests of frontal-lobe functioning and aggressive behavior in men. *Journal of Abnormal Psychology*, 103(4), 832–835.

Giedd, J. N., Blumenthal, J., Jeffries, N. O., Castellanos, F. X., Liu, H., Zijdenbos, A., Paus, T., Evans, A. C., & Rapoport, J. L. (1999). Brain development during childhood and adolescence: A longitudinal MRI study. *Nature Neuroscience*, 2(10), 861–863.

Gorenstein, E. E. (1982). Frontal lobe functions in psychopaths. *Journal of Abnormal Psychology*, 91(5), 368–379.

Goyer, P. F., Andreason, P. J., Semple, W. E., Clayton, A. H., King, A. C., Compton-Toth, B. A., Schulz, S. C., & Cohen, R. M. (1994). Positron-emission tomography and personality disorders. *Neuropsychopharmacology* 10, 21–28.

Grafman, J., Schwab, K., Warden, D., Pridgen, A., Brown, H. R., & Salazar, A. M. (1996). Frontal lobe injuries, violence, and aggression: A report of the Vietnam Head Injury Study. *Neurology*, 46, 1231–1238.

Guy, J. D., Majorski, L. V., Wallace, C. J., & Guy, M. P. (1983). The incidence of minor physical anomalies in adult male schizophrenics. *Schizophrenia Bulletin*, 9, 571–582.

Halverson, C. F., & Victor, J. B. (1976). Minor physical anomalies and problem behavior in elementary schoolchildren. *Child Development*, 47, 281–285.

Hare, R. D. (1984). Performance of psychopaths on cognitive tasks related to frontal lobe function. *Journal of Abnormal Psychology*, 93(2), 133–140.

Henry, B., & Moffitt, T. E. (1997). Neuropsychological and neuroimaging studies of juvenile delinquency and adult criminal behavior. In J. Breiling, D. M. Stoff, & J. D. Maser (Eds.), *Handbook of antisocial behavior* (pp. 280–288). New York: Wiley.

Hirono, N., Mega, M. S., Dinov, I. D., Mishkin, F., & Cummings, J. L. (2000). Left frontotemporal hypoperfusion in associated with aggression in patients with dementia. *Archives of Neurology*, 57, 861–866.

Hodgins, S., Kratzer, L., & McNeil, T. F. (2001). Obstetric complications, parenting, and risk of criminal behavior. *Archives of General Psychiatry*, 58, 746–752.

Hoffman, J. J., Hall, R. W., & Bartsch, T. W. (1987). On the relative importance of "psychopathic" personality traits and alcoholism on neuropsychological measures of frontal lobe dysfunction. *Journal of Abnormal Psychology*, 96(2), 158–160.

Hugdahl, K. (1998). Cortical control of human classical conditioning: Autonomic and positron emission tomography data. *Psychophysiology*, 35, 170–178.

Hughes, C., White, A., Sharpen, J., & Dunn, J. (2000). Antisocial, angry, and unsympathetic: "Hard-to-manage" preschoolers' peer problems and possible cognitive influences. *Journal of Child Psychology and Psychiatry and Allied Disciplines*, 41(2), 169–179.

Hux, K., Bond, V., Skinner, S., Belau, D., & Sanger, D. (1998). Parental report of occurrences and consequences of traumatic brain injury among delinquent and non-delinquent youth. *Brain Injury*, 12, 667–681.

Intrator, J., Hare, R., Stritzke, P., Brichtswein, K., Dorfman, D., Harpur, T., Bernstein, D., Handelsman, L., Schaefer, C., Keilp, J., Rosen, J., & Machac, J. (1997). A brain mapping (single positron emission computerized tomography) study of semantic and affective processing in psychopaths. *Biological Psychiatry, 42,* 96–103.

Ishikawa, S. S., & Raine, A. (2002). Psychophysiological correlates of antisocial behavior: A central control hypothesis. In J. Glicksohn (Ed.), *The neurobiology of criminal behavior publisher.* New York: Kluwer Academic/Plenum.

Ishikawa, S. S., Raine, A., Lencz, T., Bihrle, S., & LaCasse, L. (2001). Autonomic stress reactivity and executive functions in successful and unsuccessful criminal psychopaths from the community. *Journal of Abnormal Psychology, 110*(3), 423–432.

Kaufer, D. I., & Lewis, D. A. (1999). Frontal lobe anatomy and cortical connectivity. In B. L. Miller & J. L. Cummings (Eds.), *The human frontal lobes* (pp. 27–44). New York: Guilford Press.

Krakowski, M., Czobor, P., Carpenter, M. D., Libiger, J., Kunz, M., Papezova, H., Parker, B. B., Schmader, L., & Abad, T. (1997). Community violence and inpatient assaults: Neurobiological deficits. *Journal of Neuropsychiatry and Clinical Neurosciences, 9*(4), 549–555.

Kuruoglu, A. C., Arikan, Z., Vural, G., Karatas, M., Arac, M., & Isik, E. (1996). Single photon emission computerised tomography in chronic alcoholism: Antisocial personality disorder may be associated with decreased frontal perfusion. *British Journal of Psychiatry, 169*(3), 348–354.

Langevin, R., Ben-Aron, M., Wortzman, G., Dickey, R., & Handy, L. (1987). Brain damage, diagnosis and substance abuse among violent offenders. *Behavioral Sciences and the Law, 5*(1), 77–94.

LaPierre, D., Braun, C. M. J., & Hodgins, S. (1995). Ventral frontal deficits in psychopathy: Neuropsychological test findings. *Neuropsychologia, 33,* 139–151.

Laucht, M., Essser, G., Baving, L., Gerhold, M., Hoesch, I., Ihle, W., Steigleider, P., Stock, B., Stoehr, R. M., Weindrich, D., & Schmidt, M. H. (2000). Behavioral sequelae of perinatal insults and early family adversity at 8 years of age. *Journal of the American Academy of Child and Adolescent Psychiatry, 39,* 1229–1237.

Leuger, R. J., & Gill, K. J. (1990). Frontal-lobe cognitive dysfunction in conduct disorder adolescents. *Journal of Clinical Psychology, 46*(6), 696–706.

Levin, E. D., Wilkerson, A., Jones, J. P., Christopher, N. C., & Briggs, S. J. (1996). Prenatal nicotine effects on memory in rats: Pharmacological and behavioral challenges. *Developmental Brain Research, 97,* 207–215.

Lezak, M. D. (1995). *Neuropsychological Assessment* (3rd ed.). New York: Oxford University Press.

Liddle, P. F., Kiehl, K. A., & Smith, A. M. (2001). Event-related fMRI study of response inhibition. *Human Brain Mapping, 12,* 100–109.

London, E. D., Ernst, M., Grant, S., Bonson, K., & Weinstein, A. (2000). Orbitofrontal cortex and human drug abuse: Functional imaging. *Cerebral Cortex, 10,* 334–342.

Mataro, M., Jurado, A., Garcia-Sanchez, C., Barraquer, L., Costa-Jussa, F. R., & Junque C. (2001). Long-term effects of bilateral frontal brain lesion: 60 years after injury with an iron bar. *Archives of Neurolgy, 58,* 1139–1142.

Matsuzawa, J., Matsui, M., Konishi, T., Noguchi, K., Gur, R. C., Bilker, W., & Miaywaki, T. (2001). Age-related volumetric changes of brain gray and white matter in healthy infants and children. *Cerebral Cortex, 11,* 335–342.

Max, J. E., Koele, S. L., Smith, W. L., Sato, Y., Lindgren, S. D., Robin, D. A., & Arndt, S. (1998). Psychiatric disorders in children and adolescents after severe traumatic brain injury: A controlled study. *Journal of the American Academy of Child and Adolescent Psychiatry, 37,* 832–840.

Miller, B. L., Darby, A., Benson, D. F., & Cummings, J. L. (1997). Aggressive, socially disruptive and antisocial behaviour associated with fronto-temporal dementia. *British Journal of Psychiatry, 170,* 150–155.

Mittenberg, W., Wittner, M. S., & Miller, L. J. (1997). Postconcussion syndrome occurs in children. *Neuropsychology, 11,* 447–452.

Moffitt, T. E. (1993). The neuropsychology of conduct disorder. *Development and Psychopath-ology*, *5*(1–2), 135–151. [*Special Issue: Toward a Developmental Perspective on Conduct Disorder.*]

Morgan, A. B., & Lilienfeld, S. O. (2000). A meta-analytic review of the relation between antiso-cial behavior and neuropsychological measures of executive function. *Clinical Psychology Review*, *20*, 113–136.

Olds, D. (1997). Tobacco exposure and impaired development: A review of the evidence. *Mental Retardation and Developmental Disabilities Research Reviews*, *3*, 257–269.

Paulus, D. L., & Martin, C. L. (1986). Predicting adult temperament from minor physical anom-alies. *Journal of Personality and Social Psychology*, *50*, 1235–1239.

Pennington, B. F., & Bennetto, L. (1993). Main effects or transactions in the neuropsychology of conduct disorder?: Commentary on "The neuropsychology of conduct disorder." *Devel-opment and Psychopathology*, *5*, 153–164.

Pietrini, P., Guazzelli, M., Basso, G., Jaffe, K., & Grafman, J. (2000). Neural correlates of imaginal aggressive behavior assessed by positron emission tomography in healthy sub-jects. *American Journal of Psychiatry*, *157*, 1772–1781.

Pine, D. S., Wasserman, G., Coplan, J., Fried, J., Sloan, R., Myers, M., Grenhill, L., Shaffer, D., & Parsons, B. (1996). Serotonergic and cardiac correlates of aggression in children. *Annals of the New York Academy of Sciences*, *794*, 391–393.

Piquero, A., & Tibbetts, S. (1999). The impact of pre/perinatal disturbances and disadvantaged familial environment in predicting criminal offending. *Studies on Crime and Crime Pre-vention*, *8*, 52–70.

Pomeroy, J. C., Sprafkin, J., & Gadow, K. D. (1988). Minor physical anomalies as a biological marker for behavior disorders. *Journal of the American Academy of Child and Adolescent Psychiatry*, *27*, 466–473.

Raine, A. (1993). *The psychopathology of crime: Criminal behavior as a clinical disorder*. San Diego, CA: Academic Press.

Raine, A. (2002). Annotation: The role of prefrontal deficits, low autonomic arousal, and early health factors in the development of antisocial and aggressive behavior in children. *Journal of Child Psychology and Psychiatry and Allied Disciplines*, *43*(4), 417–434.

Raine, A., Brennan, P., & Mednick, S. A. (1994). Birth complications combined with early ma-ternal rejection at age 1 year predispose to violent crime at age 18 years. *Archives of Gen-eral Psychiatry*, *51*, 984–988.

Raine, A., & Buchsbaum, M. S. (1996). Violence and brain imaging. In D. M. Stoff & R. B. Cairns (Eds.), *Neurobiological approaches to clinical aggression research* (pp. 195–218). Mahwah, NJ: Erlbaum.

Raine, A., Lencz, T., Bihrle, S., LaCasse, L., & Colletti, P. (2000). Reduced prefrontal gray matter volume and reduced autonomic activity in antisocial personality disorder. *Archives of General Psychiatry*, *57*(2), 119–127.

Raine, A., Meloy, J. R., Bihrle, S., Stoddard, J., Lacasse, L., & Buchsbaum, M. S. (1998). Re-duced prefrontal and increased subcortical brain functioning assessed using positron emis-sion tomography in predatory and affective murderers. *Behavioral Sciences and the Law*, *16*, 319–332.

Raine, A., Park, S., Lencz, T., Bihrle, S., Lacasse, L., Widom, C. S., Al-Dayeh, L., & Singh, M. (2001). Reduced right hemisphere activation in severely abused violent offenders during a working memory task: An fMRI study. *Aggressive Behavior*, *27*, 111–129.

Raine, A., Stoddard, J., Bihrle, S., & Buchsbaum, M. S. (1998). Prefrontal glucose deficits in murderers lacking psychosocial deprivation. *Neuropsychiatry, Neuropsychology, and Behavioral Neurology*, *11*, 1–7.

Raine, A., Venables, P. H., & Mednick, S. A. (1997). Low resting heart rate at age 3 years predis-poses to aggression at age 11 years: Findings from the Mauritius Joint Child Health Pro-ject. *Journal of the American Academy of Child and Adolescent Psychiatry*, *36*, 1457–1464.

Rantakallio, P., Laara, E., Isohanni, M., & Moilanen, I. (1992). Maternal smoking during pregnancy and delinquency of the offspring: An association without causation? *International Journal of Epidemiology, 21*, 1106–1113.

Rasanen, P., Hakko, H., Isohanni, M., Hodgins, S., Jarvelin, M. R., & Tiihonen, J. (1999). Maternal smoking during pregnancy and risk of criminal behavior among adult male offspring in the northern Finland 1996 birth cohort. *American Journal of Psychiatry, 156*, 857–862.

Schalling, D., & Rosen, A. S. (1968). Porteus maze differences between psychopathic and non-psychopathic criminals. *British Journal of Social and Clinical Psychology, 7*(3), 224–228.

Schmitt, W. A., Brinkley, C. A., & Newman, J. P. (1999). Testing Damasio's somatic marker hypothesis with psychopathic individuals: Risk takers or risk averse? *Journal of Abnormal Psychology, 108*(3), 538–543.

Schneider, F., Habel, U., Kessler, C., Posse, S., Grodd, W., & Muller-Gartner, H. W. (2000). Functional imaging of conditioned aversive emotional responses in antisocial personality disorder. *Neuropsychobiology, 42*, 192–201.

Seguin, J. R., Boulerice, B., Harden, P. W., Tremblay, R. E., & Pihl, R. O. (1999). Executive functions and physical aggression after controlling for attention deficit hyperactivity disorder, general memory, and IQ. *Journal of Child Psychology and Psychiatry and Allied Disciplines, 40*(8), 1197–1208.

Seguin, J. R., Pihl, R. O., Harden, P. W., Tremblay, R. E., & Boulerice, B. (1995). Cognitive and neuropsychological characteristics of physically aggressive boys. *Journal of Abnormal Psychology, 104*(4), 614–624.

Soderstrom, H., Tullberg, M., Wikkelsoe, C., Ekholm, S., & Forsman, A. (2000). Reduced regional cerebral blood flow in non-psychotic violent offenders. *Psychiatry Research: Neuroimaging, 98*, 29–41.

Sowell, E. R., Thompson, P. M., Holmes, C. J., Jernigan, T. L., & Toga, A. W. (1999). In vivo evidence for post-adolescent brain maturation in frontal and striatal regions. *Nature Neuroscience, 2*(10), 859–861.

Speltz, M. L., DeKlyen, M., Calderon, R., Greenberg, M. T., & Fisher, P. A. (1999). Neuropsychological characteristics and test behaviors of boys with early onset conduct problems. *Journal of Abnormal Psychology, 108*(2), 315–325.

Spreen, O., & Strauss, E. (1998). *A compendium of neuropsychological tests: Administration, norms, and commentary* (2nd ed.). New York: Oxford University Press.

Stern, C. E., Sherman, S. J., Kirchhoff, B. A., & Hasselmo, M. E. (2001). Medial temporal and prefrontal contributions to working memory tasks with novel and familiar stimuli. *Hippocampus, 11*, 337–346.

Teicher, G., & Golden, C. J. (2000). The relationship of neuropsychological impairment to conduct disorder in adolescence: A conceptual review. *Aggression and Violent Behavior, 5*(6), 509–528.

Toupin, J., Dery, M., Pauze, R., Mercier, H., & Fortin, L. (2000). Cognitive and familial contributions to conduct disorder in children. *Journal of Child Psychology and Psychiatry and Allied Disciplines, 41*(3), 333–344.

Tremblay, R. E. (2001). The development of physical aggression during childhood and the prediction of later dangerousness. In G. F. Pinard & L. Pagani (Eds.), *Clinical assessment of dangerousness: Empirical contributions* (pp. 47–65). New York: Cambridge University Press.

Volkow, N. D., Tancredi, L. R., Grant, C., Gillespie, H., Valentine, A., Mullani, N., Wang, G. J., & Hollister, L. (1995). Brain glucose metabolism in violent psychiatric patients: A preliminary study. *Psychiatry Research—Neuroimaging, 61*, 243–253.

Wakschlag, L. S., Lahey, B. B., Loeber, R., Green, S. M., Gordon, R. A., & Leventhal, B. L. (1997). Maternal smoking during pregnancy and the risk of conduct disorder in boys. *Archives of General Psychiatry, 54*, 670–676.

Waldrop, M. F., Bell, R. Q., McLaughlin, B., & Halverson, C. F. (1978). Newborn minor physical anomalies predict short attention span, peer aggression, and impulsivity at age 3. *Science, 199,* 563–564.

Weissman, M. M., Warner, V., Wickramaratne, P. J., & Kandel, D. B. (1999). Maternal smoking during pregnancy and psychopathology in offspring followed to adulthood. *Journal of the American Academy of Child and Adolescent Psychiatry, 38,* 892–899.

Woermann, F. G., van Elst, L. T., Koepp, M. J., Free, S. L., Thompson, P. J., Trimble, M. R., & Duncan, J. S. (2000). Reduction of frontal neocortical grey matter associated with affective aggression in patients with temporal lobe epilepsy: An objective voxel by voxel analysis of automatically segmented MRI. *Journal of Neurology, Neurosurgery, and Psychiatry, 68*(2), 162–169.

# 11

# Testing Alternative Hypotheses Regarding the Role of Development on Genetic and Environmental Influences Underlying Antisocial Behavior

SOO HYUN RHEE
IRWIN D. WALDMAN

Disentangling the influences of nature and nurture is the first step toward the eventual goal of explaining the etiology of antisocial behavior. Estimating the relative magnitude of genetic and environmental influences on antisocial behavior is an important step in the search for specific candidate genes and environmental risk factors underlying antisocial behavior. Although it is not possible to disentangle genetic from environmental influences in family studies because genetic and environmental influences are confounded in nuclear families, twin and adoption studies have the unique ability to disentangle genetic and environmental influences and to estimate the magnitude of both simultaneously.

Although more than 100 twin and adoption studies of antisocial behavior have been published, it is difficult to draw clear conclusions regarding the magnitude of genetic and environmental influences on antisocial behavior given the current literature. The main reason for this difficulty is the considerable heterogeneity of the results in this area of research, with published heritability estimates (i.e., the magnitude of genetic influences) ranging from very low (e.g., .00; Plomin, Foch, & Rowe, 1981) to very high (e.g., .71; Slutske, Heath, et al., 1997). Of the various hypotheses that have been proposed to explain these heterogeneous results, some of the most interesting include those suggesting the age of the sample (e.g.,

Cloninger & Gottesman, 1987) and the age of onset of antisocial behavior (e.g., Moffitt, 1993) as moderators of genetic and environmental influences on antisocial behavior. In a recent study (Rhee & Waldman, 2002), we conducted a meta-analysis of 51 twin and adoption studies in order to provide a clearer and more comprehensive picture of the magnitude of genetic and environmental influences on antisocial behavior and to test two alternative hypotheses regarding the role of development on the magnitude of genetic and environmental influences on antisocial behavior.

## HYPOTHESIS 1: THE GENERAL DEVELOPMENTAL HYPOTHESIS

### Background

In the behavior genetics literature, there is a general finding for a variety of traits that as age increases, the magnitude of genetic and nonshared environmental influences increases, whereas the magnitude of shared environmental influences decreases (Loehlin, 1992a; Plomin, 1986). One example of such a finding is Matheny's (1989) longitudinal study of temperament. From 12 to 30 months of age, monozygotic (MZ) twins became more concordant than dizygotic (DZ) twins for age-to-age changes in temperament measures of emotional tone, fearfulness, and approach. Also, in Miles and Carey's (1997) meta-analysis of behavior genetic studies examining aggression, the magnitude of shared environmental influences decreased and the magnitude of genetic influences increased from childhood to adulthood.

### Hypothesis 1

There are causal genetic, shared environmental, and nonshared environmental influences on antisocial behavior. As twins and other relatives grow older and grow apart, the magnitude of environmental influences that make them similar (i.e., shared environmental influences) diminishes, whereas the magnitude of environmental influences that make them dissimilar (i.e., nonshared environmental influences) and genetic influences increases.

## HYPOTHESIS 2: THE DEVELOPMENTAL TAXONOMY HYPOTHESIS

### Background

The significance of age of onset and the continuity of antisocial behavior is discussed in several traditional literature reviews of behavior genetic studies examining antisocial behavior (e.g., Cloninger & Reich, 1983; DiLalla & Gottesman, 1989; Gottesman & Goldsmith, 1994). In particular, DiLalla and Gottesman (1989) hypothesized that there are three different types of offenders: *continuous antisocials*, those are who are delinquent as youths and continue to be criminal as adults; *transitory delinquents*, youths who are delinquent but not criminal as adults; and *late bloomers*, adults who are criminal but were not delinquent as adolescents. They accept the conclusion of the early twin studies (e.g., Cloninger & Gottesman, 1987) that genetic influences are minimal for juvenile delinquency, and hypothesize that many delinquents are transitory delinquents primarily affected by peer pressure.

A review by Moffitt (1993) concurs with DiLalla and Gottesman's (1989) hypothesis. Moffitt notes that although antisocial behavior shows impressive continuity over age, the prevalence of antisocial behavior increases almost tenfold during adolescence. She also suggests a subtype hypothesis for antisocial behavior, with the first subtype comprising a small group of members who are antisocial from an early age and who continue to be antisocial during adulthood, and the second subtype being a much larger group whose members have a later age of onset for antisocial behavior and are only antisocial during adolescence. She hypothesizes that the correlates and causes of persistent crime or antisocial psychopathology (e.g., genetic influences) may not characterize more transient juvenile delinquency.

There appears to be conflicting evidence regarding age as a moderator of genetic and environmental influences on juvenile delinquency versus adult criminality. In five early twin studies examining juvenile delinquency, the weighted average of concordance rates for MZ and DZ twins are .87 and .72, respectively (Cloninger & Gottesman, 1987). In comparison, in seven early twin studies examining adult criminality, the weighted average of concordance rates for MZ and DZ twins are .51 and .23, respectively (Cloninger & Gottesman, 1987). These results suggest that juvenile delinquency during adolescence, unlike criminality during adulthood, is only moderately affected by genetic influences, but very strongly affected by shared environmental influences. Given these results, researchers have theorized that genetic influences on individual differences in delinquency may be minimal because the base rate for delinquency is very high (DiLalla & Gottesman, 1989) or because environmental influences such as peer pressure are particularly strong in adolescence (Raine & Venables, 1992). Pertinent to these hypotheses, Lyons et al. (1995) assessed juvenile and adult antisocial personality disorder symptoms in the same participants using retrospective self-report. They found that the heritability for the adult antisocial traits ($h^2$ = .43) was higher than that of the heritability for the juvenile antisocial traits ($h^2$ = .07), supporting Cloninger and Gottesman's (1989) conclusions.

In contrast, Rowe (1983) examined anonymous self-reports of delinquent acts and found that both genetic and environmental influences are substantial for juvenile delinquency. Some reviewers (e.g., DiLalla &

Gottesman, 1991) attributed Rowe's contradictory finding to his use of self-reports, and suggested that the finding of genetic influences reflects the response to questionnaires rather than the construct of juvenile delinquency. They also noted that the finding of genetic influences may be a function of including items that assess aggression rather than delinquency. Other limitations of this study include a low response rate, which raises issues regarding sampling biases, and the use of a mailed questionnaire, which raises the possibility of nonindependent responses. On the other hand, Rowe and Rodgers (1989) asserted that it is premature to conclude that genetic influences are not important for delinquency, as the early twin studies had many methodological problems (e.g., haphazard sampling, small sample size, and variability in zygosity determination method). Carey (1994) admitted that the methodology of the early twin studies was generally poor, but noted that similar methodological problems did not prevent finding genetic influences on adult criminality.

Two recent twin studies report data that are relevant to the issues of age of onset and continuity of antisocial behavior. First, Slutske, Lyons, et al. (1997) found that antisocial behavior that is earlier in onset is no more heritable than later-onset antisocial behaviors, but also found that antisocial behavior that is persistent across the lifespan is more heritable than antisocial behavior that is limited to either childhood or adulthood. Slutske, Lyons, et al. (1997) cautioned that the use of retrospective reports may be a limitation of their study. Second, Waldman, Levy, and Hay (1997) examined the etiology of four types of antisocial behavior (i.e., oppositionality, aggression, property violations, and status violations) that vary monotonically in their median age of onset from 6 years old (oppositionality) to 9 years old (status violations) (Frick et al., 1993). They found that antisocial behavior with an earlier age of onset is more heritable and shows less shared environmental influences than antisocial behavior with a later age of onset.

## Hypothesis 2

There are causal genetic, shared environmental, and nonshared environmental influences on antisocial behavior. Nonetheless, there is heterogeneity in the etiology of antisocial behavior in the general population, with a larger group exhibiting adolescent-limited antisocial behavior that is influenced largely by environmental influences, and a smaller group exhibiting life-course-persistent antisocial behavior that is influenced largely by genetic influences. Therefore, the magnitude of genetic influences should be larger in children and adults than in adolescents, and the magnitude of shared and/or nonshared environmental influences should be larger in adolescents than in children and adults.

## META-ANALYSIS OF BEHAVIOR GENETIC STUDIES OF ANTISOCIAL BEHAVIOR

In a recent meta-analysis (Rhee & Waldman, 2002), we used participants' age as a moderator of the magnitude of genetic and environmental influences on antisocial behavior in order to test the two developmental hypotheses outlined above. In testing the participants' age at the time of the assessment as a moderator, we compared results for children (below age 13), adolescents (ages 13–18), and adults (above age 18). If the general developmental hypothesis is correct, the magnitude of genetic influences should be smallest in children, intermediate in adolescents, and greatest in adults, while the magnitude of shared environmental influences should be greatest in children, intermediate in adolescents, and smallest in adults. Given that so few twin studies have addressed the issue of age of onset or continuity of antisocial behavior, the present review cannot provide conclusive evidence for or against the developmental taxonomy hypothesis. If one assumes, however, that antisocial behavior in adolescents is more transitory in general (although continuous and transitory antisocial adolescents are not distinguished), under the developmental taxonomy hypothesis, the results should indicate that during adolescence the magnitude of genetic influences on antisocial behavior should be lowest, and the magnitude of shared and/ or nonshared environmental influences on antisocial behavior should be highest, relative to childhood and adulthood.

In this meta-analysis (Rhee & Waldman, 2002), we searched for published twin and adoption studies of antisocial behavior by examining the PsycInfo and Medline databases and the reference sections from relevant research studies and review papers. We also searched for relevant unpublished manuscripts or manuscripts in press by examining pertinent review papers, the Dissertations Abstracts and ERIC databases, and the abstracts of the 1995, 1996, 1997, and 1998 Behavior Genetics Association meetings.

One-hundred-forty-one twin and adoption studies examining antisocial behavior were identified. After excluding unsuitable studies according to the criteria described below (i.e., construct validity, assessment of related disorders, and inability to calculate tetrachoric or intraclass correlations), 96 studies remained. After addressing the problem of nonindependence in these studies, 51 studies remained (i.e., 10 independent adoption samples and 42 independent twin samples [two separate samples were examined in Eley, Lichtenstein, & Stevenson, 1999]).

The validity of the measures used in the studies considered for the meta-analysis was an important issue in deciding whether to include or exclude a study. Only studies examining antisocial behavior were included, and studies examining related constructs such as anger and hostility were excluded. A study was included if it clearly examined antisocial personality disorder, conduct disorder, criminality, aggression, or antisocial behavior (an ombinus operationalization including both delinquency and aggression items); if there was empirical evidence that the measure of antisocial behavior used successfully discriminated between an antisocial group and a control group; or if the measure was significantly related to a more established operationalization of antisocial behavior. Also, studies that examined another variable related to antisocial behavior (e.g., alcoholism) as well as antisocial behavior were excluded.

The effect sizes used in this meta-analysis (Rhee & Waldman, 2002) were the Pearson product moment or intraclass correlations that were reported in the studies, or the tetrachoric correlations that were estimated from the concordances or percentages reported in the studies. These effect sizes were analyzed in structural equation model fitting programs that test alternative models for the etiology of antisocial behavior and estimate the magnitude of genetic and environmental influences. Studies were excluded if these effect sizes were not reported or if there was not enough information reported to calculate these effect sizes.

In many studies considered for this meta-analysis, data from the same sample were reported more than once, causing a problem of nonindependence. Given that the sample size must be indicated in model-fitting analyses, the average of the multiple effect sizes was used if the sample size was identical across the nonindependent samples, and the effect size from the largest sample was used if the sample size was not identical across the nonindependent samples.

In behavior genetic analyses, alternative models containing different sets of causal influences are compared for their fit to the observed data (i.e., twin or familial correlations or covariances). These models posit that antisocial behavior is affected by different types of influences: additive genetic influences (A—genetic influences where alleles from different genetic loci add up to independently influence the liability for a trait), nonadditive genetic influences (D—genetic influences where alleles interact with each other to influence the liability for a trait, either at a single genetic locus or at different loci), shared environmental influences (C—environmental influences that are experienced in common by family members that make them similar to one another), and nonshared environmental influences (E—environmental influences that are experienced uniquely by family members that make them different from one another). The magnitude of additive genetic influences, nonadditive genetic influences, shared environmental influences, and non-shared environmental influences are denoted as $a^2$, $d^2$, $c^2$, and $e^2$, respectively.

Two types of adoption studies (1, parent–offspring studies comparing the correlation between adoptees and their adoptive parents and the correlation between adoptees and their biological parents; and 2, sibling adoption studies comparing the correlation between adoptive siblings and the correlation between biological siblings) and two types of twin studies (1, twin pairs reared together; and 2, twin pairs reared apart) were included in the meta-analysis (Rhee & Waldman, 2002). The effect sizes from each study were entered in separate groups in the model-fitting program *Mx* (Neale, 1995). (Stem-and-leaf plots of the effect sizes from the adoption and twin studies are shown in Rhee & Waldman, 2002, Tables 5 and 6, respectively.) In the model-fitting program, the correlations between pairs of relatives are explained in terms of the components of variance that are shared between the relatives (A, C, or D). Nonshared environmental influences, or E, do not explain any part of the correlation between relatives because, by definition, nonshared environmental influences are not shared between relatives. The correlation between different types of relatives is explained by different sets of influences and their appropriate weights. These weights reflect the genetic and environmental similarity between pairs of relatives (see Appendix B, in Rhee & Waldman, 2002).

The analyses were performed in a series of steps (Rhee & Waldman, 2002). First, we conducted the meta-analysis on data from all samples meeting the inclusion criteria and compared five alternative models (the ACDE model, the ADE model, the ACE model, the AE model, and the CE model). It is not possible to estimate $c^2$ and $d^2$ simultaneously or to test an ACDE model with data only from twin pairs reared together because the estimation of $c^2$ and $d^2$ both rely on the same information (i.e., the difference between the MZ and DZ twin correlations). In our meta-analysis, it was possible to test the ACDE model when analyzing all of the data (i.e., data from both twin and adoption studies) because the additional source of information from adoption studies allowed for the simultaneous estimation of $c^2$ and $d^2$. The fit of each model was assessed using the $\chi^2$ statistic and the Akaike Information Criterion (AIC), a fit index that reflects both the fit of the model and its parsimony (Loehlin, 1992b). Among competing models, the one with the lowest AIC and the lowest $\chi^2$ relative to its degrees of freedom is considered to be the best fitting model.

Second, we tested the moderating effects of age by contrasting the fit of a model in which the parameter estimates are constrained to be equal across children (15 samples; 54 groups; 7,807 pairs of participants), adolescents (11 samples; 31 groups; 2,868 pairs of participants), and adults (17 samples; 50 groups; 27,671 pairs of participants) to the fit of a model where the parameter estimates are free to vary by age. If the fit of the two models is significantly different, this indicates that genetic and environmental influences on antisocial behavior differ by age. If the fit of the two models does not significantly differ, this may be due to a lack of power, especially if there is little variability in the levels of a moderator. It was not possible to test moderators within the context of the ACDE model because both twin and adoption studies were not always available across different levels of age.

## THE MAGNITUDE OF GENETIC AND ENVIRONMENTAL INFLUENCES ON ANTISOCIAL BEHAVIOR

When data from all of the samples meeting the inclusion criteria ($N = 52$ samples;149 groups; 55,525 pairs of participants) were analyzed, the full ACDE model fit best as compared with the other, more restrictive models (see Table 7, in Rhee & Waldman, 2002). Based on this omnibus analysis, there were moderate additive genetic ($a^2 = .32$), nonadditive genetic ($d^2 = .09$), shared environmental ($c^2 = .16$), and nonshared environmental ($e^2 = .43$) influences on antisocial behavior.

## ASSESSMENT OF AGE AS A MODERATOR

Age was a significant moderator of the magnitude of genetic and environmental influences on antisocial behavior, $\Delta\chi^2(6) = 243.95$, $p < .001$ (Rhee & Waldman, 2002). The ACE model was the best fitting model for children ($a^2 = .46$, $c^2 = .20$, $e^2 = .34$), adolescents ($a^2 = .43$, $c^2 = .16$, $e^2 = .41$), and adults ($a^2 = .41$, $c^2 = .09$, $e^2 = .50$). The magnitude of familial influences ($a^2$ and $c^2$) decreased with age, whereas the magnitude of nonfamilial influences ($e^2$) increased with age. These findings do not support hypothesis 1 (the general developmental hypothesis), which predicts that with increasing age, $a^2$ and $e^2$ estimates should increase and $c^2$ estimates should decrease, or hypothesis 2 (the developmental taxonomy hypothesis), which predicts that the magnitude of genetic influences should be lower and the magnitude of shared and/or nonshared environmental influences should be higher in adolescence than in childhood or adulthood.

These results should be interpreted with caution for three reasons. First, although many studies examined a wide age range, either the mean or the midpoint age had to represent this range, given that access to the raw data for each study was not possible. Second, age was simplified into a categorical variable (i.e., children, adolescents, and adults) in our meta-analysis, given the difficulties of including continuous moderators in model-fitting analyses. Third, the issue of confounding between age and other possible moderators of the etiology of antisocial behavior should be considered when interpreting these results. Given that antisocial behavior is operationalized and assessed differently for children, adolescents, and adults (e.g., conduct disorder is assessed via parent report in children vs. antisocial personality disorder is assessed via self-report in adults), age of the participants tends to be substantially correlated with the operationalization of antisocial behavior and the assessment method used in the study. Indeed, we found that there was significant confounding between age and operationalization (i.e., diagnosis, criminality, aggression, or antisocial behavior [an omnibus operationalization that represents a combination of aggression and delinquency items]) and between age and assessment method (i.e., self-report, report by others, official records, reaction to aggressive material, or objective test) in the studies included in the meta-analysis (see Table 2, in Rhee and Waldman, 2002).

Thus, it is quite possible that the pattern of results we found for age may be reflecting the moderating effects of operationalization or assessment method. For example, studies examining children were more likely to use report by others, whereas studies examining adolescents and adults were more likely to use self-reports. The higher twin correlations found in studies examining children in comparison to those found in studies examining adolescents or adults thus may be due to differences in assessment method. The same individual, usually a parent, rates both twins in studies using report by others, whereas two different individuals (i.e., the twins themselves) rate the two twins separately in studies using self-report.

In fact, we found that the same pattern of results for age was also found for assessment method, with studies using report by others (used more with children) yielding higher estimates of familial influences than those using self-report (used more with adolescents and adults), as well as for operationalization, with studies examining antisocial behavior (assessed more in children) yielding higher estimates of familial influences than those examining diagnosis (assessed more in adults and adolescents).

## HYPOTHESIS 3: THE DECREASING FAMILIAL INFLUENCES HYPOTHESIS

On the other hand, these results may not be due to confounding between age and other moderators and may represent the true nature of the role of development on the magnitude of genetic and environmental influences on antisocial behavior. If this is the case, the results suggest a third, novel hypothesis for explaining developmental changes in the etiology of antisocial behavior. It is possible that the magnitude of familial influences (i.e., both genetic and shared environmental influences) on antisocial behavior is greatest during childhood and decreases with age because the salience and impact of familial influences are greatest during childhood and decrease with age. The results of the meta-analysis also are consistent with the results of McCartney, Harris, and Bernieri's (1990) meta-analysis of developmental changes in genetic and environmental influences on intelligence and several personality variables, in that the correlations for both MZ and DZ twin pairs decreased as age increased for most variables. This finding also applied to the eight twin studies examining aggression, with the MZ correlations decreasing slightly more than the DZ correlations with increasing age, suggesting that the magnitude of genetic and shared environmental influences decreased and the magnitude of nonshared environmental influences increased with age. Thus, the decreasing familial influences hypothesis appears to adequately describe the results for antisocial behavior and aggression from both the current meta-analysis and that of McCartney et al. (1990).

In general, the clarification of the role of development in the etiology of antisocial behavior should provide useful information for researchers searching for specific genetic and environmental influences on antisocial behavior, as well as those examining interventions for antisocial behavior at different stages of development. In particular, the decreasing familial influences hypothesis suggests that researchers should focus more on nonshared environmental influences when investigating the etiology of antisocial behavior, or developing interventions for it, in later stages of development.

## STUDIES NEEDED TO EXPOSE HYPOTHESES TO RISK OF REFUTATION

Both DiLalla and Gottesman (1989) and Moffitt (1993) have suggested that in order to show conclusive evidence regarding their hypotheses, future studies of antisocial behavior should include longitudinal data concerning the same individuals. A good example of such a study is Jacobson, Neale, Prescott, and Kendler's (2001) longitudinal study, where they examined the antisocial behavior of 1,070 adult male–male twin pairs during adolescence and adulthood. Jacobson et al. tested the developmental taxonomy hypothesis by examining the heritability of antisocial behavior during adolescence in two different groups: the adult antisocials and the adult nonantisocials. Heritability for antisocial behavior during adolescence was significantly higher in the adult antisocials ($h^2$ = .38; $c^2$ = .10) compared to that in adult nonantisocials ($h^2$ = .00; $c^2$ = .35), providing support for the developmental taxonomy hypothesis.

The study that will truly distinguish which (if any) of these developmental hypotheses is correct is a longitudinal twin study that examines the same individuals across the lifespan (i.e., during childhood, adolescence, and adulthood) and collects reliable information on the age of onset of antisocial behavior. In conducting such a study, the fact that antisocial behavior is often tested via different operationalizations and assessment methods at different stages of life as well as the possibility of confounding between moderators should be considered. If the general developmental hypothesis is correct, the magnitude of genetic and nonshared environmental influences should increase and the magnitude of shared environmental influences should decrease with increasing age, without regard to the age of onset of antisocial behavior. If the developmental taxonomy hypothesis is correct, the magnitude of genetic influences should be lowest and the magnitude of shared and/or nonshared environmental influences should be highest during adolescence. Also, the magnitude of genetic influences should increase, and the magnitude of shared and/or nonshared environmental influences should decrease, as the age of onset decreases. The results of the meta-analysis presented herein also suggest a third, novel developmental hypothesis regarding the etiology of antisocial behavior. If the age moderation results in the meta-analysis are not due to confounding with assessment method and/or the operationalization of antisocial behavior, and the salience and impact of familial influences on antisocial behavior do indeed decrease with age, the magnitude of genetic and shared environmental influences should decrease while the magnitude of nonshared environmental influences should increase with age.

## GENDER, RACE–ETHNICITY, AND SOCIOECONOMIC STATUS

In our meta-analysis (Rhee & Waldman, 2002), gender was not a significant moderator of the magnitude of genetic and environmental influences on antisocial behavior (males—$a^2 = .43$, $c^2 = .19$, $e^2 = .38$; females—$a^2 = .41$, $c^2 = .20$, $e^2 = .39$), $\Delta\chi^2 (3) = 1.53$, $p = .68$. There is the possibility of an interaction between gender and age of onset in the etiology of antisocial behavior, however. Silverthorn and Frick (1999) noted that antisocial girls typically have an adolescent onset of antisocial behavior despite having the correlates of the childhood-onset pathway and developing life-course-persistent antisocial behavior. Given this inconsistency, they proposed a delayed-onset pathway for girls that is analogous to the childhood-onset pathway in boys and suggested that there is no developmental pathway to antisocial behavior in girls that is analogous to the adolescent pathway in boys. Again, the study needed to expose Silverthorn and Frick's hypothesis to risk of refutation is a longitudinal twin study examining the same individuals throughout the lifespan and collecting reliable information on the age of onset of antisocial behavior. According to Silverthorn and Frick's hypothesis, age of onset should be a significant moderator of the heritability of antisocial behavior in males, with heritability being greater with earlier age of onset. In contrast, age of onset should not be a significant moderator of the heritability of antisocial behavior in females, given that for girls, adolescent onset of antisocial behavior does not necessarily mean that they have the adolescent-limited antisocial behavior that is largely influenced by environmental influences.

We were unable to test any hypotheses regarding race–ethnicity or socioeconomic status because none of the studies included in the meta-analysis presented separate results for groups differing in race–ethnicity or socioeconomic status. In addition to examining race–ethnicity or socioeconomic status as a moderator of the etiology of antisocial behavior, interesting questions regarding the potential interaction between race–ethnicity or socioeconomic status and age of onset remain unanswered. A potential limitation of both twin and adoption studies is the generalizability of the findings given reduced diversity of race–ethnicity and socioeconomic status in these types of studies. Volunteers in social science studies tend to be above average in socioeconomic status, and this limitation would pertain to twin and adoption studies just as it does to other studies. Also, the range of the adoptive home environment tends to be restricted, with adoptees having several advantages over children in the general population in terms of family stability, educational opportunities, standards of health care, material living standards, and mother–child interactions (e.g., Fergusson, Lynskey, & Horwood, 1995). Thus, it is important for future twin and adoption studies of antisocial behavior to sample individuals from a greater diversity of ethnic and socioeconomic backgrounds.

## ACKNOWLEDGMENTS

This work was supported in part by National Institute on Drug Abuse Grant No. DA-13956 and National Institute of Mental Health Grant No. MH-01818. We thank the authors who made data from unpublished studies available through personal communication. We also thank Deborah Finkel, Jenae Neiderhiser, Wendy Slutske, and Edwin van den Oord for making the data from their studies available before their publication, and Scott O. Lilienfeld, Kim Wallen, and Terrie E. Moffitt for helpful comments on earlier versions of this chapter. Portions of this chapter were presented at the meeting of the American Society of Criminology in 1996 and at the meeting of the Behavior Genetics Association in 1997, and a more extensive version has been published in Rhee and Waldman (2002).

## REFERENCES

Carey, G. (1994). Genetics and violence. In A. J. Reiss, K. A. Miczek, & J. A. Roth (Eds.), *Understanding and preventing violence* (Vol. 2, pp. 21–58). Washington, DC: National Academy Press.

Cloninger, C. R., & Gottesman, I. I. (1987). Genetic and environmental factors in antisocial behavior disorders. In S. A. Mednick, T. E. Moffitt, & S. A. Stack (Eds.), *The causes of crime: New biological approaches* (pp. 92–109). New York: Cambridge University Press.

Cloninger, C. R., & Reich, T. (1983). Genetic heterogeneity in alcoholism and sociopathy. In S. S. Kety, L. P. Rowland, R. L. Sidman, & S. W. Matthysse (Eds.), *Genetics of neurological and psychiatric disorders* (pp. 145–166). New York: Raven Press.

DiLalla, L. F., & Gottesman, I. I. (1989). Heterogeneity of causes for delinquency and criminality: Lifespan perspectives. *Development and Psychopathology, 1*(4), 339–349.

DiLalla, L. F., & Gottesman, I. I. (1991). Biological and genetic contributors to violence: Widom's untold tale. *Psychological Bulletin, 109*, 125–129.

Eley, T. C., Lichtenstein, P., & Stevenson, J. (1999). Sex differences in the etiology of aggressive and nonaggressive antisocial behavior: Results from two twin studies. *Child Development, 70*(1), 155–168.

Fergusson, D. M., Lynskey, M., & Horwood, L. J. (1995). The adolescent outcomes of adoption: A 16-year longitudinal study. *Journal of Child Psychology and Psychiatry, 36*(4), 597–615.

Frick, P. J., Lahey, B. B., Rolf, L., Tannenbaum, L., Vanhorn, Y., Christ, M. A. G., Hart, E. A., & Hanson, K. (1993). Oppositional defiant disorder and conduct disorder: A meta-analytic review of factor analyses and cross-validation in a clinic sample. *Clinical Psychology Review, 13*(4), 319–340.

Gottesman, I. I., & Goldsmith, H. H. (1994). Developmental psychopathology of antisocial behavior: Inserting genes into its ontogenesis and epigenesis. In C.A. Nelson (Ed.), *Threats to optimal development: Integrating biological, psychological, and social risk factors* (pp. 69–104). Hillsdale, NJ: Erlbaum.

Jacobson, K. C., Neale, M. C., Prescott, C. A., & Kendler, K. S. (2001). Behavioral genetic confirmation of a life-course perspective on antisocial behavior: Can we believe the results? [Abstract]. *Behavior Genetics, 31,* 456.

Loehlin, J. C. (1992a). *Genes and environment in personality development.* Newbury Park, CA: Sage.

Loehlin, J. C. (1992b). *Latent variable models: An introduction to factor, path, and structural analysis* (2nd ed.). Hillsdale, NJ: Erlbaum.

Lyons, M. J., True, W. R., Eisen, S. A., Goldberg, J., Meyer, J. M., Faraone, S. V., Eaves, L. J., & Tsuang, M. T. (1995). Differential heritability of adult and juvenile antisocial traits. *Archives of General Psychaitry, 52,* 906–915.

Matheny, A. P. (1989). Children's behavioral inhibition over age and across situations: Genetic similarity for a trait during change. *Journal of Personality, 57*(2), 215–235.

McCartney, K., Harris, M. J., & Bernieri, F. (1990). Growing up and growing apart: A developmental meta-analysis of twin studies. *Psychological Bulletin, 107,* 226–237.

Miles, D. R., & Carey, G. (1997). Genetic and environmental architecture of human aggression. *Journal of Personality and Social Psychology, 72*(1), 207–217.

Moffitt, T. E. (1993). Adolescence-limited and life-course-persistent antisocial behavior: A developmental taxonomy. *Psychological Review, 100*(4), 674–701.

Neale, M. C. (1995). *Mx: Statistical modeling.* Richmond: Virginia Commonwealth University, Medical College of Virginia, Department of Psychiatry.

Plomin, R. (1986). *Development, genetics, and psychology.* Hillsdale, NJ: Erlbaum.

Plomin, R., Foch, T. T., & Rowe, D. C. (1981). Bobo clown aggression in childhood: Environment, not genes. *Journal of Research in Personality, 15,* 331–342.

Raine, A., & Venables, P. H. (1992). Antisocial behaviour: Evolution, genetics, neuropsychology, and psychophysiology. In A. Gale & M. W. Eysenck (Eds.), *Handbook of individual differences: Biological perspectives* (pp. 287–321). New York: Wiley.

Rhee, S. H., & Waldman, I. D. (2002). Genetic and environmental influences on antisocial behavior: A meta-analysis of twin and adoption studies. *Psychological Bulletin, 128*(3), 490–529.

Rowe, D. C. (1983). Biometrical genetic models of self-reported delinquent behavior: A twin study. *Behavior Genetics, 13,* 473–489.

Rowe, D. C., & Rodgers, J. L. (1989). Behavioral genetics, adolescent deviance, and "d": Contributions and issues. In G. R. Adams, R. Montemayor, & T. P. Gullotta (Eds.), *Biology of adolescent behavior and development* (pp. 38–67). Newbury Park, CA: Sage.

Schulsinger, F. (1972). Psychopathy: Heredity and environment. *International Journal of Mental Health, 1,* 190–206.

Silverthorn, P., & Frick, P. J. (1999). Developmental pathways to antisocial behavior: The delayed-onset pathway in girls. *Development and Psychopathology, 11,* 101–126.

Slutske, W. S., Heath, A. C., Dinwiddie, S. H., Madden, P. A. F., Bucholz, K. K., Dunne, M. P., Statham, D. J., & Martin, N. G. (1997). Modeling genetic and environmental influences in the etiology of conduct disorder: A study of 2,682 adult twin pairs. *Journal of Abnormal Psychology, 106*(2), 266–279.

Slutske, W., Lyons, M., True, W., Eisen, S., Goldberg, J., & Tsuang, M. (1997, July). *Testing a developmental taxonomy of antisocial behavior.* Paper presented at the annual meeting of the Behavior Genetics Association, Toronto, Ontario, Canada.

Waldman, I. D., Levy, F., & Hay, D. A. (1997, June). *Etiological validation of a developmental taxonomy of antisocial behavior.* Paper presented at the annual meeting of the International Society for Research in Child and Adolescent Psychopathology, Paris, France.

# 12

# Prenatal and Perinatal Influences on Conduct Disorder and Serious Delinquency

PATRICIA A. BRENNAN
EMILY R. GREKIN
SARNOFF A. MEDNICK

In this chapter we evaluate the potential causal effects of perinatal factors on conduct disorder, delinquency, and other aggressive behaviors. Prenatal and perinatal problems include low birth weight, pregnancy complications such as mother's poor nutrition and viral infections, and delivery complications such as hypoxia, or lack of oxygen to the fetus during labor. They also include prenatal exposure to teratogens such as maternal cigarette smoking and substance use during pregnancy. The relationship between perinatal factors and aggression has been reviewed in detail elsewhere (Brennan, Mednick, & Raine, 1997; Tibbetts & Piquero, 1999). In contrast to reviews that simply describe this relationship, our goal is to specifically examine this area of research in terms of how previous studies reflect tests of causal relationships between perinatal factors and aggression. In addition, we propose a number of explanations for what might be in the "black box," that is, the underlying processes and mechanisms that causally link perinatal factors to aggressive and delinquent outcomes. We focus on several noncompeting moderator and mediator hypotheses, including the hypothesis that the social environment may moderate the effects of perinatal factors on aggression, as well as the hypothesis that frontal lobe damage may mediate the relationship between perinatal factors and aggression. For all of the hypotheses presented, we review existing evidence for causal connections and outline future studies designed explicitly to test them.

## PERINATAL FACTORS AND AGGRESSION

### Developmental Theory

Much of the work linking perinatal factors and aggression can be tied back into Moffitt's (1993) developmental theory of life-course-persistent antisocial behavior. Specifically, Moffitt theorizes that a combination of biological deficits and disrupted social environments work together in a transactional process to produce early-onset persistent aggression. According to the theory, prenatal and perinatal disruptions in neural development lead to neuropsychological deficits—namely, developmental impairments in executive and verbal functioning. These deficits, which may be too subtle to attract clinical attempts at remediation, cumulatively result in an infant/ toddler with a difficult temperament, poor behavioral regulation, and deficient cognitive abilities. All three deficits individually, Moffitt (1993) observes, are established predictors of later antisocial behavior. Furthermore, infants at risk for these deficits are also likely to be raised in homes that are poorly equipped, both financially and psychologically, to deal adaptively with a troublesome child. As Moffitt (1993) claims, "Vulnerable infants are disproportionately found in environments that will not be ameliorative because many of the sources of neural maldevelopment co-occur with family disadvantage or deviance" (p. 681). Thus, the stage is set for a series of maladaptive parent–child interactions, in which troublesome child behaviors evoke negative responses from parents, which in turn exacerbate the child's behavior problems. This ongoing transactional process results in an antisocial lifestyle trajectory, maintained by a combination of preexisting neuropsychological deficits, the cumulative negative consequences of ongoing antisocial behavior, and the absence of learned prosocial behavioral alternatives.

### General Findings

In accordance with Moffitt's theory, existing research suggests that perinatal factors may be more related to early-onset persistent offending and violence than to adolescent-limited delinquency or property offending. For example, violent delinquents are found to have more perinatal problems noted in their hospital records than other delinquents or controls (Lewis, Shanok, & Balla, 1979); delivery complications have been found to be related to later arrests for violence but not to arrests for property offending (Kandel & Mednick, 1991; Raine, Brennan, & Mednick, 1994); and maternal prenatal smoking has been related specifically to early-onset (Gibson, Piquero, & Tibbetts, 2000) and life-course-persistent (Brennan, Grekin, & Mednick, 1999) offending.

Research in this area also suggests that perinatal factors may be especially related to aggressive and criminal outcomes for individuals with high social risk. For example, in a prospective longitudinal study conducted in Kauai, Hawaii, Werner (1987) found that the effects of perinatal stress on delinquent outcome were strongest for children exposed to a disruptive family environment. In our research in Denmark, we have found similar biosocial interactions predicting outcomes of violent and persistent criminal behavior (Brennan et al., 1997).

It is important to note that maternal cigarette smoking during pregnancy appears to be a particularly potent perinatal risk factor for aggressive and antisocial behavior. Maternal prenatal smoking has been associated with increased risk for oppositional behavior, conduct disorder, and substance abuse outcomes in youth (Day, Richardson, Goldschmidt, & Cornelius, 2000; Wakschlag et al., 1997; Weissman, Warner, Wickramaratne, & Kandel, 1999). Statistical controls for a range of potential confounds including maternal antisocial behavior, maternal mental health, parenting behavior, socioeconomic status (SES), prenatal exposure to drugs and alcohol, and other perinatal complications do not change this general pattern of results. The effects of maternal prenatal smoking appear to be specific to externalizing or acting-out behaviors; there does not appear to be an association between maternal prenatal smoking and increased risk for internalizing problems such as depression (Orlebeke, Knol, & Verhulst, 1997).

Recent results from a prenatal intervention program designed by David Olds (Olds et al., 1998) lend further support for a relationship between perinatal factors and delinquency. In this study, women at high social risk were randomly assigned to receive nurse visitation during their pregnancy and the first 2 years of their children's lives. Nurse visitation during pregnancy focused on health promotion, including improving maternal nutrition and decreasing maternal cigarette smoking. Postnatal nurse visitation programs focused on improvements in parenting skills and abilities. At age 15, children whose mothers had received this perinatal intervention were significantly less likely to have a record of arrest or conviction or to have behavior problems associated with substance abuse.

## ESTABLISHING A CAUSAL CONNECTION

Unfortunately, the study of perinatal factors and their effect on antisocial behavior and aggression is fraught with methodological problems. The most serious methodological concern is the difficulty in establishing a causal connection due to the potential role of confounds in this process (Wakschlag, Pickett, Cook, Benowitz, & Leventhal, 2002). Research in this area is quasi-experimental. For obvious ethical reasons, women are not randomly assigned to smoke during pregnancy or to undergo particular delivery complications. Therefore, the women who do experience perinatal complications differ from the women who do not on a number of different factors, including SES, mental health, personality traits, parenting styles, and exposure to stressful life events. These factors, in turn, are associated with greater risk for problematic child aggression and antisocial behavior. Although many studies have controlled for subsets of these confounds (as noted above for the studies on maternal cigarette smoking and antisocial outcomes), no single study has been able to control for all of them.

As pointed out by Fergusson (1999), the relationship between maternal prenatal smoking and offspring antisocial outcomes could be accounted for by inherited genotypes passed down from the mother to the child. Genetically sensitive designs are needed to rule out this potential confound in the studies of perinatal factors and child aggression and antisocial behavior. As Raz, Shah, and Sander (1996) point out, twin designs can be used to control for genetic and other postnatal environmental influences, so that the effect of the perinatal complication can be separated out and examined. Of course, the basic twin design would be least effective for perinatal complications that are equivalent across twins (e.g., exposure to maternal prenatal smoking) and would be more useful for discordant perinatal risk factors such as birthweight or hypoxia. More complex twin designs (e.g., the children of twins design) or adoptee designs could, however, be used to test the genetic and environmental influences reflected in the relationship between a wide variety of perinatal problems and antisocial behavior (Rutter, Pickles, Murray, & Eaves, 2001).

Animal studies are also very useful in this area of research because they allow random assignment to particular types of perinatal problems. Animal studies are limited, however, in terms of generalizability. Intervention studies designed to reduce perinatal risks can also be useful in establishing a causal connection between perinatal factors and aggression. Unfortunately, intervention studies are limited by issues of compliance and dropout. Because compliance and dropout are related to factors predictive of aggressive outcomes, intervention studies may artificially inflate the effects of treatment (and hence the perinatal risk factor that is being treated) on these behavioral outcomes. In addition, intervention studies (such as the one described above by Olds and colleagues [1998]) typically try to promote positive change in a multitude of areas, and thus rarely provide a test of systematic change in a single independent variable such as perinatal risk. Given the inherent weaknesses in each type of study on its own, a combined set of evidence from animal studies, intervention studies, genetically sensitive designs, and longitudinal prospective studies will be necessary to establish support for a causal connection between perinatal factors and antisocial outcomes.

The establishment of a causal connection between perinatal factors and aggression would also be facilitated by a well-developed theory or set of hypotheses about the mechanisms that explain or moderate this relationship. Once these hypotheses are developed, it will be possible to examine the existing literature in support of them and to plan future studies that fill in the gap between what has been hypothesized and what is known. In this way, future research will more accurately reflect the complexities of the underlying processes that exist in the relationship between perinatal risk factors and aggression. Thus, we present moderator and mediator hypotheses that we believe are promising avenues for future study in terms of testing the causal connection between prenatal and perinatal factors and conduct disorder and serious delinquency.

## CAUSAL MODELS AND HYPOTHESES

### Moderator Hypotheses

A causal connection between perinatal risk factors and aggression may depend upon the presence of other risk factors in the child and/or his or her environment. For example, there is some evidence that family functioning, SES, and the child's gender may play a moderating role in this context. In addition, future studies are needed to examine genetic influences as a potential moderator in the relationship between perinatal risk factors and aggression.

### Social Environment

Existing research suggests that perinatal factors may be especially related to aggressive and antisocial outcomes for individuals with poor family functioning or low SES. For example, in a prospective longitudinal study conducted in Kauai, Hawaii, Werner (1987) found that the effects of perinatal stress on delinquent outcome were strongest for children exposed to a disruptive family environment. A *disruptive family environment* was defined by Werner as separation from the mother, marital discord, absence of the father, illegitimacy of the child, or parental mental health problems. These family risk factors, in combination with the risk resulting from perinatal complications, increased the likelihood for delinquent outcome in her Kauai sample. A recent study in Montreal replicated these results for violent outcomes at ages 6 and 17 years of age (Arseneault, Tremblay, Boulerice, & Saucier, 2002). Specifically Arseneault and her colleagues found that serious delivery complications interacted with family adversity in the prediction of violence during both childhood and adolescence.

Family context has also been shown to moderate the effect of maternal prenatal smoking on child outcomes (Wakschlag & Hans, 2002). In addition, a recent study of urban African American males found that low birthweight interacted with a disadvantaged social environment (i.e., low SES and weak family structure) in predicting early-onset delinquent offending (Tibbetts & Piquero, 1999). Interestingly, animal studies have also noted that the detrimental effects of prenatal stress on the hypothalamic–pituitary–adrenal (HPA) axis do not occur if the mother provides additional postbirth stimulation by stroking, grooming, or licking her newborn (Francis, Champagne, Liu, & Meaney, 1999). Thus, optimal or at least improved parenting skills may compensate for or undo the negative impact of prenatal stress in humans as well as in animals (Gunnar & Chisholm, 1999).

In our research in Denmark, we have found similar perinatal risk and family environment interactions predicting the outcomes of violent and persistent criminal behavior. For example, we examined the combined effects of early maternal rejection and delivery complications in the prediction of violent offending in adolescence in a sample of 4,169 males born at Rigshospitalet in Copenhagen between September 1, 1959, and December 31, 1961. In this study we found a significant interaction such that individuals with high maternal rejection and high delivery complications evidence the highest rates of violence during adolescence (Raine et al., 1994).

We have also examined the relationship between obstetric factors and violence with an observable indicator of fetal maldevelopment during pregnancy: the measure of minor physical anomalies (MPAs). MPAs include such measurable physical characteristics as the presence of more than one hair whorl, asymmetrical ears, attached ear lobes, curved fingers, and single palmar crease. To gain an understanding of what MPAs reflect, consider the development of the ears. Early in gestation they are seated low on the head and gradually move upward into their normal position. If the development of the fetus is disrupted, the movement of the ears could be slowed or stopped, resulting in low-set ears, a MPA. The presence of more than three MPAs suggests a disruption in fetal development. A concomitant disruption in the development of the central nervous system (CNS) is assumed. Therefore the presence of MPAs can be considered an observable indicator of CNS dysfunction resulting during the prenatal phase of life.

We examined the combined effects of MPAs and family instability on the outcome of criminal violence in a subsample of individuals from the Rigshospitalet cohort (Brennan et al., 1997). Most of the individuals in this subsample were children of psychiatrically ill parents. Seventy-two males were included in this analysis. Again, we found the same pattern of results that we noted in our analysis of delivery complications. In this high-risk sample, males with high numbers of MPAs and an unstable family upbringing evidenced higher rates of violence than other groups in the sample.

Our results from the Copenhagen cohorts consistently reveal that perinatal factors interact with each other and with other risk factors to increase the likelihood of violent outcomes in adulthood. This relationship is not simply additive. The combination of CNS damage (caused by perinatal problems) and environmental risks is a potent combination in producing the outcome of violence. Our results are consistent with Moffitt's (1993) life-course-persistent-offender theory that posits a transactional, developmental process in which biologically vulnerable individuals find themselves ensnared in social environments that do not alleviate their vulnerabilities, but rather exacerbate them. This developmental process is reflected in a lifetime characterized by aggressive, criminal, and often violent behavior.

The study of the social environment as a moderator of the effect of perinatal factors on aggression is limited by a number of methodological problems. The most significant issue is one of specificity of social risk factors. It is not clear if familial factors, SES factors, or any type of positive social environmental factors might have this moderating effect. In most of the studies that have examined the social environment as a moderator, the measurement of social environment has been rather crude and unspecified. A more specific delineation of these moderators would be useful in planning prevention or intervention studies focused on these variables. Another methodological weakness in this area is the lack of attention to developmental effects. Most of the social environment variables that have been studied have not been examined in terms of potential differential effects at particular ages or phases of development. Again, this knowledge would be useful in planning prevention or intervention programs. Finally, although these moderator effects have been noted in cross-cultural samples, there has been little research on whether or not they exist for girls as well as for boys. This is an important consideration given the fact that gender itself may play a moderating role in the relationship between perinatal factors and aggression.

*Gender*

Studies examining the moderating role of gender in the relationship between prenatal complications and antisocial behavior have yielded inconsistent results. In particular, six studies have examined gender differences in the relationship between maternal prenatal smoking and externalizing behavior. Three of these studies found no gender differences in the maternal smoking–externalizing behavior relationship (Maughan, Taylor, Taylor, Butler, & Bynner, 2001; Gibson et al., 2000; Orlebeke et al., 1997). In contrast, one study found that the relationship between maternal prenatal smoking and adolescent conduct disorder was stronger for male than for female offspring (Fergusson, Woodward, & Horwood, 1998). A second study found that maternal prenatal smoking predicted conduct disorder in male but not female offspring and drug dependence in female but not male offspring (Weissman et al., 1999). Finally, a third study found that maternal prenatal smoking predicted criminal arrest and hospitalization for substance abuse in both male and female offspring, but also found that, for female offspring, the relationship between maternal prenatal smoking and criminal arrest was no longer significant after controlling for substance-abuse hospitalizations (Brennan, Grekin, Mortensen, & Mednick, 2002).

Outside of the maternal prenatal smoking literature, one study found that the relationship between prenatal lead exposure and delinquency did not differ for males and females (Dietrich, Ris, Succop, Berger, & Bornschein, 2001). In addition, a second study found that obstetric complications interacted with inadequate parenting to predict criminal convictions for male, but not female, offspring (Hodgins, Kratzer, & McNeil, 2001).

Clearly more research is needed to clarify the role of gender in the prenatal complications–antisocial behavior relationship. In addition, future studies will need to address important methodological issues. First, studies examining gender should utilize large sample sizes. Conduct disorder, antisocial personality disorder, and criminal arrest are all fairly rare among females. Thus, failure to find a prenatal complications–externalizing behavior relationship among females may reflect low power rather than a true absence of an association. Future studies should draw from large population-based cohorts or high-risk samples in order to ensure an adequate number of antisocial female participants.

Second, it is possible that male and female antisocial behavior take different forms. For example, recent studies indicate that male aggression tends to be physical in nature (e.g., assault), while female aggression tends to be relational in nature (talking about a peer behind her back) (Crick & Bigbee, 1998). Importantly, relational aggression has been found to have detrimental psychosocial outcomes for girls, including peer rejection and depression (Crick & Grotpeter, 1995). Thus, relational aggression would seem to be a crucial outcome measure in its own right. More traditional antisocial outcome measures such as criminal arrests or number of police contacts are insensitive to female antisocial behavior of the relational aggressive type. Future studies should assess the relationship between prenatal complications and both physical and relational aggression.

Third, it is possible that gender differences in antisocial behavior depend on the type of prenatal stressor examined. The majority of studies that examine prenatal insults and antisocial behavior separately for males and females are studies of maternal prenatal smoking. It is possible that different types of prenatal stressors have different effects on the externalizing behavior of male and female offspring. Future studies should examine the antisocial behavior of males and females exposed to a variety of prenatal stressors. It is also possible that gender interacts with the timing of stressor exposure. Research indicates that fetal brain development in males is slower than fetal brain development in females (Castle & Murray, 1991). Thus, females may be more susceptible to prenatal complications early in gestation, while males are more susceptible later in gestation. Future studies should break down results by both trimester and gender, thereby allowing a meaningful analysis of gender by timing interactions.

Finally, it should be noted that males and females face vastly different postnatal stresses and expectations. Thus, it may be fruitful for future studies to explore potential interactions between gender, prenatal stressors, and postnatal environments in the prediction of antisocial behavior.

## Genetic Influences

No study to date has examined the association between perinatal factors and child aggression in a genetically sensitive design. A recent study, however, noted that a gene polymorphism moderated the effect of maternal prenatal smoking on infant birthweight (Wang et al., 2002), suggesting that this might well be a useful area of focus for future research. It interesting to consider the fact that the studies that have found family environment to be a moderator in the perinatal factor and aggression relationship may actually reflect a moderating effect of genetic influences rather than family environment per se. In other words, maternal rejection or parenting deficits may be a marker for genetic differences, which in turn interact with the perinatal risks to predict aggressive and antisocial outcomes. Studies of the potentially moderating role of genetic influences are needed to separate these genetic and environmental effects. Such studies could examine targeted genes or they could utilize twin designs. For a more thorough discussion of relevant methods, see Rhee and Waldman (Chapter 11, this volume).

## Mediator Hypotheses

Previous research has not yet established a causal connection between perinatal factors and aggression. Nevertheless, correlational data suggest that a causal connection may indeed exist. If perinatal factors are causally related to aggression, interventions designed to reduce perinatal complications would obviously be of value and importance. It is not likely, however, that any intervention can completely eliminate a child's exposure to perinatal risk factors. Therefore, an important question arises: Once exposed to these risk factors, what interventions would be useful in reducing aggressive outcomes for these children? In order to best answer this question, we need to have a more complete understanding of the process and mechanisms through which perinatal risk factors impact children's behavior. As discussed above, the family environment may moderate the effects of perinatal factors on aggressive outcomes. As such, the family may be an important focus of intervention for children who have been exposed to perinatal risks. Other important avenues of intervention would be those that focus on the mediating risk factors between perinatal complications and aggression. We hypothesize that frontal lobe dysfunction, social rejection, and stress reactivity are potential mediators in this process. Next we examine research relevant to these potential mediator hypotheses, and suggest future studies designed to more directly test them.

## Frontal Lobe Dysfunction

One possible mediator of the prenatal insults–antisocial behavior relationship is frontal lobe dysfunction. The frontal lobes are the largest and evolutionarily newest structures in the human brain. The anterior portion of the frontal lobes (the prefrontal cortex) helps control "higher" cognitive functions such as attention, planning, concept formation, and abstract reasoning. The frontal lobes also play an important role in both impulse control and the maintenance of emotional equilibrium (Fallgatter & Herrmann, 2001; Lezak, 1995). As a result, deficits in frontal lobe functioning may lead to impulsiveness, aggression, and emotional lability (Brower & Price, 2001; Chow, 2000; Miller, 1987). In order to determine whether frontal lobe dysfunction mediates the relationship between prenatal insults and antisocial behavior, three questions must be addressed. First, do prenatal stressors cause deficits in frontal lobe functioning? Second, do deficits in frontal lobe functioning cause antisocial behavior? And third, do prenatal insults continue to predict antisocial behavior after controlling for frontal lobe functioning?

*Frontal Lobe Functioning and Antisocial Behavior.* A number of researchers have hypothesized a relationship between frontal lobe dysfunction and impulsive/aggressive disorders, such as conduct disorder and antisocial personality disorder. A large body of evidence supports this hypothesis (e.g., see Ishikawa & Raine, Chapter 10, this volume; also see the recent meta-analytical review by Morgan & Lilienfeld, 2000).

It should be noted that there are a number of confounds in the frontal lobe–antisocial behavior relationship. First, it is not clear whether antisocial behavior is related specifically to frontal lobe functioning or more generally to all neuropsychological processes. Studies examining this question have yielded mixed results. For example, Wolff, Waber, Bauermeister, Cohen, and Ferber (1982) found that delinquent boys performed more poorly than age-matched, nondelinquent boys on both frontal lobe measures and tests of language and vocabulary. In addition, a recent meta-analysis found that antisocial behavior was related to both frontal lobe tests and to tests of more general neuropsychological functioning (Morgan & Lilienfeld, 2000). Thus, the issue of specificity in the antisocial behavior–frontal lobe relationship needs to be clarified.

Second, frontal lobe deficits are often difficult to detect. Neuropsychological tests are indirect measures of brain damage. In addition, more direct biological measures, such as electroenchephalogram (EEG) and positron emission technology (PET) scans, often lack the sensitivity to detect subtle brain deficits, thus diluting the findings for a frontal lobe–antisocial behavior relationship.

Third, it is not clear from previous research whether frontal lobe dysfunction precedes or follows antisocial behavior. While it is true that frontal lobe deficits caused by perinatal factors would likely precede the onset of aggressive and antisocial behavior, in many previous studies measures of frontal lobe structure and function have been taken long after a period of antisocial behavior has been established. Given the fact that certain types of antisocial behavior, such as excessive drug and alcohol use, reckless driving, and fighting may actually produce brain damage, these studies may not establish brain damage as the cause of criminal behavior but rather as the consequence of a long-standing pattern of deviance. Even a recent study noting a relationship between executive functioning and disruptive behavior in preschool boys is not immune from this temporal issue (Speltz, DeKlyen, Calderon, Greenberg, & Fisher, 1999). Already, at very young ages, aggressive children may be more likely than their nonaggressive peers to behave in ways that cause brain injuries.

These problems are partially remedied by animal studies that systematically control the timing, severity, and placement of frontal lobe lesions. It should be noted, however, that animal studies allow researchers to measure aggression, but not antisocial behavior per se. In addition, animal studies often fail to distinguish between different types of aggression (e.g., offensive and defensive) and are not ideal for examining the potentially important concept of early-onset aggression.

It is clear that further research is needed to confirm a causal relationship between frontal lobe functioning and antisocial behavior. In particular, longitudinal studies would be helpful in addressing issues of timing and specificity. Longitudinal studies with humans could utilize samples of individuals at risk for developing brain damage. These studies could follow subjects over a period of years, periodically taking functional magnetic resonance imaging (FMRI) and PET scans as well as measuring antisocial behavior with questionnaires, laboratory measures, and criminal records. In order to best clarify issues of timing, frontal lobe measures could be taken systematically from infancy, and changes in frontal lobe functioning could be compared to changes in relative rates of antisocial behavior over time.

Another method of testing the causal relationship between frontal lobe functioning and antisocial behavior is to do a random assignment treatment study that employs cognitive neurorehabilitation. Participants in this study could be assessed for rates of antisocial behavior and frontal lobe functioning before and after treatment. If posttreatment concomitant decreases are noted in frontal lobe dysfunction and antisocial behavior, this would support the hypothesis that frontal lobe dysfunction plays a causal role in aggressive behavior. Preliminary evidence for this type of effect already exists. For example, individuals who exhibit disruptive behaviors as a result of head injuries do well in cognitive neurorehabilitation programs that focus on problems with impulsivity (Stuss, Winocur, & Robertson, 1999). Further studies of this type can help to establish more concrete support for the causal role of frontal lobe functioning in aggressive behavior.

*Prenatal Stressors and Frontal Lobe Functioning.* Relatively few studies have examined the relationship between prenatal stressors and frontal lobe functioning. Those that have suggest that prenatal stressors can cause structural damage to the frontal lobes. For example, Wass, Persutte, and Hobbins (2001) found a relationship between maternal prenatal alcohol consumption and offspring frontal cortex size. Specifically, 23% of fetuses exposed to maternal alcohol consumption had a cortex size below the 10th percentile, while only 4% of nonexposed fetuses had a cortex size below the 10th percentile. Similarly, Poland et al. (1999) exposed pregnant rats to restraint stress for 2 hours per day from day 14 to day 21 of gestation. As adults, the prenatally stressed offspring showed significant neuronal loss within the left frontal cortex. Other studies have found associations between frontal lobe damage and prenatal malnutrition (Stern, Pugh, Resnick, & Morgane, 1984), as well as prenatal exposure to cocaine (Cabrera-Vera, Garcia, Pinto, & Battaglia, 2000) in rats.

It should be noted that the above studies use direct anatomical measures of frontal lobe damage (e.g., cortex size and neuronal loss). Anatomical measures are particularly informative in that they are more sensitive to structural brain damage than neuropsychological tests. In particular, some stressors have been shown to affect frontal lobe structure but not function. For example, a small group of studies has found that rats with frontal cortex lesions are behaviorally indistinguishable from control rats (Kolb, Cioe, & Muirhead, 1998). At the same time, frontal lobe damage that does not noticeably impair functioning may have limited relevance to the conduct disorder literature. In particular, crime and delinquency may be more related to complex executive functioning than to simple structural abnormalities such as cortex size. Thus, in future studies, it will be important to distinguish between stressors that cause structural impairment and those that cause functional impairment. In particular, fMRI studies would be useful in providing a relationship between function and anatomy. In addition, future studies may benefit from combining anatomical measures with neuropsychological tests.

While prenatal stressor–frontal lobe studies are informative, they are few in number and leave several research questions unanswered. For example, issues of timing in the prenatal stressor–frontal lobe relationship need to be clarified. Specifically, it is possible that only those stressors that occur within a specific time frame during gestation lead to frontal lobe deficits. Such a hypothesis is familiar to schizophrenia researchers, who propose that only prenatal stressors occurring during the second trimester are related to psychosis. It is also possible that the cortical teratogenic effects of prenatal stressors do not appear immediately. For example, Cabrera-Vera et al. (2000) found that, in a rat sample, reductions in serotonin neurons within the frontal cortex did not appear until adulthood. Finally, it is not clear which factors moderate the prenatal stressor–frontal lobe relationship. Wass et al. (2001) found that maternal age interacted with prenatal alcohol exposure to predict frontal cortex size. Few other studies, however, have examined the moderating effects of sociodemographic or other risk factors in the stressor–frontal lobe relationship.

Future studies are needed to address existing questions in the literature. Specifically, there is a need for animal studies in which the type, severity, and timing of a prenatal stressor can be controlled. Animal studies are particularly advantageous in that subjects can be randomly assigned to stressor/nonstressor conditions. It should be noted, however, that studies of brain functioning in animals may not generalize to human samples. Thus, another option may be to examine the frontal lobe functioning of human subjects who have been randomly exposed to environmental stressors, such as earthquakes or floods. This type of study would allow researchers to examine human brain functioning without the confounds of nonrandom assignment (e.g., Do mothers who choose to smoke during pregnancy care less about their children?). In future human and animal studies frontal lobe damage could be measured using ultrasound during gestation, and using fMRIs and PET scans following birth. These measurements could be followed by neuropsychological assessments later in life, allowing researchers to assess both structural and functional correlates of frontal lobe damage. It should be noted that the prenatal stressors literature may also benefit from meta-analytic studies that combine the effects sizes of small-$n$ prenatal stressor–frontal lobe studies to examine stressor type, stressor timing, and sociodemographic factors as moderators.

*Prenatal Stressors, Frontal Lobe Functioning, and Antisocial Behavior.* To show that frontal lobe functioning mediates the relationship between prenatal stressors and antisocial behavior, researchers must demonstrate that (1) prenatal stressors cause frontal lobe damage, (2) frontal lobe damage causes antisocial behavior, and (3) prenatal stressors only cause antisocial behavior when frontal lobe damage is present (Baron & Kenny, 1986). To test this model, one could conduct a longitudinal study in which individuals who had been prenatally exposed to random environmental stressors (floods, fire, earthquakes, etc.) would be assessed for frontal lobe damage during gestation with the use of ultrasound, and after birth with the use of fMRIs, PET scans, and neuropsychological tests. The offspring could also be assessed for antisocial behavior using questionnaires and laboratory measures. The frontal lobe model of prenatal stressors would predict that prenatally stressed individuals would be at increased risk of frontal lobe damage, that individuals with frontal lobe damage would be more likely to be antisocial, and that frontal lobe damage would mediate the relationship between prenatal stressors and antisocial behavior.

## Social Rejection

*Social Rejection and Antisocial Behavior.* Another factor that may mediate the relationship between prenatal insults and antisocial behavior is social rejection. Social rejection in childhood has been found to predict a variety of antisocial behaviors, including aggression, criminality, substance use, academic difficulties, and truancy (Newcomb, Bukowski, & Pattee, 1993). For example, a recent meta-analysis of 41 studies found that rejected children were more aggressive and less sociable than nonrejected children (Newcomb et al., 1993).

Unfortunately, rejection status tends to be stable across settings. For example, children who are rejected by school peers are often rejected by neighborhood peers as well (Kupersmidt, Griesler, Derosier, & Patterson, 1995). In addition, rejected children who are placed in new social settings tend to quickly reacquire their rejected status (Kupersmidt et al., 1995). It should be noted that peer rejection predicts antisocial behavior even after controlling for preexisting behavior problems. In fact, peer rejection often exacerbates preexisting antisocial behavior. For example, Bierman, Smoot, and Aumiller (1993) found that boys who were aggressive and rejected exhibited significantly more conduct problems than boys who were aggressive but not rejected. Thus, social rejection appears to be a reliable independent predictor of antisocial behavior.

Researchers have also conducted intervention studies that provide preliminary support for the causal role of social skills and social rejection in aggressive behavior. Interventions with social skills components delivered in the schools have been found to decrease aggressive and delinquent behaviors in childhood (Reid, Eddy, Fetrow, & Stoolmiller, 1999; Tremblay, Pagani-Kurtz, Masse, Vitaro, & Pihl, 1995). Unfortunately, these studies did not directly test whether social rejection or social skills changes mediated the effects of the intervention. In addition, these interventions focus on ameliorating other risk factors as well, so it is not clear whether changes in social skill per se are responsible for the decrease in behavior problems that have been noted. Future intervention studies that vary components by the inclusion or exclusion of social skills intervention would be necessary to more accurately assess their causal role in delinquent and aggressive behavior.

*Perinatal Factors and Social Rejection.* There are several ways in which prenatal insults may lead to social skills deficits and social rejection.

First, as discussed above, prenatal complications may cause fetal brain damage, which may in turn impair social skill acquisition. For example, individuals with frontal lobe damage often have difficulty identifying facial expressions (Braun, Denault, Cohen, & Rouleau, 1994; Hornak, Rolls, & Wade, 1996). In a recent study, Hornak et al. (1996) asked frontal lobe patients and non-frontal lobe patients to identify a series of emotional expressions. Results showed that frontal lobe patients had significantly more difficulty identifying facial expressions than controls. In addition, these emotion recognition impairments were correlated with subjective emotional changes and observable changes in behavior. For example, many of the individuals with impaired emotion recognition abilities reported an inability to "feel" emotions such as fear and sadness.

Such emotion recognition difficulties can interfere with the formation of meaningful relationships. For example, Nowicki and Duke (1992) found that children in elementary school with facial expression recognition difficulties were less popular and less internally controlled than were their peers. Similarly, Lancelot and Nowicki (1997) found a negative correlation between scores on a facial expression recognition test and externalizing problems among girls in elementary school receiving psychological treatment.

The inability to read facial expressions may also lead directly to antisocial behavior. For example, seeing another person's angry or sad facial expression is often a cue for us to turn on or off our own aggressive behavior. Individuals who cannot read facial expressions may not experience these cues. In addition, individuals with impaired emotion recognition abilities have difficulty feeling emotions such as fear and sadness (Hornak et al., 1996). Thus, it is possible that a reduced ability to feel fear or empathy leads to increased aggression and/or criminality among individuals who suffer prenatal frontal lobe damage. This hypothesis is supported by a recent study that found impairments in the recognition of sad and fearful facial expressions among children with psychopathic tendencies (Stevens, Charman, & Blair, 2001).

Prenatal brain damage may also lead to impulsivity. For example, patients with frontal lobe dysfunction frequently score higher than non-brain-disordered individuals on measures of impulsivity, such as the Frontal Behavioral Inventory (Kertesz, Davidson, & Fox, 1997) and the Eysenck Impulsiveness Scale (Eysenck, Easting, & Pearson, 1984). In addition, increased neurological soft signs have been found among patients with impulsive personality disorders (Stein et al., 1993).

Like emotion recognition difficulties, impulsivity can interfere with the formation of social relationships. For example, Bernfeld and Peters (1986) found that impulsive third graders were described as more aggressive and less socially skilled than their nonimpulsive peers. Similarly, in a recent meta-analysis, Newcomb et al. (1993) found that rejected children tend to be more impulsive and disruptive than nonrejected children. Other studies suggest a direct relationship between impulsivity and antisocial behavior.

For example, Cherek, Moeller, Dougherty, and Rhoades (1997) found that violent parolees were significantly more impulsive on a laboratory computer task than nonviolent parolees. Other studies have found associations between impulsivity and aggression among children (Mischel, Shoda, & Rodriguez, 1989), college students (Cherek et al., 1997), and substance abusers (Cherek et al., 1997).

The link between perinatal complications and social skills deficits has not been directly tested to date. Useful studies would compare individuals who have or have not been exposed to perinatal complications on a variety of social skills abilities and in terms of their peer social status. Intervention studies that work to reduce prenatal and perinatal complications (e.g., Olds et al., 1998) could also incorporate measures of social skill functioning and facial expression recognition in order to see whether reductions in perinatal risk factors are associated with improvements in these social functions.

*Perinatal Factors, Social Rejection, and Antisocial Behavior.* To date, it is unclear whether social rejection mediates the relationship between prenatal stressors and antisocial behavior. A mediator model could be tested in several ways. First, researchers could conduct longitudinal studies in which perinatal risk status was measured in infancy, social skills were measured in childhood, and antisocial behavior was measured in adolescence or early adulthood. Social skills measurements could include both sociometrics and specific ability tests such as tests of impulse control and facial expression recognition. A mediator model would predict that (1) prenatal insults would predict social rejection, (2) social rejection would predict antisocial behavior, and (3) the relationship between prenatal insults and antisocial behavior would no longer be significant after controlling for social rejection.

## Stress Reactivity

*Stress Reactivity and Antisocial Behavior.* Another neurophysiological process that may mediate the relationship between perinatal factors and aggression is dysregulation of the HPA axis or stress response. Preliminary evidence exists for the relationship between HPA axis functioning and aggressive behavior. Specifically, early-onset conduct disorder has been related to lower mean levels of cortisol (the final by-product of the stress response in humans) in a clinic sample of boys (McBurnett, Lahey, Rathouz, & Loeber, 2000). Similarly, in a sample of boys at high risk for alcohol abuse, aggression was related to a lower cortisol response in anticipation of a stressor (Moss, Mezzich, Yao, Gavaler, & Martin, 1995). These findings are consistent with the notion that aggressive or delinquent children may be underresponsive to stressors or stimuli in their environment, and may act aggressively either because they lack fear or because they have a physiological need to seek stimulation.

Preliminary evidence also indicates that psychosocial interventions aimed at reducing aggression might also have a positive effect on regulating HPA axis function. In a pilot study of aggressive youth in a foster care intervention program, Fisher and Stoolmiller (2002) noted that diurnal cortisol patterns change in response to the intervention. Aggressive youth had a "flat" pattern of cortisol levels (low in the morning and throughout the day) at the initiation of the intervention. Over time, their daily cortisol patterns normalized, with higher levels noted in the morning and a decrease throughout the day. Although these results are preliminary, they suggest that HPA axis responsiveness may increase in response to psychosocial interventions designed to decrease aggressive behavior.

There is preliminary evidence in the literature that the relationship between HPA axis reactivity and aggression may undergo a developmental shift, such that in younger children acting-out behaviors are associated with a hyperresponsive HPA axis, and in older children acting-out behaviors are associated with a hyporesponsive HPA axis (as noted above). In a sample of children in daycare between 39 and 106 months of age, a rise in cortisol levels throughout the day was associated with *higher* levels of aggression (Dettling, Gunnar, & Donzella, 1999). In addition, it was noted that younger children were more likely than older children to show this rise in cortisol during the day. To more fully examine the developmental effects on the relationship between aggression and HPA axis reactivity future studies in this area are necessary. As we outline below, this is a central issue in the hypothesis that HPA axis activity acts as a mediator between perinatal factors and aggression in children.

Another neglected focus in the literature on HPA axis function and aggression is the measure and comparison of different types of aggressive behaviors. For example, a relevant dimension in this regard would be the differentiation between defensive and offensive aggression. It is reasonable to hypothesize that defensive aggression may be more associated with a hyperresponsive HPA axis, and that offensive aggression is more associated with a hyporesponsive HPA axis (and stimulation-seeking behavior as described above). No studies to date have tested this distinction.

*Perinatal Factors and Stress Reactivity.* In rat populations, prenatal stress increases the response of the HPA axis after birth, specifically increasing glucocorticoids, which can have harmful effects on the developing brain (Gunnar, 1998). Prenatal and perinatal stressors such as maternal alcohol use in pregnancy and delivery complications have also been linked to increased HPA axis reactivity in human infants (Jacobson, Bihun, & Chiodo, 1999; Taylor, Fisk, & Glover, 2000). In addition, prenatal exposure to nicotine has been linked to higher basal levels of stress hormones in rats after birth (King & Strand, 1988). To date, studies of perinatal factors and HPA axis reactivity are limited in number, particularly those that focus on humans. Future studies should examine a variety of perinatal factors and control for potential confounds such as maternal psychological functioning, postnatal stressors, and family environment. Basic research is also needed to examine the relationship between perinatal factors and daily cortisol patterns, specific stress responsivity, and regulation of the HPA axis stress response. Again animal studies performed in conjunction with longitudinal studies of humans will be the most effective in terms of providing support for a causal connection in this area.

*Perinatal Factors, Stress Reactivity and Antisocial Behavior.* How might HPA axis dysregulation mediate the relationship between perinatal factors and aggressive outcomes later in childhood? There are several possible ways in which this could occur. One possibility is that individuals who are exposed to perinatal and chronic postnatal stressors may have a downregulated HPA axis. The HPA axis may downregulate in response to the chronic oversecretion of hormones in response to earlier stressors. As noted above, low baseline cortisol has been found in aggressive boys (McBurnett et al., 2000). In addition, lower anticipatory cortisol responses have been associated with cigarette smoking and marijuana use in sons of male substance abusers (Moss, Vanyukov, Yao, & Kirillova, 1999). In this latter study, the authors hypothesized that the chronic stress associated with having a substance-abusing father may have contributed to their hyporeactive cortisol responses. This suggests a potential developmental pathway leading from chronic environmental stress in childhood, to decreased HPA axis responsivity, and ultimately to an increased need for stimulation via sensation-seeking behaviors in early adolescence.

Another possibility is that an *over*responsive HPA axis could increase the risk for aggressive behavior, particularly reactive aggression. As discussed above, animal and human studies have linked perinatal risk factors to an overreactive HPA axis response. Preliminary data from our lab suggest a link between perinatal problems and a behavior pattern of high levels of fear and aggression. We examined this relationship in the context of a longitudinal study of maternal depression in Brisbane, Australia. This sample was drawn from a community cohort born between 1981 and 1984 at Mater Mother's Hospital. Mothers were interviewed and the youth were tested at ages 5 and 14 years. Based on maternal Child Behavior Checklist reports at ages 5 and 14, we categorized children as inhibited plus aggressive (above the median on both at ages 5 and 14); not inhibited, but persistently aggressive (below the median on inhibition and above the median on aggression at both ages 5 and 14); or neither inhibited nor aggressive (below the median on both at ages 5 and 14). We found that the group of children who were both inhibited and aggressive had higher rates of maternal anxiety, maternal depression, and perinatal problems than the persistently aggressive and control children. These preliminary data are consistent with the idea that perinatal complications may produce a highly reactive HPA axis, which in turn may increase the risk for aggressive behavior (in combination with high levels of inhibition). The increased risk for aggression/inhibition may result from either poor emotion regulation, high threat sensitivity, or both.

The hypothesis that HPA axis dysregulation may mediate the relationship between perinatal risk factors and aggression has only preliminary support in the literature. Future studies are needed to assess both the short-term and the long-term consequences of perinatal stressors on HPA axis regulation. Much of this work can best be done in animal studies where the timing and specificity of stressors can be controlled. Human studies can also be undertaken that examine cortisol responses in infants exposed to a variety of perinatal risk factors. Longitudinal studies are needed to assess whether or not chronic overresponsiveness of the HPA axis eventually results in a downregulation of this system. If such evidence were found, it would provide a linkage between the noted findings of perinatal stress and overresponsive HPA axis activity early in life and aggression and underresponsive HPA axis activity later in childhood. Alternatively, the role of HPA axis activity may involve a more complex relationship with different types of aggressive outcomes (e.g., defensive vs. offensive). Studies that measure and separately examine these different types of aggression will be necessary to tease out these effects.

## IMPLICATIONS FOR INTERVENTION

Frontal lobe dysfunction, social rejection, and stress reactivity have been hypothesized to be mediators and family dysfunction has been hypothesized to be a moderator of the perinatal factors–antisocial behavior relationship. If confirmed by future research, these hypotheses will have important implications for intervention. Specifically, children who have undergone perinatal risks could then be targeted for preventive interventions that are focused on cognitive rehabilitation, social skills training, and/or arousal regulation. Targeted prevention programs may also be useful if focused on potential moderators such as effective and consistent parenting.

## CONCLUSIONS

We have proposed several moderator and mediator hypotheses concerning the relationship between perinatal factors and antisocial outcomes. A review of the literature suggests that a combination of animal studies and longitudinal, genetically sensitive, and intervention studies with humans will be necessary to test these hypotheses and to determine whether or not perinatal factors play a causal role in aggression and antisocial behavior. Translational research that examines the basic science causal questions in the context of interventions would also be recommended as it allows researchers to answer these questions in a manner that provides the most immediate and direct benefit to the research participants themselves.

## REFERENCES

Arseneault, L., Tremblay, R. E., Boulerice, B., & Saucier, J. (2002). Obstetrical complications and violent delinquency: Testing two developmental pathways. *Child Development, 73*, 496–508.

Baron, R. M., & Kenny, D. A. (1986). The moderator–mediator variable distinction in social psychological research: Conceptual, strategic, and statistical considerations. *Journal of Personality and Social Psychology, 51*, 1173–1182.

Bernfeld, G. A., & Peters, R. D. (1986). Social reasoning and social behavior in reflective and impulsive children. *Journal of Clinical Child Psychology, 15*, 221–227.

Bierman, K. L., Smoot, D. L., & Aumiller, K. (1993). Characteristics of aggressive-rejected, aggressive (nonrejected), and rejected (nonaggressive) boys. *Child Development, 64*, 139–151.

Braun, C. M., Denault, C., Cohen, H., & Rouleau, I. (1994). Discrimination of facial identity and facial affect by temporal and frontal lobectomy patients. *Brain and Cognition, 24*, 198–212.

Brennan, P. A,, Grekin, E. R., & Mednick, S. A. (1999). Maternal smoking during pregnancy and adult male criminal outcomes. *Archives of General Psychiatry, 56*, 215–219.

Brennan, P. A., Grekin, E. R., Mortensen, E. L., & Mednick, S. A. (2002). Maternal smoking during pregnancy and offspring criminal arrest and hospitalization for substance abuse: A test of gender specific relationships. *American Journal of Psychiatry, 159*, 48–54.

Brennan, P. A., Mednick, S. A., & Raine, A. (1997). Perinatal and social risk factors for violence. In A. Raine, P. Brennan, D. Farrington, & S. Mednick (Eds.), *Biosocial bases of violence* (pp. 163–174). New York: Plenum Press.

Brower, M.C., & Price, B.H. (2001). Neuropsychiatry of frontal lobe dysfunction in violent and criminal behaviour: A critical review. *Journal of Neurology, Neurosurgery and Psychiatry, 71*, 720–726.

Cabrera-Vera, T. M., Garcia, F., Pinto, W., & Battaglia, G. (2000). Neurochemical changes in brain serotonin neurons in immature and adult offspring prenatally exposed to cocaine. *Brain Research, 870*, 1–9.

Castle, D. J., & Murray, R. M. (1991). The neurodevelopmental basis of sex differences in schizophrenia. *Psychological Medicine, 21*, 565–575.

Cherek, D. R., Moeller, F. G., Dougherty, D. M., & Rhoades, H. (1997). Studies of violent and nonviolent male parolees: II. Laboratory and psychometric measurements of impulsivity. *Biological Psychiatry, 41*, 523–529.

Chow, T. W. (2000). Personality in frontal lobe disorders. *Current Psychiatry Reports, 2*, 446–451.

Crick, N. R., & Bigbee, M. A. (1998). Relational and overt forms of peer victimization: A multiinformant approach. *Journal of Consulting and Clinical Psychology, 66*, 337–347.

Crick, N. R., & Grotpeter, J. K. (1995). Relational aggression, gender, and social–psychological adjustment. *Child Development, 66*, 710–722.

Day, N. L., Richardson, G. A., Goldschmidt, L., & Cornelius, M. D. (2000). Effects of prenatal tobacco exposure on preschoolers' behavior. *Journal of Developmental and Behavioral Pediatrics, 21,* 180–188.

Dettling, A. C., Gunnar, M., & Donzella, B. (1999). Cortisol levels of young children in full-day childcare centers: Relations with age and temperament. *Psychoneuroendocrinology, 24,* 519–536.

Dietrich, K. M., Ris, M. D., Succop, P. A., Berger, O. G., & Bornschein, R. L. (2001). Early exposure to lead and juvenile delinquency. *Neurotoxicology and Teratology, 23,* 511–518.

Eysenck, S. B., Easting, G., & Pearson, P. R. (1984). Age norms for impulsiveness, venturesomeness and empathy in children. *Personality and Individual Differences, 5,* 315–321.

Fallgatter, A. J., & Herrmann, M. J. (2001). Electrophysiological assessment of impulsive behavior in healthy subjects. *Neuropsychologia, 39,* 328–333.

Fergusson, D. M. (1999). Prenatal smoking and antisocial behavior. *Archives of General Psychiatry, 56,* 223–224.

Fergusson, D. M., Woodward, L. J., & Horwood, J. (1998). Maternal smoking during pregnancy and psychiatric adjustment in late adolescence. *Archives of General Psychiatry, 55,* 721–727.

Fisher, P. A., & Stoolmiller, M. (2002, April). *Investigating longitudinal trends in correlations between maltreated foster children's behavior and L-HPA axis activity.* Paper presented at the International Conference of Infant Studies, Toronto, Ontario, Canada.

Francis, D. D., Champagne, F. A., Liu, D., & Meaney, M. J. (1999). Maternal care, gene expression, and the development of individual differences in stress reactivity. In N. E. Adler, M. Marmot, B. S. McEwen, & J. Stewart (Eds.), *Socioeconomic status and health in industrial nations: Social, psychological, and biological pathways* (pp. 66–84). New York: New York Academy of Sciences.

Gibson, C. L., Piquero, A. R., & Tibbetts, S. G. (2000). Assessing the relationship between maternal cigarette smoking during pregnancy and age at first police contact. *Justice Quarterly, 17,* 519–542.

Gunnar, M. R. (1998). Quality of early care and buffering of neuroendocrine stress reactions: Potential effects on the developing human brain. *Preventive Medicine, 27,* 208–211.

Gunnar, M. R., & Chisholm, K. (1999, April). *Effects of early institutional rearing and attachment quality on salivary cortisol levels in adopted Romanian children.* Poster presented at the meeting of the Society for Research in Child Development, Albuquerque, NM.

Hodgins, S., Kratzer, L., & McNeil, T. F. (2001). Obstetric complications, parenting, and risk of criminal behavior. *Archives of General Psychiatry, 58,* 746–752.

Hornak, J., Rolls, E. T., & Wade, D. (1996). Face and voice expression identification in patients with emotional and behavioural changes following ventral frontal lobe damage. *Neuropsychologia, 34,* 247–261.

Jacobson, S. W., Bihun, J. T., & Chiodo, L. M. (1999). Effects of prenatal alcohol and cocaine exposure on infant cortisol levels. *Development and Psychopathology, 11,* 195–208.

Kandel, E., & Mednick, S. A. (1991). Perinatal complications predict violent offending. *Criminology, 29,* 519–529.

Kertesz, A., Davidson, W., & Fox, H. (1997). Frontal behavioral inventory: Diagnostic criteria for frontal lobe dementia. *Canadian Journal of Neurological Sciences, 24,* 29–36.

King, J. A., & Strand, F. L. (1988). Increased ACTH plasma levels with prenatal and postnatal nicotine administration in rats. *Annals of the New York Academy of Science, 529,* 301–303.

Kolb, B., Cioe, J., & Muirhead, D. (1998). Cerebral morphology and functional sparing after prenatal frontal cortex lesions in rats. *Behavioural Brain Research, 91,* 143–155.

Kupersmidt, J. B., Griesler, P. C., DeRosier, M. E., & Patterson, C. J. (1995). Childhood aggression and peer relations in the context of family and neighborhood factors. *Child Development, 66,* 360–375.

Lancelot, C., & Nowicki, S. Jr. (1997). The association between receptive nonverbal processing abilities and internalizing/externalizing problems in girls and boys. *Journal of Genetic Psychology*, *158*, 297–302.

Lewis, D. O., Shanok, S. S., & Balla, D. A. (1979). Perinatal difficulties, head and face trauma, and child abuse in the medical histories of seriously delinquent children. *American Journal of Psychiatry*, *136*, 419–423.

Lezak, M. D. (1995). *Neuropsychological assessment* (3rd ed.). New York: Oxford University Press.

Maughan, B., Taylor, C., Taylor, A., Butler, N., & Bynner, J. (2001). Pregnancy smoking and childhood conduct problems: A causal association? *Journal of Child Psychology and Psychiatry and Allied Disciplines*, *42*, 1021–1028.

McBurnett, K., Lahey, B. B., Rathouz, P. J., & Loeber, R. (2000). Low salivary cortisol and persistent aggression in boys referred for disruptive behavior. *Archives of General Psychiatry*, *57*, 38–43.

Miller, L. (1987). Neuropsychology of the aggressive psychopath: An integrative review. *Aggressive Behavior*, *13*, 119–140.

Mischel, W., Shoda, Y., & Rodriguez, M. L. (1989). Delay of gratification in children. *Science*, *244*, 933–938.

Moffitt, T. E. (1993). Adolescent-limited and life-course-persistent antisocial behavior: A developmental taxonomy. *Psychological Review*, *100*, 674–701.

Morgan, A. B., & Lilienfeld, S. O. (2000). A meta-analytic review of the relation between antisocial behavior and neuropsychological measures of executive function. *Clinical Psychology Review*, *20*, 113–156.

Moss, H. B., Mezzich, A., Yao, J. K., Gavaler, J., & Martin, C. S. (1995). Aggressivity among sons of substance-abusing fathers: Association with psychiatric disorder in the father and son, paternal personality, pubertal development, and socioeconomic status. *American Journal of Drug and Alcohol Abuse*, *21*, 195–208.

Moss, H. B., Vanyukov, M., Yao, J. K., & Kirillova, G. P. (1999). Salivary cortisol responses in prepubertal boys: The effects of parental substance abuse and association with drug use behavior during adolescence. *Biological Psychiatry*, *45*, 1293–1299.

Newcomb, A. F., Bukowski, W. M., & Pattee, L. (1993). Children's peer relations: A meta-analytic review of popular, rejected, neglected, controversial, and average sociometric status. *Psychological Bulletin*, *113*, 99–128.

Nowicki, S., & Duke, M. P. (1992). The association of children's nonverbal decoding abilities with their popularity, locus of control, and academic achievement. *Journal of Genetic Psychology*, *153*, 385–393.

Olds, D., Henderson, C. R., Cole, R., Eckenrode, J., Kitzman, H., Luckey, D., Pettit, L., Sidora, K., Morris, P., & Powers, J. (1998). Long-term effects of nurse home visitation on children's criminal and antisocial behavior: 15 year follow-up of a randomized trial. *Journal of the American Medical Association*, *280*, 1238–1244.

Orlebeke, J. F., Knol, D. L., & Verhulst, F. C. (1997). Increase in child behavior problems resulting from maternal smoking during pregnancy. *Archives of Environmental Health*, *52*, 317–321.

Poland, R. E., Cloak, C., Lutchmansingh, P. J., McCracken, J. T., Chang, L., & Ernst, T. (1999). Brain N-acetyl aspartate concentrations measured by H MRS are reduced in adult male rats subjected to perinatal stress: Preliminary observations and hypothetical implications for neurodevelopmental disorders. *Journal of Psychiatric Research*, *33*, 41–51.

Raine, A., Brennan, P., & Mednick, S. A. (1994). Birth complications combined with early maternal rejection predispose to adult violent crime. *Archives of General Psychiatry*, *51*, 984–988.

Raz, S., Shah, F., & Sander, C. J. (1996). Differential effects of perinatal hypoxic risk on early developmental outcome: A twin study. *Neuropsychology*, *10*, 429–436.

Reid, J. B., Eddy, J. M., Fetrow, R. A., & Stoolmiller, M. (1999). Description and immediate impacts of a preventive intervention for conduct problems. *American Journal of Community Psychology, 27,* 483–517.

Rutter, M., Pickles, A., Murray, R., & Eaves, L. (2001). Testing hypotheses on specific environmental causal effects on behavior. *Psychological Bulletin, 27,* 291–324.

Speltz, M. L., DeKlyen, M., Calderon, R., Greenberg, M. T., & Fisher, P. A. (1999). Neuropsychological characteristics and test behaviors of boys with early onset conduct problems. *Journal of Abnormal Psychology, 108,* 315–325.

Stein, D. J., Hollander, E., Cohen, L., Frenkel, M., Saoud, J. B., DeCaria, C., Aronowitz, B., Levin, A., Liebowitz, M. R., & Cohen, L. (1993). Neuropsychiatric impairment in impulsive personality disorders. *Psychiatry Research, 48,* 257–266.

Stern, W. C., Pugh, W. W., Resnick, O., & Morgane, P. J. (1984). Developmental protein malnutrition in the rat: Effects on single-unit activity in the frontal cortex. *Brain Research, 306,* 227–234.

Stevens, D., Charman, T., & Blair, R. J. R. (2001). Recognition of emotion in facial expressions and vocal tones in children with psychopathic tendencies. *Journal of Genetic Psychology, 162,* 201–211.

Stuss, D. T., Winocur, G., & Robertson, I. A. (1999). *Cognitive neurorehabilitation.* Cambridge, UK: Cambridge University Press.

Taylor, A., Fisk, N. M., & Glover, V. (2000). Mode of delivery and subsequent stress response. *Lancet, 355,* 120.

Tibbetts, S. G., & Piquero, A. (1999). The influence of gender, low birth weight, and disadvantaged environment in predicting early onset of offending: A test of Moffitt's interactional hypothesis. *Criminology, 374,* 843–877.

Tremblay, R. E., Pagani-Kurtz, L., Masse, L. C., Vitaro, F., & Pihl, R. (1995). A bimodal preventive intervention for disruptive kindergarten boys: Its impact through mid-adolescence. *Journal of Consulting and Clinical Psychology, 63,* 560–568.

Wakschlag, L. S., & Hans, S. L. (2002). Maternal smoking during pregnancy and conduct problems in high-risk youth: A developmental framework. *Development and Psychopathology, 14,* 351–369.

Wakschlag, L. S., Lahey, B. B., Loeber, R., Green, S. M., Gordon, R., & Leventhal, B.L. (1997). Maternal smoking during pregnancy and the risk of conduct disorder in boys. *Archives of General Psychiatry, 54,* 670–676.

Wakschlag, L. S., Pickett, K. E., Cook, E., Benowitz, N. L., & Leventhal, B. L. (2002). Maternal smoking during pregnancy and severe antisocial behavior in offspring: Are they causally linked? *American Journal of Public Health, 92,* 966–974.

Wang, X., Zuckerman, B., Pearson, C., Kaufman, G., Chen, C., Wang, G., Niu, T., Wise, P. H., Bauchner, H., & Xu, X. (2002). Maternal cigarette smoking, metabolic gene polymorphism, and infant birthweight. *Journal of the American Medical Association, 287,* 195–202.

Wass, T. S., Persutte, W. H., & Hobbins, J. C. (2001). The impact of prenatal alcohol exposure on frontal cortex development in utero. *American Journal of Obstetrics and Gynecology, 185,* 737–742.

Weissman, M. M., Warner, V., Wickramaratne, P. J., & Kandel, D. B. (1999). Maternal smoking during pregnancy and psychopathology in offspring followed to adulthood. *Journal of the American Academy of Child and Adolescent Psychiatry, 38,* 892–899.

Werner, E. E. (1987). Vulnerability and resiliency in children at risk for delinquency: A longitudinal study from birth to adulthood. In J. D. Burchard, & S. N. Burchard (Eds.), *Primary prevention of psychopathology* (pp. 16–43). Newbury Park, CA: Sage.

Wolff, P. H., Waber, D., Bauermeister, M., Cohen, C., & Ferber R. (1982). The neuropsychological status of adolescent delinquent boys. *Journal of Child Psychology and Psychiatry and Allied Disciplines, 23,* 267–279.

# Animal Models of the
# Causes of Aggression

# 13

# Social and Biological Mechanisms Underlying Impulsive Aggressiveness in Rhesus Monkeys

## STEPHEN J. SUOMI

Why are some individuals consistently more aggressive than others? Have they been like that since early childhood, or is their aggressiveness a recent phenomenon? Is their aggression violent—and has it always been that way? What was the basis of its origin—are these individuals violent because of something in their genes or because of something in their own history . . . or perhaps some combination of both?

During the past decade an increasing body of prospective research, some of it reviewed in various chapters in this volume, has revealed important insights regarding these questions. We now know that aggression first appears during toddlerhood in virtually all individuals, but for most (fortunately) their aggressive behaviors decline in frequency, become less likely to result in overt physical attack, and are increasingly limited to specific situations as they grow older. However, a few children continue to exhibit high levels of physical aggression well beyond toddlerhood. Many of those individuals (especially boys) who are displaying high levels of such aggression upon entry into the school system will likely continue to be highly aggressive throughout adolescence and even into adulthood. In addition, both prospective and retrospective studies have shown that such individuals are also at greatly increased risk for developing a wide range of other behavioral problems or more serious psychopathologies, including attentional difficulties and externalizing behavioral disorders in childhood and delinquency, substance abuse, violent criminality, and suicide in adolescence and adulthood (e.g., Tremblay, 1992).

A number of researchers searching for a possible biological basis of such impulsive violent aggression have focused on the apparent relationship between extreme behavioral tendencies of this nature and abnormal serotonergic functioning (cf. Coccaro & Murphy, 1990). For example, unusually low concentrations of the primary central serotonin metabolite 5-hydroxyindoleacetic acid (5-HIAA) in cerebrospinal fluid (CSF) have been found in children who are unusually aggressive toward peers and hostile toward mothers (Kruesi et al., 1990); children who torture animals (Kruesi, 1989); children and adolescents with disruptive behavior disorders (Kruesi et al., 1990); offenders convicted of violent aggressive acts and/or property destruction (Linnoila et al., 1983); men with personality disorders having extreme scores for aggression, irritability, hostility, and psychopathic deviance on standardized tests (Brown, Linnoila, & Goodwin, 1990; Linnoila, 1988); men expelled from the U.S. marines for excessive violence and psychopathic deviance (Brown, Goodwin, Ballenger, Goyer, & Major, 1979); suicide victims (e.g., Mann, Arango, & Underwood, 1990); and sons of men arrested for violence and arson (Linnoila, DeJong, & Virkkunen, 1989). The precise nature of this linkage (i.e., what causes what) and basic developmental questions concerning its initial appearance, developmental continuity, and long-term stability are all of obvious theoretical, clinical, and even societal interest, yet to date definitive answers to such questions have largely remained elusive.

## PRIMATE ANALOGUES OF IMPULSIVE AGGRESSIVENESS

### Background

Studies of impulsive violent aggression—or any other phenomena—in humans are inevitably constrained in their ability to address certain fundamental issues concerning development by some very real ethical and practical issues. Nature–nurture questions are most clearly resolved when a range of predetermined genotypes can be studied across systematically varied environmental settings, yet that is almost never ethically proper and seldom practically feasible with human subjects. Questions regarding issues of developmental continuity and stability are best studied via long-term, prospective longitudinal experiments, but such studies tend to be expensive, are often subject to nonrandom sample attrition, and inevitably take a long time to complete because humans take a long time to grow up. Many of these problems and constraints can be reduced substantially (if not eliminated) via appropriate studies with animals. Of course, the degree to which animal research can answer questions or address issues concerning human developmental phenomena is largely dependent on the degree to which the phenomena of interest generalize from the human case to the animal under study (cf. Harlow, Suomi, & Gluck, 1972). With respect to impulsive aggression—and its apparent link with 5-HIAA deficits—a growing body of evidence suggests considerable cross-species generality between humans and advanced nonhuman primates.

Investigators studying a variety of nonhuman primate species over the past two decades have reported dramatic differences in the frequency and form of aggression displayed by individuals in both captive and field settings (e.g., Bernstein, Williams, & Ramsay, 1983; Steklis, Brammen, Raleigh, & McGuire, 1985). Much of this research has been carried out with rhesus monkeys (*Macaca mulatta*), representatives of a highly successful Old World monkey species indigenous to the Indian subcontinent, who share approximately 95% of their genes with *Homo sapiens* (Lovejoy, 1981; Sibley, Comstock, & Alquist, 1990). By way of background, rhesus monkeys in their natural habitats typically reside in large social groups ("troops"), each containing several multigenerational female lineages, plus numerous immigrant adult males. This form of social organization derives from the fact that females spend their entire life in the troop in which they were born, whereas virtually all males emigrate from their natal troop around the time of puberty, when they are 4- to 6-years-old, eventually joining other nearby troops.

## Species-Normative Development of Aggression in Rhesus Monkeys

Rhesus monkey infants spend virtually all of their initial days and weeks of life in physical contact or within arm's reach of their biological mother, during which time they form a strong, specific attachment bond with her. In their second month of life, infant monkeys begin to explore their immediate physical and social environment, using their mother as a "secure base" to support such exploration (cf. Suomi, 1995). Over the next few months these infants spend increasing amounts of time engaging in extensive social interactions with other group members, especially peers. Social play with peers soon becomes their predominant social activity and remains so throughout "childhood" (i.e., the rest of their first year, all of the second, and most if not all of their third year of life). During this time play interactions become increasingly complex and involve patterns of behavior that appear to simulate virtually all adult social activities, including courtship and reproductive behaviors and dominance/aggressive interactions.

The onset of puberty is associated with major life transitions for both genders. Although rhesus monkey females remain in their natal troop throughout adolescence and thereafter, their interactions with peers decline dramatically as they redirect much of their social activities toward matrilineal kin, including the infants they subsequently bear and rear. Adolescent males, by contrast, leave their natal troop permanently and typically join all-male "gangs" for varying periods before they attempt to enter a different troop. This period of transition for adolescent and young adult males represents a time of major stress, with a mortality rate that approaches 50% in some rhesus monkey populations. Virtually all males that do survive eventually join other troops. Some of these males stay in their new troop for the rest of their lives, whereas other males may transfer from one troop to another several times during their adult years (Berard, 1989). This overall pattern of social group organization and general sequence of behavioral development is relatively common among Old World monkey species, especially within the genus *Macaca* (Lindburg, 1991).

Aggression is a normal and necessary part of every rhesus monkey's overall behavioral repertoire—indeed, most primatologists consider rhesus monkeys to be among the most aggressive of all primate species. Rhesus monkey aggression can range in intensity from mere facial threats and vocalizations to vigorous chases and actual physical aggression, including slapping, hitting, hair pulling, and biting with sufficient intensity to produce lasting tissue damage or even death. The capability for aggression is crucial for survival in the wild, not only from the standpoint of defending one's self and one's offspring from predators and conspecific competitors, but also in maintaining social order and enforcing the complex dominance hierarchies characteristic of all rhesus monkey troops. However, uncontrolled, unpredictable, and violent aggression within any troop could drive members apart and destroy the troop as a social unit. Therefore, as with humans, aggression must be *socialized*: it must be minimized or at least largely ritualized in intragroup interactions, but it also must remain a viable response in order to counter external threats or other dangers. Socialization of aggression for young rhesus monkeys involves not only learning in which circumstances and toward what targets aggressive behavior might be appropriate, but also gauging the relative intensity of the attack or response called for and the appropriate time and means for terminating an aggressive bout or for avoiding it altogether. Indeed, learning whom *not* to attack, as well as how to moderate aggressive impulses, is as important in the socialization process as honing one's fighting skills.

Aggression typically emerges in a rhesus monkey's behavioral repertoire around 6 months of age, and it initially appears in the context of rough-and-tumble play (Symonds, 1978). Biting, hair pulling, wrestling, and other forms of physical contact are basic components of rough-and-tumble play directed toward peers, which occurs with increasing frequency among males in the second half of their first year of life and becomes the predominate type of play for the rest of their juvenile years. Although some form of virtually all behavioral components of adult aggressive exchanges can be seen in the rough-and-tumble play bouts of young males, the intensity of such interactions is usually quite controlled and seldom escalates to the point of potential physical injury—if it does, the play bout is almost always terminated immediately, either via adult intervention or by one or more of the participants backing away themselves. The importance of these play bouts with peers for the socialization of aggression becomes apparent when one considers that rhesus monkey infants reared in laboratory environments that deny them regular access to peers during their initial months inevitably exhibit excessive and socially inappropriate aggression later in life (e.g., Alexander & Harlow, 1965; Harlow & Harlow, 1969).

In naturalistic settings, both prepubertal males and females readily join their mothers and other relatives in aggressive exchanges involving other families or monkeys from other troops. Such exchanges are typically precipitated by challenges to existing dominance hierarchies and usually are brief in duration and more likely to involve threats, bluffs, and chases than actual tissue-damaging physical contact. These dominance-related agonistic exchanges are a normal part of rhesus monkey everyday troop life, and it is through participation in such exchanges that most juveniles learn about the complexities of rhesus monkey dominance hierarchies and associated interactions, including the development and maintenance of social coalitions, the use of submissive responses in the face of likely defeat, and the ability to back away from or terminate rapidly escalating agonistic exchanges prior to the point of potential tissue damage. Most juveniles also eventually learn that sudden, seemingly impulsive behaviors can readily provoke aggressive reactions from more dominant troop members with obvious negative consequences, and most become increasingly proficient in inhibiting such activities in potentially dangerous social circumstances—but others do not.

## Behavioral Features of Impulsive Aggression and CSF 5-HIAA Correlates

Numerous studies of rhesus monkeys carried out in both captive and field settings over the past decade have identified a subset of individuals, mostly males, who can be characterized as basically incompetent socially. These monkeys, comprising perhaps 5–10% of field populations studied to date, seem unusually impulsive, insensitive, and overtly aggressive in their interactions with other troop members. They either fail to comprehend the complexity and social importance of dominance hierarchies, have little motivation to "follow the rules," or both. For example, they often initiate apparently spontaneous actions that are socially inappropriate and have predictably negative social consequences, such as suddenly jumping between a mother and her infant. They are disproportionately likely to harass a juvenile who is younger and physically weaker than themselves but who also belongs to a high-ranking family. Remarkably, some adolescent and young adult males have been observed to repeatedly challenge a dominant adult male, a foolhardy act that can result in serious injury, especially when they fail to exhibit appropriate submissive behavior once defeat becomes obvious and instead escalate the intensity of their aggression. The same young males also display a propensity for making dangerous leaps from treetop to treetop, occasionally with painful outcomes (Mehlman et al.,

1994). Perhaps not surprisingly, physical examinations of these males have revealed patterns of wounding and scars that are far more numerous and severe than those seen in the rest of their birth cohort (Higley et al., 1992).

As is the case with humans, numerous studies of rhesus monkeys have consistently reported an inverse relationship between measures of impulsive-like aggression and CSF 5-HIAA concentrations, not only in comparisons involving subjects of the same age, gender, and rearing background but also in more general comparisons (e.g., Higley, Suomi, & Linnnoila, 1991). For example, CSF 5-HIAA concentrations are at their highest immediately after birth, when aggression does not exist in the neonate's behavioral repertoire, and they drop by more than half over the first 5 months, a time when aggression emerges in the infant's repertoire and is typically in its least socialized form. CSF 5-HIAA concentrations continue to decline, albeit considerably more slowly, until around 18 months of age, at which point they become more or less stable until puberty. Some monkeys experience another pronounced drop in CSF 5-HIAA concentrations around puberty, and for most individuals there is a slight rise throughout the adult years. The developmental trajectory for impulsive aggression is exactly the opposite: impulsive aggression directed toward peers typically increases in frequency from 6 to 18 months of age, basically stabilizes until puberty, increases (at least in intensity) for some individuals during and shortly after puberty, and then generally declines monotonically throughout the adult years. More importantly, individual differences in impulsive aggressivity have been found to correlate negatively with individual differences in CSF 5-HIAA concentrations for monkeys at every age studied. Thus, there appears to be a strong and significant *continuity* in the inverse relationship that remains robust in the face of major developmental changes in both measures throughout the lifespan. Moreover, the inverse relationship between indices of impulsive aggression and those of central serotonin metabolism appears to generalize beyond individuals of different ages to monkeys of different genders, strains, and even species (e.g., Champoux, Higley, & Suomi, 1997; Higley et al., 1991; Raleigh & McGuire, 1994; Westergaard, Mehlman, Suomi, & Higley, 1999).

In summary, there appear to be some features common to the expressions of impulsive aggression shown by some humans and by some rhesus monkeys, most notably the inverse relationship between these behavioral patterns and CSF concentrations of the primary central metabolite of serotonin. What do we know about the developmental continuity and relative stability of individual differences in the expression of this distinctive biobehavioral response pattern shown by some rhesus monkeys? What do we know about nature–nurture issues regarding this phenomenon? And in what ways might such information inform and advance our understanding of impulsive aggression in humans? Each of these questions is addressed in the sections that follow.

## DEVELOPMENTAL CONTINUITY AND STABILITY OF INDIVIDUAL DIFFERENCES IN THE EXPRESSION OF IMPULSIVE AGGRESSIVENESS

Prospective longitudinal studies have found that young male monkeys who can be characterized as impulsively aggressive typically begin to distinguish themselves from same-sex peers in their early play interactions. They seem to lack the ability to moderate their behavioral responses to playful invitations from peers, and by late childhood their rough-and-tumble play interactions often escalate into tissue-damaging aggressive exchanges, disproportionately at their own expense. Over time most of these individuals come to be avoided by peers, and they become increasingly isolated socially. Consistent with previously cited findings, these monkeys tend to have relatively low CSF 5-HIAA concentrations (Higley, Suomi, & Linnoila, 1996).

Laboratory studies have demonstrated that monkeys who exhibit deficits in serotonin metabolism are also likely to show poor state control and visual orienting capabilities during early infancy (Champoux, Suomi, & Schneider, 1994), poor performance on delay-of-gratification tasks during childhood (Tsai, Bennett, Pierre, Shoaf, & Higley, 1999), sleep difficulties (Zajicek, Higley, Suomi, & Linnoila, 1997), and excessive cerebral glucose metabolism under mild isoflurine anesthesia as adults (Doudet et al., 1995). Recent research has shown that individual differences in both behavioral measures of impulsivity and CSF 5-HIAA values obtained during infancy are also predictive of individual differences in the propensity to consume alcohol in a "happy hour" situation. Over the past decade Higley and his colleagues have developed an experimental paradigm in which group-living rhesus monkeys are given the opportunity to consume a 7% ethanol aspartame-flavored beverage, a nonalcoholic aspartame-flavored beverage, and/or plain tap water for daily 1-hour periods within their familiar social group (e.g., Higley, Hasert, Suomi, & Linnoila, 1991). Overly impulsive and aggressive individuals tend to consume excessive amounts of alcohol when placed in the afore-mentioned "happy hour" experimental paradigm (Higley, Suomi, & Linnoila, 1996). Researchers have also demonstrated a significant relationship between degree of alcohol intoxication and serotonin transporter availability in these monkeys (Heinz et al., 1998), as well as between alcohol intake and innate tolerance, and serotonin transporter availability (Higley et al., in press). Finally, Champoux, Sponberg, Shannon, Suomi, and Higley (2002) have shown that individual differences in alcohol consumption at 5 years of age can be predicted by individual differences in measures of attention and motor maturity obtained as early as 14 days of age, suggesting that certain patterns of infant temperament may be associated with increased risk for substance abuse later in life.

Recent field studies have reported that most impulsive young males are permanently expelled from their natal group *prior* to puberty, long before the rest of their male cohort begins the normal emigration process (Mehl-man et al., 1995). These males tend to be grossly incompetent socially. Lacking the requisite social skills necessary for entry into another social group, most become solitary and typically perish within a year (Higley, Mehlman, et al., 1996). Juvenile females who exhibit excessive impulsively aggressive behavior also characteristically have chronically low CSF concentrations of 5-HIAA, and they retain these distinguishing features throughout childhood and into puberty.

In contrast to impulsive males, these females are unlikely to be expelled from their natal troop at any time thereafter, although laboratory studies indicate that they typically remain at the bottom of their social hierarchy (Higley, King, et al., 1996) and are often relatively incompetent, if not neglectful, mothers (Tsai, Lindell, Shannon, & Higley, 1998). Thus, the behavioral features of impulsive aggressiveness show substantial developmental continuity and striking interindividual stability throughout much of behavioral ontogeny. Rhesus monkeys who exhibit excessive impulsive and aggressive behavior early in life tend to follow developmental trajectories that often result in premature death among males and chronically low social status and poor parenting among females.

The developmental continuity and relative stability of CSF 5-HIAA concentrations have been found to be at least as strong as any behavioral indices of impulsivity and/or aggressiveness. As was previously mentioned, laboratory studies of rhesus monkeys across a wide age range have documented major developmental changes in CSF 5-HIAA concentrations, with levels dropping sharply during the first year and more slowly thereafter until puberty, only to typically rise slightly during the adult years. Despite these major developmental shifts, individual differences in CSF 5-HIAA remain strikingly stable, both in the short term (Higley et al., 1992; Higley, Mehlman, et al., 1996; Mehlman et al., 1995) and over the 5-year period from late infancy to early adulthood (Higley & Suomi, 1996).

## NATURE–NURTURE ISSUES REGARDING IMPULSIVE AGGRESSIVENESS IN RHESUS MONKEYS

The research reviewed in the previous section identified certain behavioral and physiological features of impulsive aggressiveness that show considerable continuity and stability of individual differences throughout much if not all of the rhesus monkey lifespan. What factors underlie these developmental phenomena—which features might be heritable, or subject to various environmental influences, or, more likely, be the product of both nature and nurture?

Several studies of rhesus monkeys raised in both laboratory and field environments have examined the relative heritability of many of the behavioral and physiological characteristics of impulsive aggressiveness. Laboratory studies utilizing half-sibling comparisons and cross-fostering rearing procedures have demonstrated significant heritability for CSF concentrations of 5-HIAA (e.g., Higley et al., 1993). Other laboratory studies comparing half-siblings or members of different genetic "strains" reared in identical nursery environments have reported suggestive evidence of heritability for a variety of infant state and temperament measures (Champoux et al., 1997; Champoux et al., 1994). Thus, there is substantial evidence that at least some of the stable individual differences seen in both behavioral and physiological indices of impulsivity throughout development can be attributed to heritable factors.

On the other hand, the fact that individual differences in various features of impulsivity tend to be quite stable in rhesus monkeys from infancy to adulthood and are at least in part heritable does not mean that these biobehavioral features are necessarily fixed at birth or are immune to subsequent environmental influence. To the contrary, an increasing body of evidence from laboratory studies has clearly demonstrated that the propensity to develop patterns of impulsive aggressiveness can be modified substantially by certain early experiences, particularly those involving early social attachment relationships.

For example, a common practice in many primate facilities over the years has been to rear monkey infants with peers instead of with their biological mother (e.g., Chamove, Rosenblum, & Harlow, 1973; Harlow & Harlow, 1969). In one form of this general rearing paradigm, infants are permanently separated from their mothers at birth, hand-reared in a neonatal nursery for their first month of life, housed with same-age, like-reared peers for the rest of their first 6 months, and then moved into larger social groups containing both peer-reared and mother-reared age-mates (e.g., Higley & Suomi, 1996). During their initial months these infants readily develop strong social attachment bonds to each other, much as mother-reared infants develop attachment relationships with their own mothers. However, because peers are not nearly as effective as a normal monkey mother in reducing fear in the face of stress or in providing a "secure base" for exploration, the attachment relationships that these peer-reared infants develop are almost always "anxious" or "insecure" in nature (Suomi, 1995). As a consequence, whereas peer-reared monkeys show completely normal physical and motor development, their early exploratory behavior is somewhat limited. They seem reluctant to approach novel objects, and they tend to be shy in their initial encounters with unfamiliar peers. Moreover, even when they interact with their same-age cage mates in familiar settings, their emerging social play repertoires are usually retarded in both frequency and complexity. For example, peer-reared monkeys are more likely to play with only one partner at a time rather than with multiple partners simultaneously, as mother-reared youngsters quickly come to prefer, and their play bouts are usually limited to relatively brief exchanges rather than the extended interactions that may go on for several minutes at a time among mother-reared peers. One explanation for their relatively poor play performance is that their cage mates must serve both as attachment objects and as playmates, a dual role that neither mothers nor mother-reared peers have to fulfill. It is also difficult for peer-reared youngsters to develop sophisticated play repertoires with basically incompetent play partners. Perhaps as a result, they typically drop to the bottom of their respective dominance hierarchies when they are grouped with mother-reared monkeys their own age (Higley, Suomi, & Linnoila, 1996).

Early peer rearing tends to make young rhesus monkeys more impulsive, especially if they are males. Like the previously described impulsive monkeys growing up in the wild, peer-reared males initially exhibit aggressive tendencies in the context of juvenile play, and as they approach puberty the frequency and severity of their aggressive episodes usually exceeds that of mother-reared group members of similar age. Peer-reared females tend to groom (and be groomed by) others in their social group less frequently and for shorter durations than their mother-reared counterparts and, as before, they usually stay at the bottom of their respective dominance hierarchies. These differences between peer-reared and mother-reared age-mates in aggression, grooming, and dominance remain relatively robust when the monkeys are subsequently moved into new social groups, and they generally are quite stable throughout the juvenile and adolescent years. Peer-reared monkeys also consistently show lower CSF concentrations of 5-HIAA than their mother-reared counterparts. These differences in 5-HIAA concentrations appear well before 6 months of age, they persist during the transition to mixed-group housing, and they remain stable at least throughout adolescence and into early adulthood. Thus, peer-reared monkeys as a group resemble the impulsive subgroup of wild-living (and mother-reared) monkeys not only behaviorally but also in terms of decreased serotonergic functioning (Suomi, 1997).

Given these findings, it should come as no surprise that peer-reared adolescent monkeys as a group consume larger amounts of alcohol under comparable *ad libitum* conditions than their mother-reared age-mates (Higley, Hasert, et al., 1991). An additional risk that peer-reared females carry into adulthood concerns their maternal behavior. Peer-reared mothers are significantly more likely to exhibit neglectful and/or abusive treatment of their firstborn offspring than are their mother-reared counterparts, although their care of subsequent offspring tends to improve dramatically (Ruppenthal, Arling, Harlow, Sackett, & Suomi, 1976). In summary, early peer rearing seems to make rhesus monkeys more impulsive, and their resulting developmental trajectories not only resemble those of naturally occurring subgroups of rhesus monkeys growing up in the wild but also persist in that vein long after their period of exclusive exposure to peers has been completed and they have been living in more species-typical social groups. Indeed, some effects of these inadequate early attachment relationships may well be passed on to the next generation via aberrant patterns of maternal care, as appears to be the case for impulsive mothers rearing infants in their natural habitat (Suomi & Levine, 1998).

## GENE–ENVIRONMENT INTERACTIONS

Studies examining the effects of peer rearing and other variations in early rearing history (e.g., Harlow & Harlow, 1969), along with the previously cited heritability findings, clearly provide compelling evidence that *both* genetic and early experiential factors can affect a monkey's capacity to regulate its expression of aggression. Do these factors operate independently, or do they interact in some fashion in shaping individual developmental trajectories? Ongoing research capitalizing on the discovery of polymorphisms in one specific gene—the serotonin transporter gene—suggests that gene–environment interactions not only occur but also can be expressed in multiple forms.

The serotonin transporter gene (5-HTT), a candidate gene for impaired serotonergic function (Lesch et al., 1996), has length variation in its promoter region that results in allelic variation in 5-HTT expression. A "short" allele (LS) confers low transcriptional efficiency to the 5-HTT promoter relative to the "long" allele (LL), raising the possibility that low 5-HTT expression may result in decreased serotonergic function (Heils et al., 1996), although evidence in support of this hypothesis in humans has been decidedly mixed to date (cf. Furlong et al., 1998, for an example of negative findings). The 5-HTT polymorphism was first characterized in humans, but it also appears in largely homologous form in rhesus monkeys and other simian primates but interestingly not in other mammalian species (Lesch et al., 1997).

Polyclonal recombinant (PCR) techniques have recently been utilized to characterize the genotypic status of monkeys in the studies comparing peer-reared monkeys with mother-reared controls described above with respect to their 5-HTT polymorphic status. Because extensive observational data and biological samples were previously collected from these monkeys throughout development, it has been possible to examine a wide range of behavioral and physiological measures for potential 5-HTT polymorphism main effects and interactions with early rearing history. Analyses completed to date suggest that such interactions are widespread and diverse.

For example, Bennett et al. (2002) found that CSF 5-HIAA concentrations did not differ as a function of 5-HTT status for mother-reared subjects, whereas among peer-reared monkeys individuals with the LS allele had significantly lower CSF 5-HIAA concentrations than those with the LL allele. One interpretation of this interaction is that mother rearing appeared to "buffer" any potentially deleterious effects of the LS allele on serotonin metabolism. Similarly, peer-reared monkeys with the LS ploymorphism exhibited much higher levels of impulsive aggression than their peer-reared counterparts with the LL polymorphism, who exhibited similarly low levels as both LL and LS mother-reared monkeys, again suggesting a "buffering" effect of maternal rearing (Barr, Newman, Becker, et al., 2002).

A different form of gene–environment interaction was revealed by the analysis of alcohol consumption data: whereas peer-reared monkeys with the LS allele consumed more alcohol than peer-reared monkeys with the LL allele, the reverse was true for mother-reared subjects, with individuals possessing the LS allele actually consuming *less* alcohol than their LL counterparts. The same pattern was found for relative levels of alcohol intoxication (Barr, Newman, Lesch, et al., 2002). In other words, the LS allele appeared to represent a risk factor for excessive alcohol consumption among peer-reared monkeys but a protective factor for mother-reared subjects. Finally, Champoux, Bennett, et al. (2002) examined the relationship between early rearing history and 5-HTT allelic status on measures of neonatal neurobehavioral development during the first month of life and found further evidence of maternal "buffering." Specifically, infants possessing the LS allele who were being reared in the laboratory neonatal nursery showed significant deficits in measures of attention, activity, and motor maturity relative to nursery-reared infants possessing the LL allele, whereas both LS and LL infants who were being reared by competent mothers exhibited normal values for each of these measures.

In sum, the consequences of having the LS allele differed dramatically for peer-reared and mother-reared monkeys: whereas peer-reared individuals with the LS allele exhibited deficits in measures of neurobehavioral development during their initial weeks of life and reduced serotonin metabolism, high levels of impulsive aggression, and excessive alcohol consumption as adolescents, mother-reared subjects with the very same allele showed normal early neurobehavioral development and serotonin metabolism, a relative absence of impulsive aggression, and reduced risk for excessive alcohol consumption. Indeed, it could be argued on the basis of these findings that having the short allele of the 5-HTT gene may well lead to psychopathology among monkeys with poor early rearing histories but might actually be adaptive for monkeys who develop secure early attachment relationship with their mothers.

## CONCLUSIONS AND IMPLICATIONS FOR UNDERSTANDING IMPULSIVE AGGRESSIVENESS IN HUMANS

At the beginning of this chapter it was argued that many of the obstacles to rigorous developmental study of nature–nurture issues, developmental continuity, and stability of individual differences issues in humans could be overcome or even avoided by investigating parallel phenomena in animals. To what extent have studies of impulsive aggressiveness in rhesus monkeys been informative with respect to each of those basic developmental issues?

First, the results of these studies have clearly demonstrated that *both* nature and nurture are at play in the development of most, if not all, biobehavioral aspects of rhesus monkey impulsive aggressiveness. On the one hand, evidence of significant heritability has been found for certain neonatal reflex and activity patterns, CSF 5-HIAA concentrations, and behavioral expressions of impulsivity and aggressiveness. On the other hand, the results of prospective longitudinal studies with rhesus monkeys have also demonstrated significant effects of differential early rearing experiences on the developmental trajectories of virtually all of these very same behavioral and physiological systems, their specific heritabilities notwithstanding. Thus, how a rhesus monkey is reared can markedly affect its pattern of neonatal reflex development, its daily distribution of activity states, its likelihood of escalating play bouts into aggressive episodes, and its chronic CSF concentrations of 5-HIAA, respectively, no matter how many genes might be involved in each instance. Clearly, both nature and nurture can contribute to the expression of impulsive aggressiveness by individual rhesus monkeys.

Perhaps the more interesting issue concerns the manner and degree to which heritable factors *interact* with environmental influences to shape individual developmental trajectories of impulsive aggressiveness. The recent findings that a specific polymorphism in the serotonin transporter gene is associated with different behavioral and biological outcomes for rhesus monkeys as a function of their early social rearing histories suggest that more complex gene–environment interactions may actually be responsible for the phenomenon. Whether comparable instances of gene–environment interactions can be demonstrated for other biobehavioral characteristics is currently the focus of ongoing research efforts. Nevertheless, even highly definitive findings from such demonstrations of gene–environment interactions would scarcely begin to address issues regarding the actual biochemical expression of the genes in question; the extent and manner in which such expression can be enhanced, blocked, or otherwise modified by specific environmental factors; and the pathways and mechanisms through which such expression might be translated into specific physiological and behavioral activities exhibited by individual monkeys. While nature and nurture can obviously interact, exactly how, when, and why has yet to be fully determined. Yet all of these issues can be translated into empirical questions that could readily be addressed in research with rhesus monkeys and other organisms, and indeed many of those empirical questions are already in the process of being formulated, if not actually tested.

Many questions regarding issues of developmental continuity and stability of individual differences in the expression of impulsive aggressiveness have been thoroughly examined in several prospective longitudinal studies with rhesus monkeys living in both laboratory and field settings, but others remain unanswered. Obvious behavioral expressions of impulsive aggressiveness are not readily apparent during infancy (although there may be some powerful predictors in certain neonatal reflex and activity state patterns; see, e.g., Champoux et al., 1997), and no study to date has looked for possible expressions of impulsive aggressiveness in aged monkeys. Moreover, while other "impulsive-like" behaviors—for example, dangerous leaps—covary with the appearance of unprovoked, escalating aggressive bouts, relatively little is presently known about other potentially impulsive "tendencies" (e.g., poor or nonexistent delay of gratification capacities) that might be shown by impulsively aggressive individuals. On the other hand, each of these patterns of behavioral expression is associated with low CSF 5-HIAA concentrations at all ages tested. Although CSF 5-HIAA concentrations change dramatically in absolute terms throughout development, at every age the lowest concentrations are always associated with the greatest prevalence of impulsive-like behavior. Furthermore, those associations with CSF 5-HIAA concentrations remain relatively unchanged regardless of the situations in which the CSF samples are obtained. All in all, there appears to be remarkable stability of individual differences in the expression of these same behavioral and physiological aspects of impulsive aggressiveness across major portions of the rhesus monkey lifespan.

What might the relevance of past, present, and proposed studies of impulsive aggressiveness in rhesus monkeys and other nonhuman primates be for advancing our understanding of phenomena associated with impulsive aggressiveness in humans? To be sure, rhesus monkeys are clearly not furry little humans with tails, and many important aspects of human impulsive aggressiveness may indeed be uniquely human (e.g., verbal expressions or written confessions of impulsive aggressive activities). Moreover, one should always be cautious in making direct comparisons between humans and other animals, even our closest phylogenetic relatives; the tendency to anthropomorphize, particularly in the face of compelling behavioral and physiological parallels, can lead to unsubstantiated assumptions of total homologies when only partial analogies or similarities actually exist. Nevertheless, the same compelling behavioral and physiological parallels between these phenomena in rhesus monkeys and in humans does argue strongly for some common principles regarding the basic issues of nature–nurture, continuity, and stability of individual differences throughout development. The research to date with rhesus monkeys strongly indicates that each of these issues is neither simple nor likely to be resolved by either–or answers. It is hard to imagine that the human phenomena would be any less complex.

# REFERENCES

Alexander, B. K., & Harlow, H. F. (1966). Social behavior of juvenile rhesus monkeys subjected to different rearing conditions during the first 6 months of life. *Zoologia Jahrb Physiologia, 60*, 167–174.

Barr, C. S., Newman, T. K., Becker, M. L., Champoux, M., Lesch, K. P., Suomi, S. J., & Higley, J. D. (2002). *The low activity varient of the serotonin transporter gene promoter is associated with decreased social play and increased aggression in rhesus macaques.* Manuscript submitted for publication.

Barr, C. S., Newman, T. K., Lesch, K. P., Suomi, S. J., Goldman, D., & Higley, J. D. (2002). *Early life stress and serotonin transporter gene variation interact to influence the level of response to alcohol in rhesus monkeys.* Manuscript submitted for publication.

Bennett, A. J., Lesch, K. P., Heils, A., Long, J., Lorenz, J., Shoaf, S. E., Champoux, M., Suomi, S. J., Linnoila, M., & Higley, J. D. (2002). Serotonin transporter gene variation, strain, and early rearing environment affect CSF 5-HIAA concentrations in rhesus monkeys (*Macaca mulatta*). *Molecular Psychiatry, 7*, 118–122.

Berard, J. (1989). Male life strategies. *Puerto Rico Health Sciences Journal, 8*, 47–58.

Bernstein, I. S., Williams, L., & Ramsay, M. (1983). The expression of aggression in Old World monkeys. *International Journal of Primatology, 4*, 113–125.

Brown, G. L., Goodwin, F. K., Ballenger, J. C., Goyer, P. F., & Major, L. F. (1979). Aggression in humans correlates with cerebrospinal fluid amine metabolites. *Psychiatry Research, 1*, 131–139.

Brown, G. L., Linnoila, M., & Goodwin, F. K. (1990). Clinical assessment of human aggression and impulsivity in relation to biochemical measures. In H. M. Van Praag, R. Plutchik, & A. Apter (Eds.), *Violence and suicidality: Perspectives in clinical and psychobiological research* (pp. 184–217). New York: Bruner/Mazel.

Chamove, A. S., Rosenblum, L. A., & Harlow, H. F. (1973). Monkeys (*Macaca mulatta*) raised only with peers: A pilot study. *Animal Behavior, 21*, 316–325.

Champoux, M., Bennett, A. J., Shannon, C., Higley, J. D., Lesch, K. P., & Suomi, S. J. (2002). Serotonin transporter gene polymorphism, differential early rearing, and behavior in rhesus monkey neonates. *Molecular Psychiatry, 7*, 1058–1063.

Champoux, M., Higley, J. D., & Suomi, S. J. (1997). Behavioral and physiological characteristics of Indian and Chinese–Indian hybrid rhesus macaque infants. *Developmental Psychobiology, 31*, 49–63.

Champoux, M., Sponberg, A., Shannon, C., Suomi, S. J., & Higley, J. D. (2002). *Neonatal behavior correlates with alcohol consumption in young adult rhesus macaques.* Manuscript submitted for publication.

Champoux, M., Suomi, S. J., & Schneider, M. L. (1994). Temperamental differences between Indian and Chinese–Indian hybrid rhesus macaques. *Laboratory Animal Science, 44*, 351–357.

Coccaro, E. M., & Murphy, D. L. (1990). *Serotonin in major psychiatric disorders.* Washington, DC: American Psychiatric Press.

Doudet, D., Hommer, D., Higley, J. D., Andreason, P. J., Moneman, R., Suomi, S. J., & Linnoila, M. (1995). Cerebral glucose metabolism, CSF 5-HIAA, and aggressive behavior in rhesus monkeys. *American Journal of Psychiatry, 152*, 1782–1787.

Furlong, R. A., Ho, L., Walsh, C., Rubinsztein, J. S., Jain, S., Pazkil, E. S., Eaton, D. F., & Rubinsztein, D. C. (1998). Analysis and meta-analysis of two serotonin transporter gene polymorphisms in bipolar and unipolar affective disorders. *American Journal of Medical Genetics, 81*, 58–63.

Harlow, H. F., & Harlow, M. K. (1969). Effects of various mother–infant relationships on rhesus monkey behaviors. In B. M. Foss (Ed.), *Determinants of infant behaviour* (Vol. 4, pp. 15–36). London: Metheun.

Harlow, H. F., Suomi, S. J., & Gluck, J. P. (1972). Generalization of behavioral data between nonhuman and human primates. *American Psychologist, 27,* 709–716.

Heils, A., Teufel, A., Petri, S., Stober, G., Riederer, P., Bengel, B., & Lesch, K. P. (1996). Allelic variation of human serotonin transporter gene expression. *Journal of Neurochemistry, 6,* 2621–2624.

Heinz, A., Higley, J. D., Gorey, J. G., Saunders, R. C., Jones, D. W., Hommer, D., Zajicek, K., Suomi, S. J., Weinberger, D. R., & Linnoila, M. (1998). *In vivo* association between alcohol intoxication, aggression, and serotonin transporter availability in nonhuman primates. *American Journal of Psychiatry, 155,* 1023–1028.

Higley, J. D., Hasert, M. L., Suomi, S. J., & Linnoila, M. (1991). A new nonhuman primate model of alcohol abuse: Effects of early experience, personality, and stress on alcohol consumption. *Proceedings of the National Academy of Sciences, 88,* 7261–7265.

Higley, J. D., Hommer, D., Lucas, K., Shoaf, S., Suomi, S. J., & Linnoila, M. (in press). CNS serotonin metabolism rate predicts innate tolerance, high alcohol consumption, and aggression during intoxication in rhesus monkeys. *Archives of General Psychiatry.*

Higley, J. D., King, S. T., Hasert, M. F., Champoux, M., Suomi, S. J., & Linnoila, M. (1996). Stability of individual differences in serotonin function and its relationship to severe aggression and competent social behavior in rhesus macaque females. *Neuropsychopharmacology, 14,* 67–76.

Higley, J. D., Mehlman, P. T., Taub, D. M., Higley, S., Fernald, B., Vickers, J. H., Suomi, S. J., & Linnoila, M. (1996). Excessive mortality in young free-ranging male nonhuman primates with low CSF 5-HIAA concentrations. *Archives of General Psychiatry, 53,* 537–543.

Higley, J. D., Mehlman, P. T., Taub, D. M., Higley, S. B., Vickers, J. H., Suomi, S. J., & Linnoila, M. (1992). Cerebrospinal fluid monoamine and adrenal correlates of aggression in free-ranging rhesus monkeys. *Archives of General Psychiatry, 49,* 436–444.

Higley, J. D., & Suomi, S. J. (1996). Reactivity and social competence affect individual differences in reaction to severe stress in children: Investigations using nonhuman primates. In C. R. Pfeffer (Ed.), *Intense stress and mental disturbance in children* (pp. 3–58). Washington, DC: American Psychiatric Press.

Higley, J. D., Suomi, S. J., & Linnoila, M. (1991). CSF monoamine metabolite concentrations vary according to age, rearing, and sex, and are influenced by the stressor of social separation in rhesus monkeys. *Psychopharmacology, 103,* 551–556.

Higley, J. D., Suomi, S. J., & Linnoila, M. (1996). A nonhuman primate model of Type II alcoholism?: Part 2. Diminished social competence and excessive aggression correlates with low CSF 5-HIAA concentrations. *Alcoholism: Clinical and Experimental Research, 20,* 643–650.

Higley, J. D., Thompson, W. T., Champoux, M., Goldman, D., Hasert, M. F., Kraemer, G. W., Scanlan, J. M., Suomi, S. J., & Linnoila, M. (1993). Paternal and maternal genetic and environmental contributions to CSF monoamine metabolites in rhesus monkeys (*Macaca mulatta*). *Archives of General Psychiatry, 50,* 615–623.

Kruesi, M. J. (1989). Cruelty to animals and CSF 5-HIAA. *Psychiatry Research, 28,* 115–116.

Kruesi, M. J., Rapoport, J. L., Hamburder, S., Hibbs, E., Potter, W. Z., Lenane, M., & Brown, G. L. (1990). Cerebrospinal fluid monoamine metabolites, aggression, and impulsivity in disruptive behavior disorders of children and adolescents. *Archives of General Psychiatry, 47,* 419–426.

Lesch, K. P., Bengel, D., Heils, A., Sabol, S. Z., Greenberg, B. D., Petri, S., Benjamin, J., Muller, C. R., Hamer, D. H., & Murphy, D. L. (1996). Association of anxiety-related traits with a polymorphism in the serotonin transporter gene regulatory region. *Science, 274,* 1527–1531.

Lesch, L. P., Meyer, J., Glatz, K., Flugge, G., Hinney, A., Hebebrand, J., Klauck, S. M., Poustka, A., Poustka, F., Bengel, D., Mossner, R., Riederer, P., & Heils, A. (1997). The 5-HT transporter gene-linked polymorphic region (5-HTTLPR) in evolutionary perspective: Alternative biallelic variation in rhesus monkeys. *Journal of Neural Transmission, 104,* 1259–1266.

Lindburg, D. G. (1991). Ecological requirements of macaques. *Laboratory Animal Science, 41,* 315–322.

Linnoila, M. (1988). Monoamines and impulse control. In J. A. Swinkels & W. Blijeven (Eds.), *Depression, anxiety, and aggression* (pp. 167–172). Houten, The Netherlands: Medidact.

Linnoila, M., DeJong, J., & Virkkunen, M. (1989). Monoamines, glucose metabolism, and impulse control. *Psychopharmacy Bulletin, 25,* 404–406.

Linnoila, M., Virkkunen, M., Scheinin, M., Nuutila, A., Rimon, R., & Goodwin, F. K. (1983). Low cerebrospinal fluid 5-hydroxyindoleacetic acid concentration differentiates impulsive from nonimpulsive violent behavior. *Life Sciences, 33,* 2609–2614.

Lovejoy, C. O. (1981). The origins of man. *Science, 211,* 341–350.

Mann, J. J., Arango, V., & Underwood, M. E. (1990). Serotonin and suicidal behavior. *Annals of the New York Academy of Science, 600,* 476–485.

Mehlman, P. T., Higley, J. D., Faucher, I., Lilly, A. A., Taub, D. M., Vickers, J. H., Suomi, S. J., & Linnoila, M. (1994). Low cerebrospinal fluid 5 hydroxyindoleacetic acid concentrations are correlated with severe aggression and reduced impulse control in free-ranging primates. *American Journal of Psychiatry, 151,* 1485–1491.

Mehlman, P. T., Higley, J. D., Faucher, I., Lilly, A. A., Taub, D. M., Vickers, J. H., Suomi, S. J., & Linnoila, M. (1995). CSF 5-HIAA concentrations are correlated with sociality and the timing of emigration in free-ranging primates. *American Journal of Psychiatry, 152,* 901–913.

Raleigh, M. J., & McGuire, M. T. (1994). Serotonin, aggression, and violence in vervet monkeys. In R. D. Masters & M. T. McGuire (Eds.), *The neurotransmitter revolution* (pp. 129–145). Carbondale: Southern Illinois University Press.

Ruppenthal, G. C., Arling, G. L., Harlow, H. F., Sackett, G. P., & Suomi, S. J. (1976). A 10-year perspective on motherless mother monkey mothering behavior. *Journal of Abnormal Psychology, 88,* 341–349.

Sibley, C. O., Comstock, J. A., & Alquist, J. E. (1990). DNA hybridization evidence of hominid phylogeny: A reanalysis of the data. *Journal of Molecular Evolution, 30,* 202–236

Steklis, H. D., Brammen, G. L., Raleigh, M. J., & McGuire, M. T. (1985). Serum testosterone, male dominance, and aggression in captive groups of vervet monkeys (*Cercopithecus aethiops sabacus*). *Hormones and Behavior, 19,* 156–165.

Suomi, S. J. (1995). Influence of Bowlby's attachment theory on research on nonhuman primate biobehavioral development. In S. Goldberg, R. Muir, & J. Kerr (Eds.), *Attachment theory: Social, developmental, and clinical perspectives* (pp. 185–201). Hillsdale, NJ: Analytic Press.

Suomi, S. J. (1997). Early determinants of behaviour: Evidence from primate studies. *British Medical Bulletin, 53,* 170–184.

Suomi, S. J., & Levine, S. (1998). Psychobiology of intergenerational effects of trauma: Evidence from animal studies. In Y. Daniele (Ed.), *International handbook of multigenerational legacies of trauma* (pp. 623–637). New York: Plenum Press.

Symonds, D. (1978). *Play and aggression: A study of rhesus monkeys.* New York: Columbia University Press.

Tremblay, R. E. (1992). The prediction of delinquent behavior from childhood behavior: Personality theory revisited. In J. McCord (Ed.), *Facts, frameworks, and forecasts: Advances in criminological theory* (Vol. 3, pp. 192–230). New Brunswick, NJ: Transaction Books.

Tsai, T., Bennett, A. J., Pierre, P. J., Shoaf, S. E., & Higley, J. D. (1999). Behavioral response to novel objects varies with CSF 5-HIAA concentrations in rhesus monkeys. *American Journal of Primatology, 49,* 109–110.

Tsai, T., Lindell, S. G., Shannon, C., & Higley, J. D. (1998). Aggression to infants and maternal competence by female rhesus monkeys with low CNS serotonin functioning. *American Journal of Primatology, 45*, 211.

Westergaard, G. T., Mehlman, P. T., Suomi, S. J., & Higley, J. D. (1999). CSF 5-HIAA and aggression in female primates: Species and interindividual differences. *Psychopharmacology, 146*, 440–446.

Zajicek, K., Higley, J. D., Suomi, S. J., & Linnoila, M. (1997). Rhesus macaques with high CSF 5-HIAA concentrations exhibit early sleep onset. *Psychiatric Research, 77*, 15–25.